PAEDIATRIC ENDOCRINOLOGY IN CLINICAL PRACTICE

PAEDIATRIC ENDOCRINOLOGY IN CLINICAL PRACTICE

Edited by

A. AYNSLEY-GREEN
James Spence Professor of Child Health
The Children's Clinic
Royal Victoria Infirmary
Newcastle upon Tyne
England

Proceedings of the Royal College of Physicians'
Paediatric Endocrinology Conference
held in London
20–21 October 1983

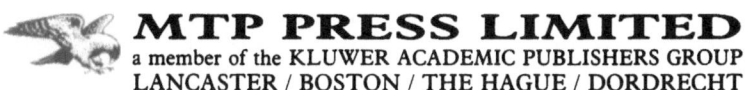

MTP PRESS LIMITED
a member of the KLUWER ACADEMIC PUBLISHERS GROUP
LANCASTER / BOSTON / THE HAGUE / DORDRECHT

Published in the UK and Europe by
MTP Press Limited
Falcon House
Lancaster, England

British Library Cataloguing in Publication Data

Paediatric endocrinology in clinical practice
  1. Pediatric endocrinology
  I. Aynsley-Green, A.
  618.92'4 RJ418

  ISBN-13:978-94-010-8974-6   e-ISBN-13:978-94-009-5610-0

  DOI: 10.1007/978-94-009-5610-0

Published in the USA by
MTP Press
A division of Kluwer Boston Inc
190 Old Derby Street
Hingham, MA 02043, USA

Library of Congress Cataloging in Publication Data

Paediatric Endocrinology Conference (1983: London, England)
  Paediatric endocrinology in clinical practice

  Includes bibliographical references and index.
  1. Pediatric endocrinology—Congresses.
I. Aynsley-Green, A. II. Royal College of Physicians of. III. Title.
[DNLM: 1. Endocrine Diseases—in infancy & childhood—congresses.
2. Endocrine Glands—physiology—congresses. WS 330 P1265c 1983]
RJ418.P34 1983 618.92'4 84-11275

CONTENTS

Page

Page

SECTION 6 MISCELLANEOUS DISORDERS
Chairman: PROFESSOR J. W. FARQUHAR

PREFACE

This book is made up of 16 papers delivered during the Paediatric Conference convened by the Royal College of Physicians of London on 20th and 21st October 1983.

The main intention of the conference was to allow each contributor to deliver a personal review of his own field, indicating recent developments and current practice. This volume, representing the proceedings of that meeting, is not intended as a comprehensive textbook of paediatric endocrinology but rather as a series of personal narratives.

I wish to express my thanks to the Chairmen, who so ably stimulated discussion, and to Miss Gillian Andrew, Conference Secretary of the Royal College of Physicians, and her colleagues, for providing invaluable help in the organization of the conference.

I am also grateful to the staff of MTP Press Limited for their help in producing the book.

A. Aynsley-Green

LIST OF CHAIRMEN

Professor R. Hoffenburg PRCP
President
Royal College of Physicians
London

Professor J. W. Farquhar MD
  FRCP(Ed)
Department of Child Life and Health
University of Edinburgh
Edinburgh

Dr C. C. Forsyth MD FRCP
Department of Child Health
University of Dundee
Dundee

Dr D. I. Johnston MD FRCP
Queen's Medical Centre
Nottingham

Dr D. A. Price FRCP
Royal Manchester Children's
  Hospital
Pendlebury
Manchester

Dr P. H. W. Rayner FRCP
Institute of Child Health
University of Birmingham
Birmingham

LIST OF CONTRIBUTORS

Dr J. Allgrove MRCP
East Birmingham Hospital
Birmingham

Professor A. Aynsley-Green
DPhil FRCP
Department of Child Health
University of Newcastle upon Tyne
Newcastle upon Tyne

Dr N. D. Barnes FRCP
Department of Paediatrics
Addenbrooke's Hospital
Cambridge

Dr J. D. Baum MD FRCP
Department of Paediatrics
University of Oxford
Oxford

Dr G. F. Bottazzo MD MRCP
Department of Immunology
The Middlesex Hospital
London

Professor Sir John Dewhurst
FRCOG
Queen Charlotte's Maternity Hospital
London

Professor D. Doniach MD FRCP
Department of Immunology
The Middlesex Hospital Medical
    School
London

Dr D. B. Grant MD FRCP
The Hospital for Sick Children
Great Ormond Street
London

Professor R. Harris MD FRCP
Department of Medical Genetics
St Mary's Hospital
Manchester

Dr I. A. Hughes MD FRCP
Department of Child Health
Welsh National School of Medicine
Cardiff

Professor R. D. G. Milner MD
    FRCP
Department of Paediatrics
University of Sheffield
Sheffield
(*Teale Lecturer*)

Dr M. A. Preece MD FRCP
Institute of Child Health
30 Guilford Street
London

Dr M. O. Savage MD MRCP
Department of Child Health
St Bartholomew's Hospital
Queen Elizabeth Hospital for
    Children
London

Dr S. M. Shalet MD MRCP
Christie Hospital and Holt Radium
  Institute
Withington
Manchester

Dr J. A. H. Wass MD MRCP
Department of Endocrinology
St Bartholomew's Hospital
London

Professor P. C. Sizonenko MD
Division de Biologie de la Croissance
  et de la Reproduction
Hôpital Cantonal Universitaire
Geneva
Switzerland

SECTION 1

Neonatal Endocrinology

Chairman: THE PRESIDENT

1

THE EFFECTS OF MATERNAL ENDOCRINE DISEASE ON THE FETUS AND NEONATE

J. A. H. WASS

INTRODUCTION

During the past 10 years or so there have been widespread studies of maternal, fetal and neonatal endocrine physiology and our knowledge has expanded considerably. This is due in part to the development of sensitive and specific radioimmunoassays and also to the availability and use of radiolabelled hormones. These newly developed techniques have been applied successfully to study human fetuses, some newborn infants and to studies of other primate species. Studies of fetal and neonatal pathology in mothers with endocrine disease have provided important clues not only to normal physiology, but have also given insight as to how these conditions may be treated successfully, thereby reducing maternal and neonatal mortality and morbidity. It is clear that much work still needs to be done, not least because many of the conditions to be described are very rare.

Most of the work quoted in this review will relate to man or to studies carried out in mammalian or primate species. A discussion of some of the rarer maternal conditions affecting the fetus and neonate will be preceded by a review of the placental transfer of hormones and, finally, thyroid disease will be discussed in more detail, as this is one of the commonest endocrine diseases to affect mother and child.

PLACENTAL TRANSFER OF HORMONES

In assessing data on the placental transfer of hormones and the placental barrier, several points have to be borne in mind. First, the production rates of the hormone in question may vary in the mother and fetus, and consideration must be given to fetal hormone metabolism. Secondly, it is clear that there may be transfer both from the mother to the fetus and vice versa. Thirdly, binding of the hormone may be different in mother and fetus[1].

Polypeptide hormones

Data from a variety of species, including man, suggest that the placenta is completely impermeable to the majority of polypeptide hormones (Table 1). Thus, it is impermeable to growth hormone (GH)[2,3], adrenocorticotrophic hormone (ACTH)[4], thyrotrophin (TSH)[5] and the gonadotrophins, luteinizing hormone (LH) and follicle-stimulating hormone (FSH). With the smaller polypeptide hormones there is less available evidence in man. However, based on minimal data, there appears to be no transfer of oxytocin and vasopressin[6]. Transfer of insulin[7,8] and glucagon[9], parathyroid hormone (PTH) and calcitonin also do not occur to a significant extent.

Table 1   Placental transfer of polypeptide hormones

Impermeable
Growth hormone
Adrenocorticotrophic hormone
Thyroid-stimulating hormone
Luteinizing hormone
Follicle-stimulating hormone
Oxytocin
Vasopressin
Insulin
Glucagon
Parathyroid hormone
Calcitonin

The development of fetal endocrine control systems in particular, as it relates to some polypeptide hormones, is also relevant to a sound knowledge of the effect of maternal endocrine disease on the neonate. By 8–10 weeks of gestation the fetal hypothalamus has significant concentrations of thyrotrophin-releasing hormone (TRH), gonadotrophin-releasing hormone (LHRH), and growth hormone release-inhibiting hormone (somatostatin) and the human fetal adenohypophysis and neurohypophysis are embryologically intact by 11–12 weeks when secretory granules can be identified. Anterior pituitary hormone content gradually rises with gestational age. In the serum, however, concentrations of hormones also change but differently with gestational age. Thus there is a rise in circulating growth hormone to a peak at around 20–24 weeks.

4

Mid-gestational levels of the gonadotrophins, TSH and ACTH, are also higher than at term. On the other hand, fetal serum prolactin, largely because of the progressive increase in the maternal–fetal oestrogen levels, rises until term. At term, levels of GH, prolactin, TSH and ACTH are all higher than those seen postpartum[10], and this may be relevant to biochemical tests undertaken early in the neonatal period.

The endocrine control of anterior pituitary function gradually develops and there are progressive changes in anterior pituitary hormone secretion which correlate with brain maturation. These occur in the third trimester of pregnancy. Thus, there is a progressive maturation of negative feedback control systems for ACTH, TSH, LH and FSH secretion, and these are relatively mature at birth[10]. Shortly thereafter there are surges in ACTH and TSH secretion which result, respectively, in a rise in cortisol within 12 hours, and a rise in thyroxine 24–48 hours after birth. These concentrations fall and are stable 36–72 hours (cortisol) and 3 days (thyroxine) after birth[11–13].

On the other hand, the homeostatic mechanisms controlling calcium are less well developed at term and this accounts for the greater frequency of hypocalcaemia in infants, especially those that are premature. This is the case since, *in utero*, levels of calcium are high because of active transport across the placenta[14]. Moreover, in the early neonatal period parathormone secretion[15] is suppressed and, because of this, there may be a delayed response to hypocalcaemia.

Steroid hormones

The placenta is freely permeable to the passage of adrenocorticosteroids as well as to aldosterone, progesterone, and androgenic and oestrogenic steroids[16]. However, levels of cortisol are normally lower in the fetus, in part because of faster and different fetal metabolism[17].

Catecholamines

Adrenaline and noradrenaline can traverse the placental barrier and it is clear that the maternal injection of noradrenaline produces a transient fetal bradycardia, while maternal adrenaline infusion results in fetal tachycardia and cardiac irregularities[18]. This bradycardia with noradrenaline has been shown to be due to placental transfer by the injection of the radiolabelled catecholamine[19].

Thyroid hormones

It is clear that very little thyroid hormone crosses the placental barrier from mother to fetus when it is present in the maternal circulation in physiological concentrations[5]. Thus, there are marked maternal–fetal serum concentration gradients of thyroxine (T_4) and free T_4 because concentrations are low in the human fetus, especially before 11 weeks gestation. There is thereafter a progressive increase in T_4 so that at term concentrations are similar in mother and fetus. Fetal serum tri-iodo-thyronine (T_3) and free T_3 levels are low throughout gestation.

If large quantities of thyroid hormone, either T_4 or T_3, are given to the mother, there is only minimal maternal–fetal transfer[20,21]. It is possible that T_3 is transferred across the placenta to a greater extent than T_4, but these differences are marginal and of no significance unless large supraphysiological doses are used[21].

It is clear from the foregoing discussion that, amongst other things, the molecular weight of the hormones under discussion is important (Table 2)[22]. Thus, the larger polypeptide hormones of molecular weight between 1100 and 30000, as well as the thyroid hormones of molecular weight around 800, do not cross the placenta significantly, while the steroid hormones of molecular weight 350 and the catecholamines of molecular weight 180 do.

Table 2 Placental hormone transfer as related to molecular weight

Hormone	Approximate molecular weight	Placental transfer
Polypeptide hormones	1100–30000	no
Thyroid hormones	800	no
Steroid hormones	350	yes
Catecholamines	180	yes

FETAL AND NEONATAL COMPLICATIONS OF MATERNAL ENDOCRINE DISEASE

Hyperpituitarism (including acromegaly and prolactinoma)

It is obvious that there are no fetal complications of pituitary hyper-secretory syndromes because these hormones are not transferred across the placenta. Thus, there are no known effects on the fetus of high maternal prolactin or growth hormone levels. Cushing's disease due to a pituitary tumour secreting ACTH may result in high fetal cortisol levels and this is discussed later.

Hyperparathyroidism in pregnancy

Primary hyperparathyroidism is commoner in women and most fre-quently affects females in the older age group who are past their child-bearing years. If diagnosed during pregnancy, maternal primary hyperparathyroidism should be treated in its own right, if possible by mid-trimester parathyroidectomy, thus avoiding perinatal problems[23]. However, neonatal tetany may be the first clue that the mother has primary hyperparathyroidism[24].

In the infants of these mothers there is a high incidence of spontaneous abortion, stillbirth and neonatal death[23,25]. Indeed, the risk of perinatal death and neonatal hypocalcaemia and tetany have been considered to be as high as 25 and 50%, respectively[26]. The marked hypocalcaemia in infants is probably due to suppression of fetal parathyroid glands by the prolonged intra-uterine hypercalcaemia. It usually responds to the administration of calcium salts but, rarely, vitamin D may be necessary. Usually the symptoms decline so that treatment may be ceased by 3 months. If diagnosed early and treated adequately the infant should recover completely with no long-term sequelae.

Familial hypocalciuric hypercalcaemia

Familial hypocalciuric hypercalcaemia is a rare autosomal dominant condition in which there is an elevation of serum calcium due, in part, to increased renal absorption of calcium, and which is almost invariably picked up by chance[27]. In adults it runs a benign course and affected patients develop none of the usual complications of hypercalcaemia. In patients presenting with hypercalcaemia it is an important differential diagnosis which is, in contrast to primary hyperparathyroidism, associated with hypocalciuria.

Recently, babies born to patients with hypocalciuric hypercalcaemia have been described as having neonatal hypercalcaemia. In infants born to these patients, however, the course is far from benign. Marked hypercalcaemia may continue, and this is associated with failure to thrive, anorexia, constipation, muscular hypotonia and skeletal undermineralization[28,29]. Untreated, these infants have a high mortality and may require urgent total parathyroidectomy in the neonatal period to control hypercalcaemia[28,30]. Although no treatment for the mother is indicated, awareness of the potential neonatal problems will assist in the early correct management of neonatal hypercalcaemia. The reason for hypercalcaemia, which is associated with parathyroid hyperplasia, is unclear.

Glucocorticoids and pregnancy

Exogenous

In early publications assessing the risks of the administration of glucocorticoids given for non-endocrine conditions during pregnancy, it is said that there is a low rate of fetal abnormality and, in fact, only two

7

fetuses out of 260 born to mothers taking them during pregnancy had cleft palates; both of these patients had received glucocorticoids before the 14th week[31]. This evidence stands in marked contrast to that gained in other mammals where there is a high incidence of cleft palate. Furthermore, adrenal insufficiency is not seen in these infants[32].

Endogenous

Pregnancy in patients with untreated Cushing's syndrome is uncommon. Usually, mothers with this condition are amenorrhoeic and anovulatory. However, in the small number of cases that have been reported, there is a low incidence of normal pregnancy and delivery[33]. In this, the largest series of 21 cases reported, there was a spontaneous abortion rate of 15%, 4% had a therapeutic abortion, 23% of infants were born prematurely and 15% were stillborn. Only 42% of infants were born normally at term.

Because of its rarity, there are no data on the optimum management of a pregnant mother with Cushing's syndrome.

Although ACTH does not cross the placental barrier it is clear that cortisol does. From the theoretical point of view, therefore, there may be either fetal or neonatal adrenal suppression. In the infants reported, however, this is not at all a problem and in fact only one infant with hypoadrenalism has been reported, born to a mother with Cushing's syndrome[34]. The reasons for this elude adequate explanation at present, but it seems that routine steroid cover is not necessary in infants born to mothers with Cushing's syndrome.

Phaeochromocytoma in pregnancy

Phaeochromocytoma in pregnancy is also exceedingly rare. If it occurs it presents a serious threat to the life of both mother and fetus. The high maternal and fetal mortality, which is particularly marked if the condition is undiagnosed, is caused by catecholamines which cross the placental barrier. Thus, in a review of 89 cases, maternal mortality falls from 48 to 17% if the condition is diagnosed, but fetal mortality remains little changed (54 and 50%)[35]. Early diagnosis of this rare condition in pregnancy is therefore of paramount importance.

Although there is a high incidence of spontaneous abortion (55%), in part accounted for by early separation of the placenta, a large proportion of fetal deaths occur during or shortly after birth. It seems that the rise in catecholamines is associated with placental vasoconstriction and fetal hypoxia.

For this reason, if diagnosed, the patient should be delivered by Caesarian section rather than allowed to deliver vaginally. Labour and vaginal delivery have been followed by maternal or fetal death due to a sudden discharge of catecholamines resulting from mechanical interference with the tumour. During Caesarian section the maternal blood pressure should be controlled either with intravenous nitroprusside or combined alpha and beta blockade. While drugs inducing adequate control of hypertension in the mother may affect the fetus, this must be a secondary consideration in view of the high maternal mortality of untreated phaeochromocytoma in pregnancy.

Early diagnosis of patients with phaeochromocytoma is essential to decrease mortality and morbidity of this rare, but very serious condition of pregnancy.

THYROID DISEASE IN PREGNANCY

Maternal–fetal considerations

There is no change in thyroid homeostasis during pregnancy, but a large number of parameters change consequent upon the rise in oestrogen secreted by the placenta. Thus, thyroid-binding globulin levels produced by the liver rise by 4–8 weeks of pregnancy and this is associated with a fall in thyroid-binding pre-albumin[36]. This results in an increase in the extrathyroidal pool of T_4 and T_3 and levels of total T_4 and total T_3 rise, though concentrations of free T_4 and T_3 do not rise and may fall slightly[37, 38]. The TSH level is unchanged[39]. However, human chorionic gonadotrophin (hCG), which is biochemically closely related to TSH, has thyroid-stimulating properties, and further may cross-react in the TSH assay, thus giving falsely elevated values during pregnancy.

In terms of the maternal–fetal unit, while TSH and the thyroid hormones do not significantly cross the placenta, a number of compounds that affect thyroid function do. These include the human thyroid-stimulating immunoglobulins which cause Graves' disease, as well as thyroid-blocking antibodies which, rarely, may cause hypothyroidism in the fetus, and antithyroid drugs like carbimazole, propranolol and iodine (Table 3)[5].

Lastly, the diagnosis of neonatal thyroid disease may be initially complicated by changes in circulating TSH, T_4 and reverse T_3 in the

Table 3   The passage across the placenta of compounds affecting thyroid function

Good	Poor
TRH	TSH
Human thyroid-stimulating immunoglobulins	T_4
Antithyroid drugs, e.g. carbimazole	T_3
Propranolol	reverse T_3
Iodine	

9

first days of life. At birth, there is a rise in TSH, detectable after 30 minutes, probably stimulated by extra-uterine cooling, which causes T_3 and T_4 to rise and peak 24–48 hours postpartum[12,13].

Maternal hypothyroidism

Hypothyroidism presenting during pregnancy is exceedingly rare, because this condition reduces fertility. Available data, however, suggest that maternal hypothyroidism has little or no detrimental effect on the fetus since the fetal thyroid functions autonomously.

Management of maternal thyrotoxicosis

The diagnosis of hyperthyroidism in pregnancy is complicated by the fact that in normal pregnancy there is an increase in metabolic rate, altered routine thyroid function tests, including an increase in serum thyroxine and tri-iodothyronine, and sometimes an increase in the size of the thyroid gland itself. Biochemically, the diagnosis is made with a free thyroxine measurement, but this is not widely available; the technology is difficult and so mostly the free thyroxine index is used. Provided the clinician has access to both the total T_4 and uptake test measurement he can assess the contribution of high-binding proteins to total T_4. Thyrotoxicosis affects 0.2% of pregnant mothers[40], and it is clear that treatment using drugs which can cross the placenta may affect the fetus, though the disease *per se* does not.

If diagnosed in pregnancy, thyrotoxicosis should be treated with antithyroid drugs, either carbimazole or propylthiuracil (PTU). Both drugs have their advocates. Theoretically, PTU decreases peripheral conversion of T_4 to T_3 and may have a more rapid onset of action. No formal comparisons have been made. Radio-iodine is clearly contra-indicated.

Thyrotoxicosis should be carefully supervised clinically and biochemically so that thyroid function tests remain in the upper part of the normal range using the lowest possible dose of antithyroid drug[41]. Some have advocated the concurrent use of thyroxine given to the mother, in case of the development of maternal hypothyroidism[42]. This has little to commend it and may result in the administration of excess antithyroid drug. However, there are no formal comparisons published of antithyroid drugs with and without concomitant thyroxine. As soon as possible, the dose should be reduced below the equivalent of carbimazole 30 mg daily[41]. If diagnosed in early pregnancy, mid-trimester thyroidectomy may be indicated, but this is usually reserved for patients whose thyrotoxicosis is fluctuant or difficult to control. Antithyroid drugs can cross the placenta and therefore there is a risk of fetal goitre which occurs in 10% of children born to mothers taking 30–80 mg/day carbimazole.

This may interfere with labour by causing extension of the head. Neonatal hypothyroidism is very rare indeed and of short duration[24, 36]. No treatment is usually required.

The cause of neonatal thyrotoxicosis

It is now clear that fetal and neonatal thyrotoxicosis are caused by the transplacental passage of human thyroid-stimulating immunoglobulins. These are usually immunoglobulins of the IgG class which, when produced, cause Graves' disease and thyrotoxicosis. What is the evidence? First, neonatal thyrotoxicosis usually occurs in babies born to women with high titres of the thyroid-stimulating immunoglobulins LATS or LATS-P[43]. Munro et al. (1978) have looked at paired maternal and cord sera and found similar levels in both (Figure 1), thus confirming their transplacental passage. In this study, neonatal thyrotoxicosis was invariably associated with levels above 20 units/ml. Secondly, neonatal thyrotoxicosis is usually a self-limiting illness, which would fit in with the known half-life of maternal immunoglobulins in the fetal circulation. Lastly, neonatal thyrotoxicosis has an equal sex ratio in the newborn, in contrast to Graves' disease in the adult which has a marked female preponderance.

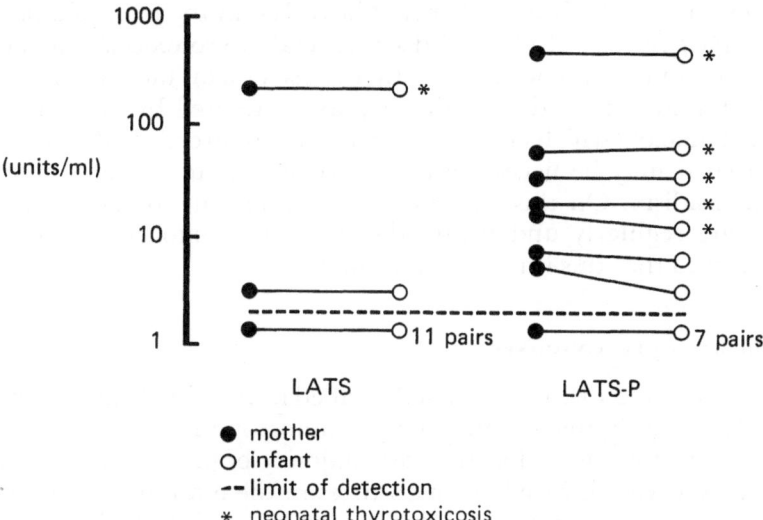

Figure 1 LATS and LATS-P activities in paired maternal and cord sera (Munro et al., 1978, reproduced with permission)

For these reasons, it is important to screen all mothers with current Graves' disease, or a past history of Graves' disease, be they euthyroid or even hypothyroid on thyroxine after radio-iodine or thyroidectomy, since thyroid-stimulating immunoglobulins may persist in these patients. Clearly, if in the past there is any question of a previous baby developing neonatal thyrotoxicosis, this also merits careful screening during any subsequent pregnancy (Table 4).

Table 4 Fetal and neonatal hyperthyroidism—mothers at risk

(1) Current Graves' disease

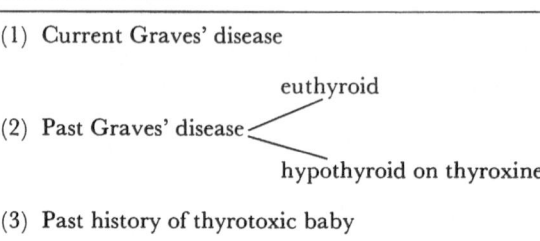

(2) Past Graves' disease ⟨ euthyroid / hypothyroid on thyroxine

(3) Past history of thyrotoxic baby

Fetal thyrotoxicosis

Data are scanty, but it is probable that thyrotoxicosis can develop *in utero*. It is, therefore, important to carefully assess, throughout pregnancy, the fetal heart rate[44]. Although this falls in normal pregnancy between the 20th and 30th week[45] it is abnormal for it to rise above 160 beats/minute. If the heart rate rises above 160 in the fetus of a patient with a past history of Graves' disease, fetal thyrotoxicosis should be considered in the absence of any other cause of fetal tachycardia.

If it develops, fetal thyrotoxicosis may be treated by administering oral carbimazole which crosses the placenta (Figure 2). If the mother is euthyroid it may be necessary to give thyroxine to prevent maternal hypothyroidism. On this treatment it is important to assess the fetal heart rate regularly and titrate the dose of carbimazole or propylthiouracil so that this is rendered normal.

Neonatal thyrotoxicosis

Neonatal Graves' disease was first described in 1912 by White *et al.*[46] and first related to thyroid-stimulating immunoglobulins by McKenzie in 1964[47]. It is now clear that the vast majority of patients who develop neonatal Graves' disease have high titres in the maternal serum of the thyroid-stimulating immunoglobulins LATS or LATS-P, and these should therefore by measured in every pregnant mother with a history of Graves' disease. LATS-P levels fall during pregnancy[43], but whether this means that the time during the pregnancy at which LATS-P is measured is important is not known.

Characteristically, neonatal thyrotoxicosis is a transient illness with a delayed onset of several days. This delay is particularly marked if the mother was taking carbimazole during pregnancy, but may occur in the absence of this history. In these cases, the reason for this delay is unclear.

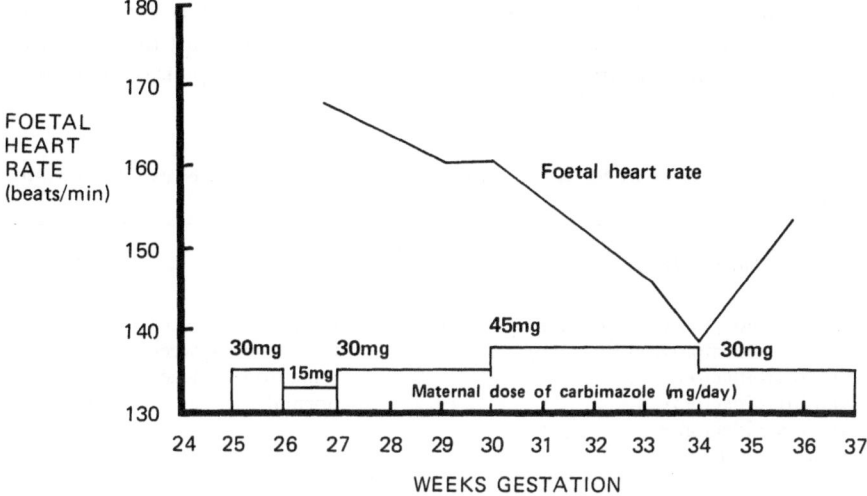

Figure 2 Variations of fetal heart rate related to maternal daily dose of oral carbimazole (Robinson *et al.*, 1979, reproduced with permission)

It is not clear how frequently neonatal thyrotoxicosis occurs. Its diagnosis may be missed because of this delay in onset sometimes to the second week of life. In the series reported by Munro *et al.*[43], 12 out of 96 children were diagnosed as having neonatal thyrotoxicosis, but in a careful prospective study over 3 years we have found, at St Bartholomew's Hospital, that 20% of children born to mothers with a known history of Graves' disease have subsequently developed fetal or neonatal thyrotoxicosis, so that it may be that the previous estimates of its frequency have not been accurate (Table 5).

At birth, 39% of infants are premature or of low birth weight and 57% have a goitre[48]. A smaller proportion have an accelerated bone age, frontal bossing and lymphadenopathy.

Untreated, there is a mortality of some 16% in these children, so that awareness and early diagnosis and treatment are essential.

Clinical manifestations of neonatal thyrotoxicosis include irritability and restlessness, failure to gain weight, feeding problems like vomiting and diarrhoea, and tachypnoea and tachycardia due to congestive cardiac failure associated, in some cases, with a very wide pulse pressure. Neonates may also have hepatosplenomegaly. Goitre may rarely cause respiratory obstruction. Exophthalmos and periorbital oedema may be present. Often these symptoms do not develop until 2 weeks postpartum, so that all children of mothers with a history, past or present, of Graves' disease should be carefully screened at this time.

13

Although usually a transient illness, these children need careful follow-up as, in 35% of cases, symptoms last 2–6 months, 17% have symptoms of longer duration than 6 months and hyperactivity may persist for 5 years or more[48]. Furthermore, there is an increased risk of cranio-synostosis and developmental impairment, so that five out of nine children born to thyrotoxic mothers who were followed up had impaired intelligence[49].

Table 5   Experience at St Bartholomew's Hospital over 3 years (20 women, 24 pregnancies)

Thyroid status	LATS-P (U/ml)	Fetus	Neonate
Partial thyroidectomy on thyroxine	120	toxic from 36 weeks	toxic
Partial thyroidectomy on thyroxine	209	toxic from 28 weeks	toxic
Partial thyroidectomy	29	toxic from 35 weeks	normal
Partial thyroidectomy	<2	normal	toxic
Partial thyroidectomy on carbimazole 10 mg daily	<8	normal	toxic

Diagnosis and treatment of this condition is therefore of paramount importance. These children should be given small amounts of carbimazole (0.5–1.0 mg/kg/day in divided doses 8-hourly) or propylthiouracil and propranolol (2 mg/kg/day in divided doses 8-hourly). If cardiac failure develops, digitalis may also need to be used. During this time, the pulse and blood sugar are carefully monitored.

It is not known at present whether breast milk contains thyroid-stimulating immunoglobulins.

Several problems persist in the management of neonatal thyrotoxicosis. Diagnosis is difficult and may be missed because of the delayed onset. If it develops, it seems that although it is a self-limiting disease, treatment is necessary because in a few patients a hyperkinetic state may persist and, further, intelligence may be adversely affected.

In summary, in mothers with a history of thyrotoxicosis, it is essential to monitor thyroid function during pregnancy. Maternal thyroid-stimulating immunoglobulins should be measured and careful monitoring of fetal heart rate should be carried out during the gestation. The neonate should be assessed at birth and after 2 weeks.

CONCLUSIONS

An increase in knowledge has occurred in the last 10 years and as a result a great deal more is known about maternal, fetal and neonatal endocrinology. This knowledge, together with careful treatment of both the mother, fetus and neonate can, and has, resulted in decreased mortality and a decrease in morbidity.

However, as many of these syndromes in pregnancy remain rare, it is important for the paediatrician to be wary of their presence as there is no doubt that early diagnosis and treatment can improve the prognosis both for the mother and her child.

References

1. Josimovich, J. B. (1973). The passage of hormones through the placenta. In *Handbook of Physiology, Section 7, Vol. 2, Part 2, Female Reproductive System*. pp. 277–84. (Baltimore: American Physiological Society)
2. Gitlin, D., Kumate, J. and Morales, C. (1965). Metabolism and materno-fetal transfer of human growth hormone in the pregnant woman at term. *J. Clin. Endocrinol. Metab.*, **25**, 1599–1608
3. King, K. C., Adam, P. A. J., Schwartz, R. and Teramo, K. (1971). Human placental transfer of human growth hormone-I[125]. *Pediatrics*, **48**, 534–9
4. Miyakawa, I., Ikeda, I. and Maeyama, M. (1974). Transport of ACTH across the human placenta. *J. Clin. Endocrinol. Metab.*, **39**, 440–2
5. Roti, E., Gnudi, A. and Braverman, L. E. (1983). The placental transport, synthesis and metabolism of hormones and drugs which affect thyroid function. *Endocr. Rev.*, **4**, 131–49
6. Chard, T., Hudson, C. N., Edwards, C. R. W. and Boyd, M. R. H. (1971). Release of oxytocin and vasopressin by the human foetus during labour. *Nature (London)*, **234**, 352–3
7. Wolf, H., Sabata, V., Frerichs, H. and Stubbe, P. (1969). Evidence for the impermeability of the human placenta for insulin. *Horm. Metab. Res.*, **1**, 274–5
8. Adam, P. A. J., Teramo, K., Raiha, N., Gitlin, D. and Schwartz, R. (1969). Human fetal insulin metabolism early in gestation. Response to acute elevation of the fetal glucose concentration and placental transfer of human insulin I[131]. *Diabetes*, **18**, 409–16
9. Adam, P. A. J., King, K. C., Schwartz, R. and Teramo, K. (1971). Human placental barrier to ^{125}I-glucagon early in gestation. *J. Clin. Endocrinol. Metab.*, **34**, 772–82
10. Kaplan, S. L., Grumbach, M. M. and Aubert, M. L. (1976). The ontogenesis of pituitary hormones and hypothalamic factors in the human fetus: maturation of central nervous system regulation of anterior pituitary functions. *Recent Prog. Horm. Res.*, **32**, 161–243
11. Reynolds, J. W. (1976). Feto-placental and neonatal steroid endocrinology. In Smith, C. A. and Nelson, N. M. (eds.) *The Physiology of the Newborn Infant*. 4th Edn., pp. 664–735. (Springfield, Illinois: Charles C. Thomas)
12. Erenberg, A., Phelps, D. L., Lamb, R. and Fisher, D. A. (1974). Total and free thyroxine and triiodothyronine concentrations in the newborn period. *Pediatrics*, **53**, 211–16
13. Sack, J., Fisher, D. A. and Wang, C. C. (1976). Serum thyrotropin, prolactin and growth hormone levels during the early neonatal period in the human infant. *J. Pediatr.*, **89**, 298–300
14. Delivoria Papadopoulos, M., Battaglia, F. C., Bruns, P. D. and Meschia, G. (1967). Total, protein-bound and ultra filterable calcium in maternal and fetal plasmas. *Am. J. Physiol.*, **213**, 363–6
15. David, L. and Anast, C. S. (1974). Calcium metabolism in newborn infants. *J. Clin. Invest.*, **54**, 287–96

16. Solomon, S. and Friesen, H. G. (1968). Endocrine relations between mother and fetus. *Annu. Rev. Med.*, **19**, 399–430
17. Bashore, R. A., Smith, F. and Gold, E. M. (1970). Placental transfer and metabolism of 4-¹⁴C-cortisol in the pregnant monkey. *Nature (London)*, **228**, 774–5
18. Beard, R. W. (1962). Response of the human foetal heart and maternal circulation to adrenaline and noradrenaline. *Br. Med. J.*, **1**, 443–6
19. Sandler, M., Ruthven, C. R. J., Contractor, S. F., Wood, C., Booth, R. T. and Pinkerton, J. H. M. (1963). Transmission of noradrenaline across the human placenta. *Nature (London)*, **197**, 598
20. Fisher, D. A., Lehman, H. and Lackey, C. (1964). Placental transport of thyroxine. *J. Clin. Endocrinol. Metab.*, **24**, 393–400
21. Raiti, S., Holzman, C. B., Scott, R. L. and Blizzard, R. M. (1967). Evidence for the placental transfer of triiodothyronine in human beings. *N. Engl. J. Med.*, **277**, 456–9
22. Fisher, D. A. (1979). Fetal endocrinology: endocrine disease and pregnancy. In De Groot. L. J., Cahill, G. F., Martini, L., Nelson, D. H., Odell, W. D., Potts, J. T., Steinberger, E. and Winegrad, A. I. (eds.) *Endocrinology*. pp. 1649–63. (New York: Grune and Stratton)
23. Ludwig, G. D. (1962). Hyperparathyroidism in relation to pregnancy. *N. Engl. J. Med.*, **267**, 637–42
24. Fisher, D. A. (1976). Endocrine physiology II. In Smith, C. A. and Nelson, N. M. (eds.) *The Physiology of the Newborn Infant*. 4th Edn., pp. 624–41. (Springfield, Illinois: Charles C. Thomas)
25. Pedersen, N. T. and Permin, H. (1975). Hyperparathyroidism in pregnancy. *Acta Obstet. Gynaecol. Scand.*, **54**, 281–3
26. Better, O. S., Levi, J., Greif, E., Tuma, S., Gellei, B. and Erlik, D. (1973). Prolonged neonatal parathyroid suppression. *Arch. Surg.*, **106**, 722–4
27. Menko, F. H., Bijvoet, L. M., Fronen, J. L. H. H., Sandler, L. M., Adami, S., O'Riordan, J. L. H., Schopman, W. and Heynen, G. (1983). Familial benign hypercalcemia. *Q. J. Med.*, **52**, 120–40
28. Matsuo, M., Okita, K., Takemine, H. and Fujita, T. (1982). Neonatal primary hyperparathyroidism in familial hypocalciuric hypercalcemia. *Am. J. Dis. Child.*, **136**, 728–31
29. Marx, S. J., Attie, M. F., Spiegel, A. M., Levine, M. A., Lasker, R. D. and Fox, M. (1982). The association between neonatal severe primary hyperparathyroidism and familial hypocalciuric hypercalcemia in three kindreds. *N. Engl. J. Med.*, **306**, 257–64
30. Sopwith, A. M., Burns, C., Grant, D. B., Taylor, G. W., Wolf, E. and Besser, G. M. (1984). Familial hypocalciuric hypercalcaemia: association with neonatal primary hyperparathyroidism, and possible linkage with HLA haplotype. *Clin. Endocrinol.* (In press)
31. Bongiovanni, A. M. and McPadden, A. J. (1960). Steroids during pregnancy and possible fetal consequences. *Fertil. Steril.*, **11**, 181–6
32. Kulin, H. E., Metzl, K. and Peterson, R. (1966). Urinary tetrahydrocortisone and tetrahydrocortisol in infants born of mothers treated with corticosteroids during pregnancy. *J. Pediatr.*, **69**, 648–51
33. Grimes, E. M., Fayez, J. A. and Miller, G. L. (1973). Cushing's syndrome and pregnancy. *Obstet. Gynecol.*, **42**, 550–9
34. Kreines, K. and De Vaux, W. D. (1971). Neonatal adrenal insufficiency associated with maternal Cushing's syndrome. *Pediatrics*, **47**, 516–19
35. Schenker, J. G. and Chowers, I. (1971). Pheochromocytoma and pregnancy. *Obstet. Gynecol. Surv.*, **26**, 739–47
36. Selenkow, H. A. (1975). In Fisher, D. A. and Burrow, G. N. (eds.) *Perinatal Physiology and Disease*. pp. 145–61. (New York: Raven Press)

37. Whitworth, A. S., Midgley, J. E. M. and Wilkins, T. A. (1982). A comparison of free T_4 and the ratio of total T_4 to T_4-binding globulin in serum through pregnancy. *Clin. Endocrinol.*, **17**, 307–13

38. Franklyn, J. A., Sheppard, M. C. and Ramsden, D. B. (1983). Serum free thyroxine and free triiodothyronine concentrations in pregnancy. *Br. Med. J.*, **287**, 394

39. Hershman, J. M., Kenimer, J. G., Higgins, P. and Patillo, R. A. (1975). Placental thyrotropins. In Fisher, D. A. and Burrow, G. N. (eds.) *Perinatal Thyroid Physiology and Disease*. pp. 11–20. (New York: Raven Press)

40. Burrow, G. N. (1978). Maternal–foetal considerations in hyperthyroidism. *Clin. Endocrinol. Metab.*, **7**, 115–25

41. Cheron, R. G., Kaplan, M. M., Larsen, P. R., Selenkow, H. A. and Crigler, J. F. (1981). Neonatal thyroid function after propylthiuracil therapy for maternal Graves' disease. *N. Engl. J. Med.*, **304**, 525–8

42. Solomon, D. H. (1981). Pregnancy in PTU. *N. Engl. J. Med.*, **304**, 538–9

43. Munro, I. S. S. M., Humphries, I. E. S. H., Smith, T. and Broadhead, G. D. (1978). The role of thyroid-stimulating immunoglobulins of Graves' disease in neonatal thyrotoxicosis. *Br. J. Obstet. Gynaecol.*, **85**, 837–43

44. Robinson, P. L., O'Mullane, N. M. and Alderman, B. (1979). Prenatal treatment of fetal thyrotoxicosis. *Br. Med. J.*, **1**, 383–4

45. Visser, G. H. A., Dawes, G. S. and Redman, G. W. G. (1981). Numerical analysis of the normal human antenatal fetal heartrate. *Br. J. Obstet. Gynaecol.*, **88**, 792–802

46. White, C. (1912). A foetus with congenital hereditary Graves' disease. *J. Obstet. Gynaecol. Br. Emp.*, **21**, 231–3

47. McKenzie, M. J. (1964). Neonatal Graves' disease. *J. Clin. Endocrinol. Metab.*, **24**, 660–8

48. Hollingsworth, D. R. and Mabry, C. C. (1976). Congenital Graves' disease. *Am. J. Dis. Child.*, **130**, 148–55

49. Daneman, D. and Howard, N. J. (1980). Neonatal thyrotoxicosis: intellectual impairment and craniosynostosis in later years. *J. Pediatr.*, **97**, 257–9

2

NORMAL AND ABNORMAL PANCREATIC ENDOCRINE FUNCTION IN THE NEONATE

A. AYNSLEY-GREEN

The purpose of this chapter is to review some aspects of normal and abnormal pancreatic endocrine function in the newborn period. In order to understand fully the importance of the endocrine pancreas at this time of life and the metabolic derangements caused by abnormal function, it is necessary to review first the control of blood glucose homeostasis in the fetus and neonate.

THE ROLE OF THE ENDOCRINE PANCREAS IN THE CONTROL OF BLOOD GLUCOSE HOMEOSTASIS IN THE FETUS AND NEONATE

For obvious reasons, far less is known of the precise mechanisms controlling blood glucose concentrations in the human fetus at different stages of gestation than in adult subjects, and current concepts of fetal glucose homeostasis have been derived primarily from studies in experimental animals.

The fetus receives a constant intravenous supply of glucose across the placenta and this makes the major contribution to determining fetal blood glucose concentration. Although little is known of the changes in delivery rate in relation to maternal feeding and fasting, it is unlikely that the normal fetus experiences intrauterine 'starvation'.

Insulin is the main fetal anabolic hormone, and it can be identified in the human pancreas early in gestation. The orderly anatomical and functional development of the cell types secreting hormones is of crucial

19

importance for coping with the metabolic crisis to be faced by the fetus at birth.

Discrete endocrine cells arise from acinar buds around the 10th week of gestation. The cells migrate to form the functional unit of the endocrine pancreas, the islet of Langerhans. By the 22nd week, well-formed mature islets can be recognized as discrete structures in close association with the ducts from which they have budded. The relevance of these developmental changes for human pathology is emphasized by the observation that the characteristic budding of pancreatic islets from exocrine ducts in nesidioblastosis (*vide infra*) is reminiscent of the embryogenesis of normal pancreatic islets. The factors controlling the anatomical and functional development of the endocrine pancreas are not understood, and much work is needed to define the regulation of fetal pancreatic endocrine development. Nonetheless it can be said that the net effect of these developments is to ensure that there is, *in utero*, a high circulating insulin:glucagon ratio which favours anabolism and the formation of glycogen and adipose tissue.

Recent findings in relation to receptor numbers and affinity further support the predominance of anabolism. Glucagon receptors in the fetal liver are markedly decreased[1], but the insulin receptor number and/or affinity in several fetal tissues are markedly higher than those of corresponding adult tissue[2,3].

Glucose is the most important substrate for brain metabolism, and a continuous supply of glucose is essential for normal neurological function. At delivery the constant supply of glucose received from the mother ceases abruptly, and the neonate has to face an immediate metabolic crisis, namely the need to maintain normoglycaemia.

The normal infant born at term shows an immediate fall in blood glucose concentration during the first 4–6 h[4], from values close to maternal levels to around 2.5 mmol/l (45 mg/100 ml), suggesting that one or more of the mechanisms required for fasting adaptation are not fully developed at birth. During the first hours after birth the maintenance of normal blood glucose levels is dependent upon several factors: adequate stores of glycogen, a functioning glycogenolytic enzyme system, normal functioning gluconeogenic enzymes, an adequate supply of endogenous gluconeogenic substrates (amino acids, lactate and glycerol), and finally, and of greatest importance in triggering these processes, the integrated secretion of metabolic hormones.

Postnatal hormonal changes have a central role in regulating glucose mobilization through glycogenolysis and gluconeogenesis[5]. Of particular importance is the abrupt increase in plasma glucagon which occurs within minutes to hours of birth in the neonates of all mammalian species studied[5,6]. This initial glucagon surge is the key adaptive change which triggers the switch to glucose production. Plasma insulin levels, on the other hand, remain low for several days[5]. Evidence to support the importance of glucagon is the severe hypoglycaemia which occurs if glucagon secretion is prevented in lambs by infusion of somatostatin: normoglycaemia is maintained if sufficient exogenous glucagon is infused with somatostatin to restore plasma glucagon levels to those of the normal animal[5].

Although adrenaline and noradrenaline concentrations increase markedly[7], and circulating growth hormone concentrations are also high at birth[4], the available evidence suggests that they have a relatively small role in the initial stabilization of blood glucose levels. The role of cortisol is at present enigmatic, and further work is needed to define the individual importance of all of these hormones in the adaptive process. Nonetheless, the net effect of these postnatal endocrine inter-relations is to ensure the 'switching on' of new glucose production.

The neonate born at term responds to the first feed of milk with an increase in blood glucose in the order of 1.0 mmol/l (18 mg/100 ml), associated with a small increase in plasma insulin; plasma growth hormone, gastrin and enteroglucagon concentrations also rise[8]. Although the preterm infant fails to show a change in any intermediary metabolite or hormone concentration after the first feed[9], by 2 days after birth feed-induced metabolic and endocrine surges can be defined[10].

During the first days after birth the healthy term and preterm infant show progressive increments in basal (prefeed) concentrations of glucose and a number of enteroinsular hormones, including enteroglucagon, gastrin, pancreatic polypeptide and neurotensin[9, 11–14]. In addition, a progressive postprandial increase in the release of enteroinsular hormones in response to feeds occurs during the first days, the change in insulin secretion appearing to be related to the development of gastric inhibitory polypeptide secretion[13]. Thus enteral feeding, through stimulating enteroinsular hormone release, may trigger morphological and functional changes in the neonatal pancreas, alimentary tract and liver.

ABNORMAL PANCREATIC ENDOCRINE FUNCTION

The most common and important abnormality caused by deranged neonatal islet cell function is hyperinsulinaemic hypoglycaemia. Hyperinsulinism causes hypoglycaemia as a result of both increased utilization of blood glucose and decreased rate of endogenous glucose production[15–17]. The causes of hyperinsulinism in the neonate can be classified according to whether the resulting hypoglycaemia is a transient phenomenon or one which recurs or persists.

TRANSIENT NEONATAL HYPERINSULINISM

Transient neonatal hypoglycaemia due to hyperinsulinism is seen commonly in infants of diabetic mothers (IDMs), infants with erythroblastosis fetalis and in those with the Beckwith–Wiedemann syndrome. It has also been observed after the administration of some drugs to the mother, after intrapartum maternal glucose infusions and in sporadic cases with unknown aetiology ('idiopathic').

The infant of a diabetic mother

Infants born to mothers with poorly controlled diabetes mellitus have a characteristic appearance. They are overweight for gestational age, with increased body fat and increased length. There is a clear association between the severity and control of the maternal diabetes and the development of hypoglycaemia in the infant[18]. Postnatally most infants have a 1–4 h transient period of asymptomatic hypoglycaemia before a spontaneous increase in blood glucose level occurs. Others have a more prolonged period of severe symptomatic hypoglycaemia, while a minority develop late hypoglycaemia after an initial benign course. All, however, regain normal blood glucose control within the first few days after birth.

IDMs have hyperinsulinism at birth due to increased placental transfer of glucose and other nutrients stimulating hyperplasia of the islets of Langerhans in the fetus[19]. Umbilical plasma has an elevated level of C-peptide, the connecting peptide of the proinsulin molecule[20], with increased levels after glucose, confirming increased insulin production[21]. Insulin receptor number is, paradoxically, 'up-regulated' in these infants, so that they have an unexpected increase in receptor number[2].

The infants also fail to develop the normal increase in plasma glucagon at 2 h of age[6,22], so that the development of hypoglycaemia is due to a combination of hyperinsulinaemia and hypoglucagonaemia. The effect of this on the liver has been confirmed by demonstrating decreased glucose production with stable isotope methods[15].

The dominance of insulin also affects other metabolic fuels. Thus plasma free fatty acid levels are low, with a diminished increase during the first few hours, and blood ketone body concentrations are also significantly lower than in normal infants. Plasma amino acid concentrations are less affected than in organic hyperinsulinism, and the characteristic low blood level of branched chain amino acids is not an invariable finding[23–25], possibly due to other transient disturbances in postnatal metabolic adaptation. The glycaemic response to alanine, for example, is blunted at 3 h of age, but alanine is readily converted into glucose at 16–24 h of age[26]. This observation implies delayed development of hepatic gluconeogenesis.

The pancreas shows hyperplasia and hypertrophy of the islets of Langerhans[27,28] without evidence of nesidioblastosis. An increase of the glucagon and PP cell fractions in the pancreas has recently also been shown by modern immunocytochemical methods[29].

In relation to management, meticulous control of the maternal diabetes throughout pregnancy is essential. Venous blood glucose values should be obtained from mother and cord at delivery and from the infant at least 1, 2, 4 and 6 h after birth. Transient asymptomatic hypoglycaemia may be prevented by giving enteral feeds with milk within 1–2 h after delivery, since it has been shown that a feed of 10 mg/kg of human milk will cause an increase of blood glucose in the order of 1 mmol/l at this time[10].

Should hypoglycaemia occur despite feeding, a single injection of glucagon (0.03–0.1 mg/kg body weight) will cause an increase in blood glucose and may suffice to prevent recurrence. Sick infants unable to tolerate enteral feeding should receive an intravenous infusion of glucose at an initial rate of 4–8 mg/kg/min to prevent the development of hypoglycaemia. Symptomatic hypoglycaemia in any infant, however, warrants immediate correction by a bolus injection of 0.2–0.5 g/kg glucose followed by glucose infusion, the rate being adjusted as necessary to maintain normoglycaemia. Occasionally, hypoglycaemia persists despite these measures, and then 5 mg/kg cortisol can be given intravenously or intramuscularly at 12 h intervals.

Enteral feeds can be increased and parenteral glucose decreased after the blood glucose concentration has been stable for 12 h or so. Reactive hypoglycaemia may occur if the glucose infusion is decreased too quickly.

The long-term prognosis after transient hypoglycaemia in the IDM is generally good, although very few prospective studies are available[30–32].

It should be emphasized that in the vast majority of infants of strictly controlled, euglycaemic, diabetic mothers, hypoglycaemia is rarely a problem. Normal C-peptide levels have been found in the cord blood of such infants[33], and the glucose production rate, measured by stable isotope methods, is normal[34].

Erythroblastosis fetalis

There is a well-recognized association between hypoglycaemia and moderate to severe erythroblastosis fetalis due to rhesus incompatibility. A frequency of 18% was reported in one study by Raivio and Osterlund[35] in infants with a cord blood haemoglobin below 10 g/dl.

The postnatal hypoglycaemia is due to hyperinsulinism, which may be present before birth[36]. Thus these infants have elevated plasma insulin concentrations[37], and low levels of circulating free fatty acids. Interestingly, they also have increased plasma glucagon concentrations[38] and increased clearance of administered glucose[39]. Exchange transfusion for hyperbilirubinaemia with acid, citrate dextrose (ACD) blood causes an increase in blood glucose and plasma insulin, but insulin secretion is slow to decrease when the exchange is stopped, leading to rebound hypoglycaemia.

The pathophysiology of the hyperinsulinism is not completely understood. The pancreas contains increased extractable insulin[40], and there is hyperplasia of the islets of Langerhans, the appearance differing from that of IDMs[41]. Using modern immunocytochemical methods, Milner et al.[42] have shown that the volume fractions of all four cell types were greater in the PP-rich (ventral lobe) part of the pancreas, with no change in the PP-poor (dorsal lobe) islets. The stimulus which causes islet hyperplasia is unknown: various hypotheses have been suggested, including insulin destruction during intravascular haemolysis leading to compensatory hypertrophy of the beta cells, and release of amino acids or other products of haemolysis which are trophic to the islets.

Blood glucose levels should be monitored carefully in all infants with erythroblastosis before and particularly after exchange transfusions. The management of more prolonged hypoglycaemia is identical to that of the IDM.

Beckwith–Wiedemann syndrome

The syndrome, described independently by Beckwith[43] and Wiedemann[44], is characterized by exomphalos, macroglossia, visceromegaly, gigantism and hyperinsulinaemic hypoglycaemia. Over 80 cases have been reported[45] and a number of endocrine abnormalities have been described. Symptomatic hypoglycaemia occurs in up to 50% of cases, which may explain the mental retardation reported in many survivors. Because of this, the diagnosis must be considered and blood glucose levels monitored in any infant with exomphalos or gigantism at birth, since the full constellation of signs may not be evident.

Islet cell hypertrophy has been described[43,46], although a deficiency of glucagon has been proposed as an alternative explanation for the hypoglycaemia[47]. Using modern immunocytochemical methods, we have shown, in collaboration with Dr J. M. Polak, a marked increase in total area occupied by endocrine tissue and by islets in the pancreas without evidence of nesidioblastosis. There was a reduction in the area occupied by somatostatin cells and a decrease in extractable somatostatin, but it is not known whether this is a primary or secondary change. Since others[48,49] have documented some features of nesidioblastosis in pancreata from such infants, it must be concluded that the hyperinsulinism may be associated with different histological appearances of the pancreatic abnormalities. Further work is needed to clarify these aspects.

It is not clear why hyperinsulinism develops. The mothers do not have glycosuria during pregnancy, nor do they have any other known metabolic abnormality. Elevated concentrations of plasma growth hormone and somatomedin have been detected at birth[50,51], suggesting that there is an abnormality in the production of fetal growth-regulating peptides.

The hypoglycaemia of the Beckwith–Wiedemann syndrome is usually transient but may occasionally be prolonged and severe, lasting for several months[52]. Frequent small feeds, glucagon, diazoxide, corticosteroids and adrenaline alone or in various combinations have been used in the latter circumstance, and in one very severe case partial pancreatectomy was necessary[48]. The diagnosis and management of hyperinsulinism are described below.

Transient neonatal hyperinsulinism due to maternal drug and glucose therapy

The majority of drugs given to the pregnant woman readily cross the placenta and can affect the fetus. Drugs causing fetal and neonatal hyperinsulinism can act in two ways: they may either stimulate the fetal beta cell directly (e.g. sulphonylureas), or cause fetal hyperinsulinism which is in part due to the fetal hyperglycaemia caused by the drug (e.g. beta-sympathomimetic drugs).

Of much greater practical importance is the induction of hyperinsulinism due to maternal glucose therapy during labour. It has long been demonstrated that fetal insulin secretion can be induced by maternal glucose infusions[53–56]. The effect of 'routine' intravenous infusion of glucose during delivery has also been studied. Lucas et al.[57] found that if mothers were given 10–20 g glucose/h intravenously for over 4 h before delivery, cord blood plasma insulin values were significantly increased compared with those infants whose mothers had either received no glucose before delivery or had been given a glucose infusion supplying less than 10 g glucose/h.

'Idiopathic' hyperinsulinism

Cornblath et al.[58] reported that relatively high levels of plasma insulin were present in neonatal infants with transient symptomatic hypoglycaemia when compared with asymptomatic controls. Similar results were found by Pildes et al.[59] in a mixed group of neonates with transient neonatal hypoglycaemia. Furthermore, Le Dune[60] showed that some hypoglycaemic small-for-gestational-age (SGA) infants also had high plasma insulin levels. Although in the majority of SGA infants the hypoglycaemia is part of a multifactorial phenomenon, functional hyperinsulinism may be an additional and determinant mechanism responsible for the hypoglycaemia.

Severe hyperinsulinaemic hypoglycaemia can also develop immediately after birth in full-term, appropriate-for-gestational-age babies born after apparently normal pregnancy and delivery with no history of maternal diabetes, drug therapy or antenatal maternal glucose infusion. We have observed three such babies recently[61] who regained normal glucose homeostasis spontaneously.

Spontaneous remission of severe neonatal hyperinsulinaemic hypoglycaemia has also been described by Landau et al.[62]. We conclude that transient hyperinsulinaemic hypoglycaemia is an enigmatic entity, and it is possible that it represents a regulatory disturbance in insulin secretion immediately after birth.

PERSISTENT OR RECURRENT HYPERINSULINISM

The conditions described above are usually associated with a transient disturbance, the hypoglycaemia eventually resolving with restoration of normal insulin control. Of much greater importance are conditions leading to recurrent or persistent hypoglycaemia, particularly since the hyperinsulinism may be exceedingly difficult to control.

This type of hyperinsulinism is the most common cause of severe persistent hypoglycaemia in infants during the first year of life[63]. It has previously masqueraded under various names, including 'idiopathic hypoglycaemia of infancy'[64], leucine-sensitive hypoglycaemia, neonatal insulinoma, microadenomatosis, focal hyperplasia and nesidioblastosis.

The vast majority of cases present with the classical symptoms of hypoglycaemia developing in many of them within minutes of birth. In 13 of the 18 cases of organic hyperinsulinism we have reviewed recently[61], the infants presented with hypoglycaemia within 3 days of birth. One child presented as an averted death on the first day[65]. The importance of hypoglycaemia as a cause of early neonatal death is further emphasized by Polak and Wigglesworth[66], who reported the occurrence of nesidioblastosis in the pancreas of such an infant. It is clear, therefore, that hyperinsulinism is a potent cause not only of severe persistent hypoglycaemia during the first days after birth, but also of sudden early neonatal death. Whether pancreatic nesidioblastosis can cause fatal hypoglycaemia in an older infant without any previous symptom suggestive of hypoglycaemia has yet to be proved, although Cox et al.[67] reported that 36% of pancreata from cases of sudden infant death in the first year of life showed pancreatic nesidioblastosis.

Equal numbers of male and female infants and children seem to be affected. Analysis of the neonatal cases reveals that only a few of the reports give details of the pregnancies, but none of these mothers suffered from diabetes mellitus and the pregnancies had been completely uneventful. There are a few reports of siblings being affected with severe neonatal nesidioblastosis[68], suggesting an autosomal recessive mode of inheritance.

Many of the babies have a striking similar physical appearance, resembling that of the IDM, with chubby cheeks, generalized adiposity and increased birth weight. The clinical presentation of an infant with a localized pancreatic abnormality (insulinoma) can be identical to that of a baby with a more diffuse abnormality (nesidioblastosis).

DIAGNOSTIC CRITERIA FOR HYPERINSULINISM FROM METABOLIC AND ENDOCRINE STUDIES

The most important diagnostic point is the demonstration of an inappropriate plasma insulin value for the level of glycaemia. Insulin release normally falls to very low or undetectable levels when blood glucose concentration decreases[69], and the demonstration of even normal fasting levels of plasma insulin during severe hypoglycaemia implies a defect in the control of basal insulin release. It must be emphasized that a plasma insulin value can only be interpreted when the blood glucose level in the same blood sample is known.

In healthy individuals, fasting elicits lipolysis and ketogenesis, related to the fall in blood glucose and plasma insulin levels. Hyperinsulinism prevents ketogenesis through a decrease in adipose tissue lipolysis and hence a diminution of fatty acid substrate supply to the liver. Baker and Stanley[63] were the first to emphasize the importance of documenting a lack of ketosis as a diagnostic point for hyperinsulinism in childhood (as opposed to 'ketotic' hypoglycaemia), and this has been shown also to apply to the neonate[70].

The coexistence of hypoglycaemia and hypoketonaemia in hyperinsulinism is of major clinical significance. On the one hand, the brain is deprived of glucose as a primary fuel, whilst on the other hand, ketone bodies as alternative fuels are not available. Thus, the central nervous system is apparently left with no fuels to maintain normal metabolism. The importance of the hypoketonaemia is further emphasized by the clinical observation that brain damage in children suffering from other causes of hypoglycaemia with ketosis is usually less frequent and less severe than in hyperinsulinism[71]. With the exception of rare defects of fatty acid metabolism, all conditions causing hypoglycaemia in childhood are associated with endocrine counter-regulation, lipolysis and ketogenesis ('ketotic' hypoglycaemia). The occurrence of hypoglycaemia with ketosis ('non-ketotic' hypoglycaemia) must be regarded as being due to hyperinsulinism until proved otherwise.

The plasma levels of branched chain amino acids are sensitive indicators of the circulating plasma insulin concentrations. Thus these acids are elevated in diabetic ketosis (insulin deficiency) and decreased in both adults and children with hyperinsulinism[72–74].

The high glucose disappearance rate measured during an intravenous glucose tolerance test can be regarded as one of the biochemical characteristics of hyperinsulinism. However, the diagnostic value of the intravenous glucose tolerance test is limited by the danger of inducing reactive hypoglycaemia. The calculation of the glucose infusion rate in terms of mg/kg/min needed to maintain a blood glucose level above 2.0 mmol/l is a safer method of assessing glucose clearance. A mean glucose infusion rate of 16.1 ± 2.1 mg/kg/min was needed to achieve this level of glycaemia in newborn infants with hyperinsulinism[61]; the normal glucose production rate in neonates is of the order of 6 mg/kg/min[75].

An important and predictable effect of hyperinsulinism is the inappropriate conservation of liver glycogen during fasting. Inhibition of liver glycogenolysis by insulin probably accounts for this inappropriate preservation of hepatic glycogen stores. This is clearly demonstrated by the characteristically large increase in blood glucose levels when glucagon is administered during hyperinsulinaemic hypoglycaemia[61,70,76]. As a result of the glycogenic effect of insulin hypersecretion in hyperinsulinaemic newborns receiving continuous glucose infusion, there is a progressive increase in the size of the liver and its glycogen content when measured by biopsy[70].

A decrease in the concentration of glucose and an increase in that of insulin after the administration of leucine has long been used as a test for excessive secretion of insulin[77,78]. It has also been shown, however, that a considerable proportion of patients[61,79] do not respond. It should also be noted that when the result is positive, the increased release of insulin may cause profound symptomatic hypoglycaemia. The results of the arginine infusion test are even more disappointing[77], and we do not recommend the use of these two provocative tests in the diagnosis of hyperinsulinism in children.

The ability of somatostatin to decrease endogenous insulin secretion has led to its use as a diagnostic tool to demonstrate organic hyperinsulinism. In contrast to the variable results in adults[79], somatostatin infusion in infants and children with hyperinsulinism invariably has increased blood glucose and decreased plasma insulin concentrations[80–83,91]. This effect has led to its use as therapy of hyperinsulinism (*vide infra*).

Since there is no reliable biochemical or hormonal marker for the nature of the underlying pancreatic abnormality, several procedures, including selective coeliac angiography and ultrasonography, have been used in the preoperative localization of insulin-secreting tumours in adults and older children[10,61,79]. There are technical limitations in the small neonate, but nonetheless Kirkland et al.[84] reported a case in which the preoperative diagnosis of an insulinoma in a neonate was established by selective angiography. We recommend coeliac angiography only in the older child.

MANAGEMENT OF HYPERINSULINAEMIC HYPOGLYCAEMIA

Medical therapy

The immediate priority is to increase blood glucose concentrations to prevent convulsions and neurological damage. Glucose administration is clearly the first therapeutic measure, but very high infusion rates (>15 mg/kg/min) may only alleviate symptoms without restoring normoglycaemia. Most reports have emphasized the extreme difficulty in controlling blood glucose concentrations in these infants, particularly vulnerable periods occurring during the resiting of glucose infusions.

Diazoxide induces an increase in glycaemia by interfering with three basic mechanisms controlling carbohydrate metabolism: it inhibits insulin release from the pancreas, it enhances the secretion of adrenaline from the adrenal medulla and from sympathetic nerve endings, and it stimulates glycogenolysis[85].

The first report of diazoxide administration in children was that of Drash and Wolff[86], who initiated diazoxide treatment to control hypoglycaemia in a child with 'leucine sensitivity' who had previously undergone a subtotal pancreatectomy. During the last 20 years diazoxide has been used widely in the treatment of different forms of hyperinsulinism, with variable results[71,87]. In none of 20 documented cases in a more recent analysis[88] was diazoxide entirely effective, although in some it had an initial beneficial effect with subsequent return to hypoglycaemia. This was, of course, a highly selected series of infants, since all came to laparotomy because of a failure of medical therapy. In our series of 18 children[61], five infants with neonatal nesidioblastosis responded to diazoxide only initially, but improvement was not maintained, and all infants eventually underwent total pancreatectomy. Two other infants in the same series with onset of symptoms at 5 days and 6 months responded to and remain on diazoxide, whereas another two infants responded only after partial pancreatectomy. In one of these cases it was possible to stop diazoxide treatment after 5 years, the child remaining normoglycaemic thereafter.

It is not clear why improvement is not maintained in some infants who may respond extremely well initially to diazoxide and it must be concluded that the response to diazoxide is unpredictable and that continuing close supervision is needed for any infant who appears to respond well to the introduction of diazoxide therapy.

Diazoxide is usually given in doses of up to 25 mg/kg/day and in combination with a thiazide diuretic. The addition of the latter not only reduces the incidence of side-effects, especially water retention, but also potentiates the hyperglycaemic effect of diazoxide.

Although several minor complications of diazoxide therapy have been observed, the most commonly seen is hypertrichosis of the languo type (hypertrichosis lanuginosa), which is observed in almost all cases treated for periods longer than a few months. More important side-effects are fluid retention and oedema and the development of blood dyscrasias. However, dose dependency of these side-effects has been reported[89], and most resolve with a decrease or discontinuation of therapy.

Although recommended by some as part of an initial diagnostic therapeutic trial, hydrocortisone rarely improves blood glucose concentration, and once its ineffectiveness has been demonstrated it should be discontinued to prevent the development of hyperadrenocorticism and delay in wound healing.

Glucagon appears to be effective through mobilizing glucose directly from glycogen. The normal short-acting glucagon has only a transient effect, lasting usually less than 1–2 h, but it is particularly useful for emergency situations, e.g. to cover the time needed for resiting an intravenous glucose infusion. A long-acting preparation, zinc-protamine glucagon, was used with transient success by Aynsley-Green et al.[70]. One major disadvantage of glucagon is that in addition to mobilizing glucose it also stimulates insulin release through a direct effect on the beta cells[90]. Prolonged use could theoretically exacerbate the underlying hyper-insulinism and may contribute to a regeneration of the endocrine pancreas after partial pancreatectomy through the continuous stimulation of insulin release[88].

Somatostatin has an inhibitory effect on insulin release and has been used in both diagnosis and therapy of hyperinsulinism in neonates and infants (for review, see reference 91). At present, however, this drug can only be used as a temporary measure, since it inhibits other endocrine systems and the long-term effects of prolonged treatment are unknown.

Cornblath and Schwartz[71] recommended long-acting adrenaline (Susphrine) in the initial diagnostic therapeutic evaluation of severe neonatal hypoglycaemia. Propranolol, a drug which has been tried in adults in pancreatic insulinomas, has also been tried in infants, with no beneficial effect[74,88].

Phenytoin has a direct inhibitory effect on insulin secretion and has been used in adult patients with insulinomas, but no beneficial effect was observed when this drug was used in one newborn infant[70].

Finally, an attempt was made by Aynsley-Green et al.[70] to provide an increase in alternative fuels to glucose by increasing blood ketone body concentrations by means of a diet rich in medium chain triglycerides and by injections of human growth hormone. No beneficial effect was seen with either form of therapy. However, direct infusion of ketone bodies has recently been shown to increase hepatic glucose production[17].

It is concluded that the underlying endocrine abnormality may be remarkably resistant to drugs which have powerful effects on inhibiting insulin secretion, both in vitro from pancreatic islets with normal architecture, and in vivo from adenomas in adults.

One other aspect of medical treatment deserves mention, and this is the use of potent antimitotic beta cell poisons in the form of alloxan and streptozotocin, drugs which have been used for many years to induce diabetes in experimental animals and in adults with malignant insulinomas. We have discounted their use in childhood in view of their toxicity and the uncertainty of their effect on other tissues and potential long-term sequelae. The latter are of particular importance, not only because of the potential effects on rapidly developing organs, but also because of the possibility of inducing malignant insulinomas, as can occur in experimental animals given stretozotocin[92]. Nonetheless, a recent paper has reported two children treated with alloxan with apparently good result[121].

The role of surgery

Not all infants and children who develop hyperinsulinaemic hypoglycaemia require surgery. Five infants with 'idiopathic transient neonatal hyperinsulinism' have been reported recently[61]. In this series two infants improved spontaneously after 3–4 days glucose therapy alone, the other three responded well to diazoxide. This treatment was withdrawn after a few days without subsequent recurrence of hypoglycaemia. Two other patients in the same series responded to and remain on diazoxide.

Many other infants have been reported who require longer periods of diazoxide therapy but maintain satisfactory blood glucose concentrations with the use of this drug. In the absence of histological data it is impossible to know the nature of the underlying pancreatic pathology in these children. Some caution is necessary, therefore, before proceeding to surgery, and the need for this major step must be considered in the context of each patient and his or her particular management problems.

Surgical treatment of hyperinsulinism, however, is indicated as a matter of urgency during the first days of life when the biochemical criteria for the diagnosis are met, and when the infant remains glucose-drip dependent despite diazoxide (20–25 mg/kg/day) and chlorothiazide. The biochemical data do not provide information as to whether the lesion causing the hyperinsulinism is a discrete adenoma or a more widespread and diffuse form of nesidioblastosis; the successful pre-operative diagnosis and localization of an adenoma by angiography in the newborn is exceptionally rare.

Moreover, the palpation of the pancreas at operation may not reveal the presence of a small tumour. So even if a localized lesion cannot be found preoperatively or at surgery in the resected pancreas, then a tissue diagnosis must be established by using insulin-specific and immunohistochemical methods. In the absence of a detectable adenoma a subtotal pancreatectomy should be performed, in the first instance removing

75–80% of the pancreas. Practical aspects of the surgery have been reviewed by Thomas et al.[93] and Fonkalsrud et al.[94]. Resection of a localized lesion is likely to result in cure of the hyperinsulinism.

The outcome of 26 infants after operation was recently analysed by Aynsley-Green[88]. Nineteen (73%) remained hypoglycaemic after partial pancreatectomy, and 11 were submitted to total or near-total pancreatectomy thereafter, at intervals ranging from 2 weeks to 10 months after the first operation.

In our series of eight children with severe hyperinsulinaemic hypoglycaemia[61], a localized lesion was found in three, but in the remaining five, who had nesidioblastosis, subtotal pancreatectomy failed to control hypoglycaemia, and all subsequently underwent further surgery. It is noteworthy that pancreatic regeneration had occurred in two of these cases.

Subtotal pancreatectomy alone also failed to control hypoglycaemia in all of the six infants with diffuse pancreatic pathology reported by Baker and Stanley[63], but it was beneficial in that it allowed better control with diazoxide in five of them. Two of our patients[61] also responded to diazoxide after pancreatectomy.

In the absence of an insulinoma, partial pancreatectomy alone is rarely a definitive treatment for nesidioblastosis. In a review of 44 cases[88], only five infants were said to have normal blood glucose concentrations after partial pancreatectomy. A few infants subjected to 'total' pancreatectomy became normoglycaemic without insulin therapy, the majority developed diabetes. Presumably enough pancreatic endocrine tissue was left behind in the former infants to prevent hyperglycaemia.

There are theoretical long-term risks to the child following total removal of the pancreas, particularly in the control of complications of diabetes. There is no information on the incidence of such long-term complications of diabetes induced by pancreatectomy in early life. Nonetheless, the theoretical and practical risks of long-term post-pancreatectomy diabetes (including the requirement for pancreatic exocrine supplementation) must be balanced against the probability that permanent brain damage will result from recurrent hypoglycaemic convulsions.

PATHOPHYSIOLOGY AND AETIOLOGY OF PERSISTENT HYPERINSULINISM

Until recently, persistent hyperinsulinaemic hypoglycaemia in early life had been attributed not only to pancreatic nesidioblastosis, but also to a number of other pathologies, including diffuse beta cell hyperplasia[95], microadenomatosis[96], focal islet cell adenomatosis[97] and 'functional' beta cell disorders without histological abnormalities. It has not been possible to differentiate these conditions clinically or biochemically, and the morphological classification has usually been based on imprecise histological grounds. However, recent developments in immunohisto-chemistry and morphometry have led to the challenge of the view that the different morphological patterns noted above are discrete entities; they seem rather to be all variants of nesidioblastosis, the end result of inappropriate control of pancreatic endocrine development during fetal life[98]. However, this conclusion is not universally accepted, and it must be stated immediately that much remains to be learned of the aetio-logical and functional significance of various histological abnormalities.

Brown and Young[99] and Yakovac et al.[100] were the first to draw attention to the presence of an unusual histological feature in pancreata removed from children with severe hypoglycaemia. The latter authors reported that although only a minority of pancreata looked abnormal when stained conventionally, all showed individual and grouped insulin-secreting cells lying in duct epithelium and in acinar tissue outside islets of Langerhans when insulin-specific staining methods were used. This abnormality was termed 'nesidioblastosis'.

Structural and morphometric analyses were performed by Kloppel et al.[97] on a single case of nesidioblastosis, while Sovik et al.[101] analysed three cases of profound hyperinsulinism. Heitz et al.[98], in a more detailed study, examined seven pancreata from children submitted to lapar-otomy because of persistent hyperinsulinaemic hypoglycaemia. The latter authors concluded that the most important feature common to all cases was a five-fold increase in mean total area occupied by endocrine tissue compared with control pancreata, a feature which could only be recognized by precise quantification of the endocrine cells. The presence of 'budding off' from the ductular epithelium, with interposition of individual or clusters of insulin, glucagon, somatostatin and PP cells lying between ductal epithelium cells, was also noted in some cases.

Polak and Bloom[102] and Bishop et al.[103] in a further analysis commented that in the islets of these infants the somatostatin cells appeared to be decreased in number and size and, when compared with control somatostatin cells, had fewer secretory granules. The normal ratio of approximately two insulin cells to one somatostatin cell seen in fetal and normal neonatal pancreas was changed to five insulin cells to one somatostatin cell, all cells appearing scattered throughout the pancreas rather than in islets.

Polak and Bloom[102] suggested from this that an additional important feature of nesidioblastosis was the lack of the normal close anatomical relationship of the insulin and somatostatin cells. Radioimmunoassay of tissue extracts from pancreata showed a substantial increase in insulin content, and of considerable interest and supporting the morphological results was the observation that somatostatin content was only half that found in the controls[102]. This substantiates the clinical observations (*vide supra*) on the effectiveness of exogenous somatostatin in increasing blood glucose concentrations.

The hypothesis that the above histological features are pathological has been questioned by more recent studies[104–106]. In essence, these authors have shown that the nesidioblastosis-like picture also occurs in control pancreata from children dying without hypoglycaemia in the first months after birth. Falkmer *et al.*[105] raised the question of whether there were specific types of endocrine cell in pathological pancreata with a nesidioblastosis-like appearance which were not present in normal pancreata. The appearance of an 'intermediate' endocrine cell type was also described by Gould *et al.*[106]. It is possible that subtle abnormalities in paracrine or neurocrine activity of regulatory peptides may also be responsible for the uncontrolled insulin secretion in these cases.

In addition to the histological controversy described above, there appears to be a functional abnormality in insulin secretion in islets which may appear structurally normal. Thus we have demonstrated a loss of the normal glucose dependency of insulin release in islets isolated and incubated *in vitro* from the pancreas removed from a newborn infant with hyperinsulinaemic hypoglycaemia[61, 70]. Whether this is due to a decrease in somatostatin cells in these clusters or to a primary abnormality of glucose recognition by the beta cell is unknown.

Clearly there are many questions which need to be answered in relation to the control of both fetal pancreatic endocrine development and neonatal islet regulation. Further research may clear up several paradoxes which seem inexplicable at present, particularly in the context of the spectrum of presentation and the response to treatment. Such research may also reveal why some children 'outgrow' hyperinsulinism. The lack of information inevitably means that present management can only be pragmatic and empirical, with early recourse to surgery as a definitive treatment.

In contrast to the controversies surrounding the concept of diffuse nesidioblastosis, there is incontrovertible evidence that isolated adenomas exist in the neonate and that resection is curative.

Whilst organic hyperinsulinism during the early neonatal period is usually due to nesidioblastosis, many cases of insulinoma (congenital islet cell adenoma) have been described in neonates[84, 107–113], resection of which is curative of the hypoglycaemia.

The aetiology of the pancreatic abnormalities causing hyperinsulinism in early life is unknown. Heitz *et al.*[98] suggested that the histological resemblance of nesidioblastosis pancreata to those from the fetus early in gestation arises as a result of inappropriate control during the earliest phases of endocrine pancreatic development. Whether the adverse influence causing the endocrine malfunction is primarily a genetic defect or the result of interplay of various external factors cannot be decided until more is known of the factors regulating fetal pancreatic development. That there may be a genetic component with an autosomal recessive inheritance pattern is shown by the familial occurrence of neonatal nesidioblastosis[67,68,101] and by nesidioblastosis in familial endocrine adenomatosis[114].

LEUCINE-SENSITIVE HYPOGLYCAEMIA

The entity of leucine-sensitive hypoglycaemia was first suggested by Cochrane et al.[115]. Many patients have been reported subsequently who developed hypoglycaemia during leucine administration[95] and who improved on a low-leucine diet. However, leucine administration stimulates insulin secretion in normal children and adults, suggesting that leucine sensitivity is not a specific diagnostic entity, but only one manifestation of an underlying tendency to hyperinsulinism. Thus patients with hypoglycaemia after leucine may also demonstrate increased insulin release after tolbutamide or glucagon[95].

In instances where such patients have been subjected to pancreatectomy or pancreatic biopsy, beta cell hyperplasia or evidence for nesidioblastosis has been found[95]. Conversely, most patients with less severe leucine sensitivity have not been subjected to pancreatic exploration, and there are no histological data on the pancreata of those mildly affected children who respond to a low-leucine diet. It remains to be proved that there exists a disorder in which the beta cells are specifically sensitive to leucine alone. It is likely that infants diagnosed in the past as suffering from this condition have had a form of nesidioblastosis, and this is supported by the fact that the majority of reported cases have presented during the neonatal period of the first 6 months after birth with symptoms identical to those of infants with proven nesidioblastosis.

GLUCAGON DEFICIENCY

The suggestion that a deficiency of glucagon can be the cause of childhood hypoglycaemia was first made as early as 1950[116]. This was followed by case reports based upon histological evidence of a reduced number of pancreatic alpha cells[117,118]. However, these observations have not been confirmed by modern immunohistochemical techniques, which alone are capable of distinguishing the various types of endocrine cells. In addition, the glucagon 'deficiency' was not verified by measurement of pancreatic glucagon in the plasma.

There are only two cases in the literature where the diagnosis of glucagon deficiency was based on low plasma glucagon concentrations[119,120].

Both patients presented with severe and recurrent neonatal hypogly-caemia, had low plasma glucagon levels at the time of hypoglycaemia, and improved markedly during treatment with glucagon. In the case of Vidnes and Oyasaeter[119] the glucagon response to alanine was absent, but the response of glucagon to other provocative stimuli was not investigated. Although it seemed very likely that hypoglycaemia was due to glucagon deficiency in both cases, the role of insulin could not be completely discounted. In addition, there was no information on the histology of the pancreas in either case. That insulin release was not normal is suggested by an abnormal disappearance rate of glucose, with a K value of 7.5% min[119]; incomplete suppression of plasma insulin levels was evident, and blood ketone levels were abnormally low in both patients. It remains to be proved, therefore, that there exists a specific entity of glucagon deficiency.

CONCLUSION

The endocrine pancreas has a central role to play in the neonatal regulation of normoglycaemia. Deranged function leading to hyper-insulinism is of particular importance, since it can cause transient hypo-glycaemia in the newborn period as well as being the most common cause of persistent hypoglycaemia in infancy.

The classical symptoms of hypoglycaemia in a large-for-dates new-born with a characteristic appearance of generalized adiposity are highly suggestive of hyperinsulinism. However, in many other infants there is no pathognomic abnormal physical sign.

Hyperinsulinism, however, causes a specific and diagnostic profile of circulating hormones and intermediary metabolite concentrations, and the condition can be identified from a single blood sample by recog-nition of hypoglycaemia with inappropriately elevated plasma insulin and low blood ketone body and branched chain amino acid concen-trations.

Apart from the transient forms of neonatal hyperinsulinism, in the majority of cases the underlying endocrine abnormality is remarkably resistant to medical therapy, and most children require surgery.

Hyperinsulinism carries serious implications if unrecognized or when the diagnosis and effective treatment are delayed. On the other hand, however, the outlook is excellent if the condition is promptly and appropriately treated.

References

1. Vinicor, F., Higdon, J. F., Clark, J. F. and Clark, C. M. (1976). Development of glucagon sensitivity in the neonatal rat liver. *J. Clin. Invest.*, **58**, 571–8
2. Kaplan, S. A. (1981). The insulin receptor. *Pediatr. Res.*, **15**, 1156–62

3. Sinha, M. K., Ganguli, S. and Sperling, M. A. (1981). Disappearance of erythrocyte insulin receptors during maturation in sheep. *Diabetes*, **30**, 411–15
4. Cornblath, M., Parker, M. L., Reisner, S. H., Forbes, A. E. and Daughaday, W. (1965). Secretion and metabolism of growth hormone in premature and full-term infants. *J. Clin. Endocrin. Metab.*, **25**, 209–18
5. Sperling, M. A. (1982). Integration of fuel homeostasis by insulin and glucagon in the newborn. In *Monographs in Paediatrics*, Vol. 16, pp. 39–58. (Basel: Karger)
6. Bloom, S. R. and Johnston, D. I. (1972). Failure of glucagon release in infants of diabetic mothers. *Br. Med. J.*, **4**, 453–4
7. Lagercrantz, H. and Bistoletti, P. (1973). Catecholamine release in the newborn infants at birth. *Pediatr. Res.*, **11**, 889–93
8. Aynsley-Green, A., Bloom, S. R., Williamson, D. H. and Turner, R. C. (1977). Endocrine and metabolic response in the human newborn to first feed of breast milk. *Arch. Dis. Child.*, **52**, 291–5
9. Lucas, A., Bloom, S. R. and Aynsley-Green, A. (1978). Metabolic and endocrine events at the time of the first feed of human milk in preterm and term infants. *Arch. Dis. Child.*, **53**, 731–6
10. Aynsley-Green, A. (1982). The control of the adaptation to postnatal nutrition. In *Monographs in Paediatrics*, Vol. 16, pp. 59–87. (Basel: Karger)
11. Lucas, A., Adrian, T. E., Bloom, S. R. and Aynsley-Green, A. (1980). Plasma secretin in neonates. *Acta Paediatr. Scand.*, **69**, 205–10
12. Lucas, A., Adrian, T. E., Christofides, N. D., Bloom, S. R. and Aynsley-Green, A. (1980). Plasma motilin, gastrin and enteroglucagon and feeding in the human newborn. *Arch. Dis. Child.*, **55**, 673–7
13. Lucas, A., Sarson, D. L., Bloom, S. R. and Aynsley-Green, A. (1980). Developmental aspects of gastric inhibitory polypeptide (GIP) and its possible role in the enteroinsular axis in neonates. *Acta Paediatr. Scand.*, **69**, 321–5
14. Lucas, A., Aynsley-Green, A., Blackburn, A. M., Adrian, T. G. and Bloom, S. R. (1981). Plasma neurotensin in term and preterm infants. *Acta Paediatr. Scand.*, **70**, 201–6
15. Kalhan, S. C., Savin, S. M. and Adam, P. A. J. (1977). Attenuated glucose production rate in newborn infants of insulin-dependent diabetic mothers. *N. Engl. J. Med.*, **296**, 375–6
16. Rizza, R. A. (1981). Pathogenesis of hypoglycaemia in insulinoma patients: suppression of hepatic glucose production by insulin. *Diabetes*, **30**, 377–81
17. Bougneres, P. F. and Chaussain, J. L. (1984). Glucose production and utilization in hypoglycaemic infants with hyperinsulinism. *Pediatr. Res.* (Abstr.) (In press)
18. Kuhl, C., Molsted-Pedersen, L., Pedersen, J., Skouby, S. O. and Winkel, S. (1980). Plasma insulin, glucagon and the molar insulin:glucagon ratio in newborn infants of diabetic mothers. In Andreani, D., Lefebvre, P. J. and Marks, J. (eds.) *Current Views of Hypoglycaemia and Glucagon*, pp. 397–407. (New York: Academic Press)
19. Pedersen, J., Bojsen-Moller, B. and Poulsen, H. (1954). Blood sugar in newborn infants of diabetic mothers. *Acta Endocrin.*, **15**, 33–5
20. Block, M. B., Pildes, R. S., Mossabhoy, N. A., Steiner, D. F. and Rubenstein, A. (1974). C-peptide immunoreactivity: a new method of studying infants of insulin-treated diabetic mothers. *Pediatrics*, **53**, 923–8
21. Phelps, R. L., Freinkel, N., Rubenstein, A. H., Kuzuya, H., Metzger, B. E., Boehm, J. J. and Molsted-Pedersen, L. (1978). Carbohydrate metabolism in pregnancy. XV. Plasma C-peptide during IVGTT in neonates from normal and insulin-treated mothers. *J. Clin. Endocrin. Metab.*, **46**, 61–8
22. Williams, P. R., Sperling, M. A. and Racasa, Z. (1979). Blunting of spontaneous and alanine-stimulated glucagon secretion in newborn infants of diabetic mothers. *Am. J. Gynecol.*, **133**, 51–6

23. Cockburn, F., Blagden, A., Michie, E. A. and Forfar, J. C. (1971). The influence of pre-eclampsia and diabetes mellitus on plasma-free amino acids in maternal umbilical vein and infant blood. *J. Obstet. Gynaecol. Br. Commonw.*, **78**, 215–31

24. Vejtorp, H., Pedersen, J., Klebbe, J. G. and Lund, F. (1977). Low concentration of plasma amino acids in newborn babies of diabetic mothers. *Acta Paediatr. Scand.*, **66**, 53–8

25. Soltesz, G., Schultz, K., Mestyan, G. and Horvath, M. (1978). Blood glucose and plasma-free amino acid concentrations in infants of diabetic mothers. *Pediatrics*, **61**, 77–82

26. Taylor, R., Felig, P. and Warshaw, D. B. (1976). Glycaemic response following alanine infusion in infants of diabetic mothers. *Pediatr. Res.*, **10**, 416 (Abstr.)

27. Cardell, B. S. (1953). Hypertrophy and hyperplasia of the pancreatic islets in newborn infants. *J. Path.*, **66**, 335–41

28. Steinke, J. and Driscoll, S. G. (1965). The extractable insulin content of pancreas from fetuses and infants of diabetic and control mothers. *Diabetes*, **14**, 573–88

29. Milner, R. D. G., Wirdham, P. K. and Tsanakas, J. (1981). Quantitative morphology of B, A, D and PP cells in infants of diabetic mothers. *Diabetes*, **30**, 271–4

30. Farquar, J. W. (1969). Prognosis for babies born to diabetic mothers in Edinburgh. *Arch. Dis. Child.*, **44**, 36–47

31. Francois, R., Picaud, J. J., Ruitton-Ugliengo, A., David, L., Cartal, M. Y. and Bauer, D. (1974). The newborn of diabetic mother. *Biol. Neonate*, **24**, 1–31

32. Yssing, M. (1974). Oestriol excretion in pregnant diabetics related to long-term prognosis of surviving children. *Acta Endocrinol.*, **75** (Suppl. 185), 95–102

33. Gëro, L., Baranyi, E., Bekefi, D., Dimeny, E. and Szalay, J. (1982). Investigation on serum C-peptide concentrations in pregnant diabetic women and in newborns of diabetic mothers. *Horm. Metab. Res.*, **14**, 516–20

34. King, C. K., Tserng, K. and Kalhan, S. C. (1982). Regulation of glucose production in newborn infants of diabetic mothers. *Pediatr. Res.*, **16**, 608–12

35. Raivio, K. O. and Osterlund, K. (1969). Hypoglycaemia and hyperinsulinaemia associated with erythroblastosis fetalis. *Pediatrics*, **43**, 217–25

36. Brown, G., Brown, R. and Hey, E. (1978). Fetal hyperinsulinism in rhesus isoimmunisation. *Am. J. Obstet. Gynecol.*, **131**, 682–6

37. From, G. A. L., Driscoll, S. G. and Steinke, J. (1960). Serum insulin in newborn infants with erythroblastosis fetalis. *Pediatrics*, **44**, 549–53

38. Milner, R. D. G., Fekete, M. and Assan, R. (1972). Glucagon, insulin and growth hormone response to exchange transfusion in premature and term infants. *Arch. Dis. Child.*, **47**, 186–9

39. Molsted-Pedersen, L., Trautner, H. and Jorgensen, K. R. (1973). Plasma insulin and *K* values during intravenous glucose tolerance test in newborn infants with erythroblastosis fetalis. *Acta Paediatr. Scand.*, **62**, 11–16

40. Driscoll, S. G. and Steinke, J. (1967). Pancreatic insulin content in severe erythroblastosis. *Pediatrics*, **39**, 448–50

41. Molsted-Pedersen, L. and Tygstrup, I. (1968). Cell infiltration in the pancreas of newborn infants of diabetic mothers. *Acta Pathol. Scand.*, **75**, 537–48

42. Milner, R. D. G., Dinsdale, F., Wirdham, P. K. and Van Assche, F. A. (1983). Pancreatic endocrine cell fractions in erythroblastosis fetalis. *Diabetes*, **32**, 313–15

43. Beckwith, J. B. (1963). Extreme cytomegaly of the adrenal fetal cortex, omphalocoele, hyperplasia of kidneys and pancreas, and Leydig cell hyperplasia. Another syndrome? *Proceedings of the Western Society for Pediatric Research*

44. Wiedemann, H. R. (1974). Complex malformatif familial avec hernie onbilicael et macroglossie. Un 'syndrome nouveau'? *J. Genet. Hum.*, **13**, 223–32

45. Ichiba, Y. and Gardner, L. T. (1975). In Gardner, L. T. (ed.) *Metabolic and Genetic Diseases of Childhood and Adolescence*, pp. 1314–38. (Philadelphia: Saunders)

46. Combs, J. T., Grund, J. A. and Brandt, I. K. (1966). New syndrome of neonatal hypoglycaemia: association with visceromegaly, macroglossia, microcephaly and abnormal umbilicus. *N. Engl. J. Med.*, **275**, 236–43

47. Lazarus, L., Young, J. D. and Friend, J. C. M. (1968). EMG syndrome and carbohydrate metabolism. *Lancet*, **1**, 1347–8

48. Roe, T. F., Kershnar, A. K., Weitzmann, J. J. and Madrigal, L. S. (1973). Beckwith's syndrome with extreme organ hyperplasia. *Pediatrics*, **52**, 373–81

49. Dammaco, F., Carnevale, F. and Albrizio, M. (1975). Nesidioblastosis in Beckwith syndrome. *J. Pediatr.*, **86**, 647–8

50. Ashton, I. K. and Aynsley-Green, A. (1978). Somatomedin in an infant with Beckwith's syndrome. *Early Hum. Dev.*, **1**, 357–66

51. Schabel, F. and Fritsch, H. (1979). Erhönte Somatomedin-Aktivität beim Beckwith–Wiedemann Syndrome. *Paediatr. Paedol.*, **14**, 249–57

52. Moncrief, M. W., Lacey, K. A. and Malleson, P. N. (1977). Management of prolonged hypoglycaemia in Beckwith's syndrome. *Postgrad. Med. J.*, **53**, 159–61

53. Milner, R. D. G. and Hales, C. N. (1965). Effect of intravenous glucose on concentration of insulin in maternal and umbilical cord plasma. *Br. Med. J.*, **1**, 284–6

54. Tobin, J. D., Roux, J. F. and Soeldner, J. S. (1969). Human fetal insulin response after acute maternal glucose administration during labour. *Pediatrics*, **44**, 668–71

55. Coltart, T. M., Beard, R. W., Turner, R. C. and Oakley, N. W. (1969). Blood glucose and insulin relationships in the human mother and fetus before onset of labour. *Br. Med. J.*, **4**, 17–19

56. Obenshain, S. S., Adam, P. A. J., King, P. C., Teramo, K., Raivio, K. O., Raiha, N. and Schwartz, R. (1970). Human fetal insulin response to sustained maternal hyperglycaemia. *N. Engl. J. Med.*, **283**, 566–70

57. Lucas, A., Adrian, T. E., Aynsley-Green, A. and Bloom, S. R. (1980). Iatrogenic hyperinsulinism at birth. *Lancet*, **1**, 144–5

58. Cornblath, M., Joassin, G., Weisskopf, B. and Swlatek, K. R. (1966). Hypoglycaemia in the newborn. *Pediatr. Clin. N. Am.*, **13**, 905–28

59. Pildes, R. S., Patel, D. A. and Nitzan, M. (1973). Glucose disappearance rate in symptomatic neonatal hypoglycaemia. *Pediatrics*, **52**, 75–82

60. Le Dune, M. A. (1972). Intravenous glucose tolerance and plasma insulin studies in small-for-dates infants. *Arch. Dis. Child.*, **47**, 111–14

61. Soltesz, G., Jenkins, P. A. and Aynsley-Green, A. (1984). Hyperinsulinaemic hypoglycaemia in infancy and childhood: a practical approach to diagnosis and medical treatment based on experience of 18 cases. *Acta Paediatr. Acad. Sci. Hung.* (In press)

62. Landau, H., Perlman, M., Meyer, S., Isacsohn, M., Krausz, M., Mayan, H., Lijovethky, G. and Schiller, M. (1982). Persistent neonatal hypoglycaemia due to hyperinsulinism: medical aspects. *Pediatrics*, **70**, 440–6

63. Baker, L. and Stanley, C. A. (1977). Hyperinsulinism in infancy: a pathophysiological approach to diagnosis and treatment. In Chiumello, G. and Laron, Z. (eds.) *Recent Progress in Pediatric Endocrinology*, pp. 89–100. (New York: Academic Press)

64. McQuarrie, I. (1954). Idiopathic spontaneously occurring hypoglycaemia in infants. Clinical significance of problems and treatment. *Am. J. Dis. Child.*, **87**, 399–428

65. Aynsley-Green, A., Polak, J. M., Keeling, J., Gough, M. H. and Baum, D. (1978). Averted neonatal death due to nesidioblastosis of the pancreas. *Lancet*, **1**, 550–1

66. Polak, J. M. and Wigglesworth, J. (1976). Islet-cell hyperplasia and sudden infant death. *Lancet*, **2**, 570–1 (Letter)

67. Cox, J. N., Guelpa, G. and Terrapon, M. (1976). Islet-cell hyperplasia and sudden infant death. *Lancet*, **2**, 739–40 (Letter)

68. Woo, D., Scopes, J. W. and Polak, J. M. (1976). Idiopathic hypoglycaemia in sibs with morphological evidence of nesidioblastosis of the pancreas. *Arch. Dis. Child.*, **51**, 528–31
69. Turner, R. C. and Johnson, P. C. (1973). Suppression of insulin release by fish insulin-induced hypoglycaemia. *Lancet*, **1**, 1483–5
70. Aynsley-Green, A., Polak, J. M., Gough, M. H., Keeling, J., Ashcroft, S. H., Turner, R. C. and Baum, D. (1981). Nesidioblastosis of the pancreas: definition of the syndrome and the management of the severe neonatal hyperinsulinaemic hypoglycaemia. *Arch. Dis. Child.*, **56**, 496–508
71. Cornblath, M. and Schwartz, R. (1976). *Disorders of Carbohydrate Metabolism in Infancy*, 2nd edn. (Philadelphia: Saunders)
72. Berger, M., Zimmermann-Telschow, H., Berhold, P., Doest, H., Muller, W. A., Gries, F. A. and Zimmermann, H. (1978). Blood amino acid levels in patients with insulin excess (functioning insulinoma) and insulin deficiency (diabetic keto-acidosis). *Metabolism*, **27**, 793–9
73. Chaussain, J. L., Georges, P., Gendrel, D., Donnadieu, M. and Job, J. C. (1980). Serum branched-chain amino acids in the diagnosis of hyperinsulinism in infancy. *J. Pediatr.*, **97**, 923–6
74. Soltesz, G., Molnar, D., Pinter, A. and Nemeth, A. (1980). Hyperinsulinism. *Acta Paediatr. Acad. Sci. Hung.*, **21**, 1–8
75. Bier, D. M., Leake, R. D., Haymond, M. W., Arnold, K. J., Gruenke, L. D., Sperling, M. A. and Kipnis, D. M. (1977). Measurement of 'true' glucose production rates in infancy and childhood with 6-6-dideutero-glucose. *Diabetes*, **26**, 1016–23
76. Finegold, D. N., Stanley, C. A. and Baker, L. (1980). Glycaemic response to glucagon during fasting hypoglycaemia: an aid in the diagnosis of hyperinsulinism. *J. Pediatr.*, **96**, 257–9
77. Fajans, S. S. (1967). Diagnostic tests for functioning pancreatic islet cell tumours. *Excerpta Medica*, **172**, 894
78. Grant, D. B. (1968). Serum-insulin changes following administration of L-leucine to children. *Arch. Dis. Child.*, **43**, 69–72
79. Marks, V. and Rose, F. C. (1981). *Hypoglycaemia*, 2nd edn. (Oxford: Blackwell Scientific Publications)
80. Hirsch, H. J., Loo, S., Evans, N., Crigler, J. F., Filler, R. M. and Gabbay, K. H. (1977). Hypoglycaemia of infancy and nesidioblastosis. Studies with somatostatin. *N. Engl. J. Med.*, **296**, 1323–6
81. Becker, K., Wendel, U., Przyrembel, H., Tsotsalas, M., Munterfering, H. and Bremer, H. J. (1978). Beta cell nesidioblastosis. *Eur. J. Pediatr.*, **127**, 75–89
82. Bloomgarden, Z. T., Sundell, H., Rogers, L. W., O'Neill, L. A. and Liljenquiest, S. E. (1980). Treatment of intractable neonatal hypoglycaemia with somatostatin plus glucagon. *J. Pediatr.*, **69**, 148–51
83. Kitson, H. F., McCrossin, R. B., Jimenez, M., Middleton, A. and Silink, M. (1980). Somatostatin treatment of insulin excess due to B-cell adenoma in a neonate. *J. Pediatr.*, **96**, 145–8
84. Kirkland, J., Ben-Menachem, Y., Akhtar, M., Marschall, R. and Dudrick (1978). Islet cell tumour in a neonate: diagnosis by selective angiography and histological findings. *Pediatrics*, **61**, 790–1
85. Peters, G. and Roch-Ramel, F. (1969). Thiazide diuretics and related drugs. In Herken, H. (ed.) *Diuretica. (Handbook of Experimental Pharmacology*, Vol. 24). (Berlin: Springer)
86. Drash, A. L. and Wolff, F. E. (1964). Drug therapy in leucine-sensitive hypoglycaemia. *Metabolism*, **13**, 487–93
87. Drash, A. L., Kenny, F., Field, F., Blizzard, R., Langs, H. and Wolff, F. (1968). The therapeutic application of diazoxide in pediatric hypoglycaemic states. *Ann. N.Y. Acad. Sci.*, **150**, 377–455

88. Aynsley-Green, A. (1981). Nesidioblastosis of the pancreas in infancy. In Randle, P. J., Steiner, D. F. and Whelan, W. J. (eds.) *Carbohydrate Metabolism and its Disorders*. (London: Academic Press)

89. Victorin, L. H. and Thorell, J. I. (1974). Plasma insulin and blood glucose during long-term treatment with diazoxide for infant hypoglycaemia. *Acta Paediatr. Scand.*, **63**, 302–6

90. Samols, E., Marri, G. and Marks, V. (1965). Promotion of insulin secretion by glucagon. *Lancet*, **2**, 415–16

91. Aynsley-Green, A., Barnes, N. D., Kingston, J., Boyes, S. and Bloom, S. R. (1981). The effect of somatostatin infusion on intermediary metabolism and enteroinsular hormone release in infants with hyperinsulinaemic hypoglycaemia. *Acta Paediatr. Scand.*, **70**, 889–95

92. Volk, B. W., Wellman, P. and Brancato, P. (1974). Fine structure of rat islet cell tumours induced by streptozotocin and nicotinamide. *Diabetologia*, **10**, 37–43

93. Thomas, C. G., Jr, Underwood, L. E., Carney, C. N., Cokourt, J. L. and Whitt, J. J. (1977). Neonatal and infantile hypoglycaemia due to insulin excess: new aspects of diagnosis and surgical management. *Ann. Surg.*, **185**, 505–17

94. Fonkalsrud, E. W., Trout, H. H., Lippe, B., La Franchi, S. and Dakake, C. (1974). Idiopathic hypoglycaemia in infancy: surgical management. *Arch. Surg.*, **108**, 801–4

95. Zuppinger, K. A. (1975). Hypoglycaemia in childhood. In *Monographs in Paediatrics*, Vol. 4. (Basel: Karger)

96. Schwartz, J. F. and Zwiren, G. T. (1971). Islet cell adenomatosis and adenoma in an infant. *Pediatrics*, **79**, 232–8

97. Kloppel, G., Altenahr, E. and Manke, B. (1975). The ultrastructure of focal islet adenomatosis in the newborn. *Virchows Arch. (Path. Anat.)*, **366**, 223–36

98. Heitz, P. U., Kloppel, G., Hack, W. H., Polak, J. M. and Pearse, A. G. E. (1977). Nesidioblastosis: the pathologic basis of persistent hypoglycaemia in infants. *Diabetes*, **26**, 632–42

99. Brown, R. E. and Young, R. B. (1970). A possible role for the exocrine pancreas in the pathogenesis of neonatal leucine-sensitive hypoglycaemia. *J. Am. Digest. Dis.*, **15**, 65–72

100. Yakovac, W. C., Baker, L. and Hummeler, K. (1971). Beta cell nesidioblastosis in idiopathic hypoglycaemia of infancy. *J. Pediatr.*, **79**, 226–31

101. Sovik, V., Vidnes, J. and Falkmer, S. (1975). Persistent neonatal hypoglycaemia. *Acta Path. Microb. Scand.*, **83**, 155–6

102. Polak, J. R. and Bloom, S. R. (1980). Decrease of somatostatin content in persistent neonatal hyperinsulinaemic hypoglycaemia. In Andreani, D., Lefebvre, P. J. and Marks, V. (eds.) *Current Views on Hypoglycaemia and Glucagon*, pp. 367–78. (New York: Academic Press)

103. Bishop, A. E., Polak, J. M., Garin Chesa, P., Timson, D. M., Bryant, M. G. and Bloom, S. R. (1981). Decrease of pancreatic somatostatin in neonatal nesidioblastosis. *Diabetes*, **30**, 122–6

104. Jaffe, R., Hashida, Y. and Yunis, E. (1980). Pancreatic pathology in hyperinsulinaemic hypoglycaemia of infancy. *Lab. Invest.*, **42**, 356–65

105. Falkmer, S., Sovik, O. and Vidnes, J. (1981). Immunohistochemical, morphometric and clinical studies of the pancreatic islets in infants with persistent neonatal hypoglycaemia of familial type with hyperinsulinism and nesidioblastosis. *Acta Biol. Med. Germ.*, **40**, 39–54

106. Gould, V. E., Memoli, V. A., Dardi, L. E. and Gould, N. S. (1981). Nesidiodysplasia and nesidioblastosis of infancy. Ultrastructural and immunohistochemical analysis of islet cell alterations with and without associated hyperinsulinaemic hypoglycaemia. *Scand. J. Gastroenterol.*, **16** (Suppl. 70), 129–42

107. Garces, L. Y., Drash, A. and Kenny, F. M. (1968). Islet cell tumour in the neonate. Studies in carbohydrate metabolism and therapeutic response. *Pediatrics*, **41**, 789–96

108. Salinas, E. D., Jr, Mangurten, H. H., Robert, S. S., Simon, W. H. and Cornblath, M. (1968). Functioning islet cell adenoma in the newborn. Report of a case with failure of diazoxide. *Pediatrics*, **41**, 646–53
109. Grant, D. B. and Barbor, P. R. H. (1970). Islet-cell tumour causing hypoglycaemia in a newborn infant. *Arch. Dis. Child.*, **45**, 434–6
110. Robinson, M. J., Clarke, A. M., Gold, H. and Connelly, J. F. (1971). Islet cell adenoma in the newborn: report of two patients. *Pediatrics*, **48**, 232–6
111. Todd, R. M., Rickham, P. P. and Coulter, J. B. S. (1972). Islet cell tumour in the newborn. *Helv. Paediatr. Acta*, **27**, 131–7
112. Fischer, G. W., Vazquez, A. M., Buist, N. R. M., Campbell, J. R., McCarty, E. and Egan, E. T. (1974). Neonatal islet cell adenoma: case report and literature review. *Paediatrics*, **53**, 753–6
113. Carney, C. N. (1976). Congenital insulinoma (nesidioblastoma). *Arch. Path. Lab. Med.*, **100**, 352–6
114. Vance, J. E., Stoll, R. W., Kitabchi, A. E., Williams, R. H. and Wood, F. C. (1969). Nesidioblastosis in familial endocrine adenomatosis. *J. Am. Med. Assoc.*, **207**, 1679–82
115. Cochrane, W. A., Payne, W. W., Simpkiss, M. J. and Woolf, L. I. (1956). Familial hypoglycaemia precipitated by amino acids. *J. Clin. Invest.*, **35**, 411–22
116. McQuarrie, I., Bell, E. T., Zimmermann, B. and Wright, W. S. (1950). Deficiency of alpha cells of pancreas as possible etiologic factor in familial hypoglycaemosis. *Fed. Proc.*, **9**, 337
117. Wagner, T., Spranger, J. and Brunck, H. J. (1969). Kongenitaler Alpha-Zellmangel als Ursache einer chronischen infantilen Hypoglykaemia. *Monatsschr. Klinderheilk*, **117**, 236–8
118. Gotlin, R. W. and Silver, H. K. (1970). Neonatal hypoglycaemia, hyperinsulinism and absence of pancreatic alpha cells. *Lancet*, **1**, 1346 (Letter)
119. Vidnes, J. and Oyasaeter, S. (1977). Glucagon deficiency causing severe neonatal hypoglycaemia in a patient with normal insulin secretion. *Pediatr. Res.*, **11**, 943–9
120. Kollee, L. A., Monnens, L. A., Cejka, V. and Wilms, R. H. (1978). Persistent hypoglycaemia due to glucagon deficiency. *Arch. Dis. Child.*, **53**, 422–4
121. Davidson, P. M., Young, D. G., Logan, R. W. and Patrick, W. J. A. (1984). Alloxan therapy for nesidioblastosis. *J. Paediatr. Surg.*, **19**, 87–9

SECTION 2

The Thyroid Gland

Chairman: D. I. JOHNSTON

3

CONGENITAL HYPO-THYROIDISM: PATHOGENESIS, SCREENING AND PROGNOSIS

D. B. GRANT

During the last two decades there have been great advances in our understanding of fetal and neonatal thyroid function. This information has played a vital role in the development of screening methods for congenital hypothyroidism and will be reviewed briefly before the pathogenesis and prognosis in congenital hypothyroidism are considered.

THYROID FUNCTION IN THE FETUS AND NEWBORN

The development of fetal thyroid function and the changes in thyroid hormone levels which take place soon after birth have been fully reviewed by Fisher et al.[1,2].

It is generally recognized that the human placenta is virtually impermeable to thyroid hormones and that development of the fetal thyroid–pituitary axis is independent of maternal thyroid function. By the 12th week of fetal life the thyroid gland has developed its characteristic structure and immunoreactive TSH can be detected in the fetal pituitary. Maturation of the fetal–pituitary axis during the second trimester causes a progressive rise in plasma T_4 and TSH, and release of pituitary TSH after injection of TRH has been shown to occur by the 26–28th weeks of gestation. Plasma T_3 remains low in the fetal circulation, probably because of selective deiodination of T_4 to reverse T_3 (rT_3). Shortly after birth there is an abrupt rise in plasma TSH which reaches a peak within 4–6 hours. Thermal stress after delivery is thought to be the main stimulus for this TSH surge.

There are also marked changes in the circulating levels of thyroid hormones soon after birth. These changes seem to be initiated by cessation of blood flow in the umbilical vessels, but the exact mechanism is still obscure. Plasma T_3—and to a lesser extent T_4—rise to levels which would normally indicate hyperthyroidism in adult life, and it is important to appreciate that a normal plasma T_4 by adult standards can indicate significant hypothyroidism in the newborn period. High plasma T_4 and T_3 persist for some time after birth, before slowly falling into the normal adult range. Values in the first weeks of life have been given by Cuestas[3] (Table 1).

Table 1   Serum T4 values according to age and gestation, mean (± SD)

Age at test	Estimated gestational age (weeks)				
	30–31	32–33	34–35	37–37	Term
Cord blood	84 (13)	97 (27)	86 (15)	97 (36)	106 (23)
12–72 hours	148 (27)	159 (41)	160 (40)	200 (34)	245 (27)
3–10 days	99 (23)	110 (25)	129 (31)	164 (32)	205 (39)
11–20 days	97 (23)	107 (21)	135 (23)	144 (37)	157 (26)
21–45 days	101 (19)	103 (22)	120 (17)	147 (54)	156 (19)
	(30–37 weeks)				
46–90 days	124 (22)				132 (25)

T₄ measurements made using radioimmunoassay commercial kit by Beckman.
Data adapted from Cuestas[3].
Serum T₄ values are given in nmol/l.

CONGENITAL HYPOTHYROIDISM

In Europe and the rest of the Western world, defects in thyroid embryogenesis and defects in thyroid hormone biosynthesis are the two main causes of congenital hypothyroidism. Maternal iodine deficiency during pregnancy, once an important cause of congenital hypothyroidism in areas of endemic goitre, is now confined to a few countries in the Third World. Pituitary (secondary) and hypothalamic (tertiary) hypothyroidism appear to be relatively uncommon and will not be considered in detail.

The different types of defect in thyroxine biosynthesis which can lead to hypothyroidism are listed in Table 2. All are associated with the presence of a goitre, although this is often difficult to identify during the neonatal period, and all but the 'trapping' defect cause increased radioiodine uptake by the thyroid gland. Often the enzyme defect may be incomplete and the plasma levels of T_3 (and sometimes T_4) are normal but the circulating TSH level is moderately elevated.

In the past, fairly sophisticated laboratory methods have been required to identify some of these enzyme defects, but the introduction of new techniques has simplified this task—for example, radioimmunoassay for thyroglobulin (Tg) is now becoming fairly widely available and demonstration of undetectable levels of plasma Tg in a patient with a palpable thyroid gland points to a defect in Tg synthesis[4,5]. From the practical point of view, identifying the nature of the enzyme defect has no real effect on treatment as all these patients are managed by giving replacement therapy with thyroxine.

Table 2   Disorders of thyroid biosynthesis

Iodide trapping defect
Peroxidase defect
Deiodinase defect
Coupling defect
Defect in Tg synthesis

Most of the disorders are probably inherited as recessive conditions and carry the recurrence risk of 1 : 4 in any future child born to the same parents. However, in some families with goitrous hypothyroidism the condition has appeared in two or more generations, suggesting a dominant pattern of inheritance. Inspection of Table 3 suggests that these abnormalities of hormone biosynthesis account for between 10 and 20% of all cases of congenital hypothyroidism.

Table 3   Isotope scanning

	A (67)	B (43)	C (33)	D (127)	E (100)
Absent	31%	51%	12%	46%	45%
Hypoplastic	5%	21%	15%	2%	7%
Ectopic	36%	12%	48%	41%	27%
Normal or enlarged	28%	16%	24%	10%	21%

Mäenpää, 1972; Jacobsen, 1980; Hulse, 1982; Fisher, 1979; MRC Register, 1983.

The great majority of cases with congenital hypothyroidism have either aplasia (or hypoplasia) of the gland or have an ectopic thyroid. As seen in Table 3, the ratios between these different development defects varies in different series of patients. It is likely that these discrepancies are due both to the scanning techniques used and the age at which the patients were investigated. The different anatomical types of thyroid dysplasia are associated with different degrees of hypothyroidism and cases with large ectopic glands may maintain normal thyroid hormone levels more or less indefinitely[6].

47

While the cause of thyroid gland dysgenesis is not known, it is twice as common in girls and there have been a few reports of its occurrence in siblings[7,8], suggesting that there is a genetic component. There is also evidence to suggest that the incidence of the disorder differs in different ethnic groups; for example, it is very uncommon in black people[9].

Although the placenta is virtually impermeable to thyroid hormones other substances such as antithyroid drugs can pass from mother to fetus and cause transient neonatal hypothyroidism. Maternal antibodies which cross the placenta usually cause neonatal hyperthyroidism, but in a few cases may have been associated with transient hypothyroidism[10,11], which is not due to maternal treatment with antithyroid drugs. Transient hypothyroidism has also been reported in normal neonates exposed to iodine-based disinfectants[12].

Extreme prematurity is associated with low levels of circulating T_4 and T_3 which rise with increasing age and which are not associated with elevated TSH values. Similar low T_4/T_3 and TSH levels are also found in severely ill neonates. In some series significant numbers of infants with mildly raised TSH levels and low T_4 values have been reported. These latter abnormalities, which usually return to normal soon after delivery, may be related to a low maternal iodine intake[13].

To date, there is no real evidence that these transient states of hypo-thyroxinaemia or hyperthyrotrophinaemia are of clinical importance.

CONGENITAL HYPOTHYROIDISM AND BRAIN DEVELOPMENT

The importance of thyroid hormones on brain development is well known and will only be outlined briefly. In experimental animals, neonatal or prenatal hypothyroidism is associated with a variety of disorders of brain development. For example, in the rat neonatal hypo-thyroidism produces reduced cell size in the cerebrum and cerebellum[14], delayed myelination[15], and a marked reduction in the number of dendritic connections[16]. These changes can be prevented if thyroxine replacement is started before the 10th day of life[17].

In man, the observation that early treatment leads to a better prognosis for subsequent intelligence[18–20] also suggests that there is a critical period after which treatment is less effective in preventing or reversing the effects of thyroid deficiency. However, all the reported studies on intelligence and the age at which treatment was started have shown considerable overlap of intelligence in the early- and late-treated groups, and most paediatricians will be familiar with the late-diagnosed case who does surprisingly well. These discrepancies are probably partly related to the wide range of biochemical severity which occurs in congenital hypothyroidism: for example, cases with agenesis of the gland have been reported to have a poor outcome compared to patients with ectopic glands[21]. However, other factors, such as social class or the age at which patients were tested[22], have an important role in the outcome. In a retrospective study, Hulse[23] found that the mean IQ in cases from social class I + II families was 90.5, while the figure in social class IV + V was 64.2.

In addition to poor intelligence, congenital hypothyroidism is associated with other neurological symptoms, and these may be more of a handicap than the mental impairment. Restlessness, poor concentration and behaviour disorders are common, as are other features such as impaired speech, squint and general clumsiness[24-26]. Impaired hearing has also been reported in some cases. In a minority of patients, congenital hypothyroidism is associated with cerebral palsy.

The extent of disability caused by congenital hypothyroidism can be judged from Hulse's[23] findings in a recent retrospective study in the London area. Out of 112 schoolchildren in his survey, 32 attended special schools and, of the 80 children attending normal schools, 23 required remedial teaching in at least one subject.

There have been very few neuropathological studies in congenital hypothyroidism, but increased head size is a very typical feature[27]. CT scans carried out in a small number of hypothyroid children with large heads showed no abnormal features, in particular, no evidence of ventricular dilation (unpublished communication).

Congenital hypothyroidism is known to cause other features of delayed fetal maturation. For example, a high proportion of cases are postmature, suggesting that development of the mechanism which initiates labour has been delayed. Persistent jaundice in the neonatal period is very common and is probably due to immaturity of liver enzymes[28], and a similar mechanism probably accounts for the high levels of fetoprotein (AFP) which have been described in congenital hypothyroidism[29].

SCREENING FOR CONGENITAL HYPOTHYROIDISM

In the early 1970s advances in understanding of fetal and neonatal thyroid function opened up the possibility of routine screening of the newborn and, in 1974, Klein et al.[30] in Pittsburgh described a pilot programme using TSH assay on cord blood. In the following year Dussault et al.[31] described their findings in a screening programme in the State of Quebec based on measurement of T_4 in dried blood spots on filter paper. Subsequently, it was shown that it was possible to assay TSH on dried blood spots[32] and this method was rapidly introduced in several European countries, Australia and Japan.

By 1979, Fisher et al.[33] could report the results of screening in a million North American infants and, at the end of 1982, more than 11 million newborn had been screened in Europe and over 3000 cases of hypo-thyroidism identified[34] (see Table 4). In the United Kingdom, pilot schemes for screening for hypothyroidism were launched in East Anglia, Scotland and the North Thames Region in 1977–8. By the end of 1982 virtually all children born in the UK were being screened, most commonly by regional screening centres which worked in close co-operation with the centres for screening for phenylketonuria. Returns for 1982 from the 23 screening laboratories in England, Wales and Northern Ireland indicated that 600000 newborns had been screened and 181 cases of hypothyroidism identified (unpublished communication).

Table 4   Neonatal thyroid screening: Europe 1982

More than 90% newborn		
Finland	United Kingdom	France
Sweden	Eire	Austria
Norway	Netherlands	Switzerland
Denmark	Belgium	Israel
West Germany	Luxemburg	
50–90% newborn		
Italy	Spain	Greece

In general, the early North American screening programmes were based on T_4 assay while TSH assay was chosen in most European programmes, and for some years there was considerable debate on the relative merits of the two systems. T_4 assay had the advantage of measuring the active hormone, thereby detecting secondary or tertiary hypothyroidism as well as primary hypothyroidism. However, it also detected cases of thyroxine-binding globulin (TBG) deficiency, which was of no clinical importance, but missed 'compensated' cases due to a large ectopic gland or partial enzyme deficit. More important, as the normal neonatal plasma T_4 values show a bell-shaped distribution curve, and as many of the hypothyroid cases had T_4 values in the lower part of the normal range, 2–3% of patients had to be recalled for repeat tests of thyroid function until TSH assay was introduced into the programme[35] to eliminate most of these 'false positives'.

In contrast, when TSH assay was used for screening there was little overlap between the hypothyroid and normal subjects so that recall rates for second blood samples were very low. Although the method could not detect secondary or tertiary hypothyroidism this low recall rate was considered an overwhelming advantage by many screening laboratories in Europe.

An interesting aspect of the different screening programmes is related to the incidence of congenital hypothyroidism. Retrospective studies in Sweden[36], Denmark[37] and the Netherlands[38] have suggested that congenital hypothyroidism occurs in one in every 6500–7500 births. This figure is very close to that reported in some of the North American screening programmes using T_4 assay and is much lower than the figure of around 1:3500 which has been reported in most of the European programmes using TSH assay[34]. The most likely explanation for these discrepancies probably lies in the fact that 'compensated' cases due to an ectopic gland are identified by TSH assay and that before screening these cases would have presented as cases of 'juvenile hypothyroidism' in later childhood.

It is very unlikely that any newborn screening programme will be 100% effective and there have been at least two published reports of missed cases[39, 40], usually due to technical or clerical errors, and it is very important that the possibility of a 'missed case' is still kept in mind in any infant with clinical features of hypothyroidism. In some programmes repeat thyroid function tests have been introduced to detect any cases of hypothyroidism missed in the newborn period, but this strategy would appear to be very difficult to justify in 'cost-effective' terms.

EFFECT OF EARLY TREATMENT IN PATIENTS DETECTED BY SCREENING

Relatively few screening programmes have been in being for long enough to enable the potential benefits of early treatment to be assessed in any detail. For example, the programme at The Hospital for Sick Children, London, was started in the autumn of 1978 and the earliest cases detected are just approaching an age at which estimates of intelligence can be made with any degree of confidence. Preliminary results using the Griffiths test at the age of 1 year are very encouraging (Hulse et al.[41]): out of 36 children tested at the age of 1 year all but two had general quotients above 90 and the mean score was normal at 104. Very similar results have been obtained using the McCarthy test and a behaviour screening questionnaire at the age of 3 years (Murphy, 1982, unpublished communication). The mean score was 96.6 (normal 100) and only four children had scores below 90 on the general quotient, with only one child having a score above 10 on the behaviour questionnaire. These results are in keeping with results given by Glorieux et al.[42] and those from the New England Collaborative Study[43]—in the latter group of 71 patients diagnosed by screening the distribution of IQ scores was similar to that in a normal population. In seven patients the score was at or below the normal limits—three of these patients had clinical features of hypothyroidism very soon after birth, suggesting that they had severe prenatal hypothyroidism, and four came from families who had not been co-operative over treatment.

It seems likely that similar results will be obtained in other centres and that one of the challenges for the future will be to recognize cases who are at risk for mental retardation despite early diagnosis and treatment. In addition, there is at present very little information on the effects of early diagnosis and treatment on other neurological symptoms such as clumsiness, squint, or speech difficulties, although there is some indirect evidence that they may not be completely prevented by early treatment[26]. Another challenge will be the development of methods of quantitating such symptoms, thereby allowing analysis of the prenatal and postnatal factors which may be important in their pathogenesis.

Finally, perhaps the greatest challenge will be to use the epidemiological and clinical information provided by neonatal screening to try to unravel the different factors which are involved in the aetiology of dysgenesis of the thyroid gland.

References

1. Fisher, D. A., Dussault, J. H., Sack, J. and Chopra, D. (1977). Ontogenesis of hypothalamic–pituitary–thyroid function and metabolism in man, sheep and rat. *Recent Prog. Horm. Res.*, **33**, 59–116
2. Fisher, D. A. and Klein, A. H. (1981). Thyroid development and disorders of thyroid function in the newborn. *N. Engl. J. Med.*, **304**, 702–12
3. Cuestas, R. A. (1978). Thyroid function in healthy premature infants. *J. Pediatr.*, **92**,, 963–7
4. Black, E. G., Bodden, S. J., Hulse, J. A. and Hoffenberg, R. (1982). Serum thyroglobulin in normal and hypothyroid neonates. *Clin. Endocrinol.*, **16**, 267–74
5. Czernichow, P., Schlumberger, M., Pomarede, R. and Fragu, P. (1983). Plasma thyroglobulin measurements help determine the type of thyroid defect in congenital hypothyroidism. *J. Clin. Endocrinol. Metab.*, **56**, 242–5
6. Neinas, F. W., Gorman, C. A., Devine, K. D. and Woolner, L. B. (1973). Lingual thyroid: clinical characteristics of 15 cases. *Ann. Int. Med.*, **79**, 205–10
7. Orti, E., Castells, S., Qazi, Q. H. and Inamdar, S. (1971). Familial thyroid disease: lingual thyroid in two siblings and hypoplasia of a thyroid lobe in a third. *J. Pediatr.*, **78**, 671–7
8. Kaplan, M., Kauli, R., Raviv, U., Lubin, E. and Laron, Z. (1977). Hypothyroidism due to ectopy in siblings. *Am. J. Dis. Child.*, **131**, 1264–5
9. Brown, A. L., Fernhoff, P. M., Milner, J., McEwen, C. and Elsas, L. S. (1981). Racial differences in the incidence of congenital hypothyroidism. *J. Pediatr.*, **99**, 934–6
10. Iseki, M., Shimizu, M., Oikawa, T., Mojo, H., Arikawa, K., Ichikawa, Y., Moinotani, N. and Ito, K. (1983). Sequential serum measurements of thyrotropin-binding inhibitor immunoglobulin G in transient familial neonatal hypothyroidism. *J. Clin. Endocrinol. Metab.*, **57**, 384–7
11. Ritzen, E. M., Mahler, H. and Alveryd, A. (1981). Transitory congenital hypothyroidism and maternal thyroiditis. *Acta Paediatr. Scand.*, **70**, 765–6
12. Lyen, K. R., Finegold, D., Orsini, R., Herd, J. E. and Parks, J. S. (1982). Transient thyroid suppression associated with topically applied povidine–iodine. *Am. J. Dis. Child.*, **136**, 369–70
13. Delange, F., Dodion, J., Wolter, R., Bourdoux, P., Dalhem, A., Glinoer, D. and Ermans, A-M. (1978). Transient hypothyroidism in the newborn infant. *J. Pediatr.*, **92**, 974–6
14. Lewis, P. D., Patel, A. J., Johnston, A. L. and Balazs, R. (1976). Effect of thyroid deficiency on cell acquisition in the postnatal rat brain: a quantitative histological study. *Brain Res.*, **104**, 49–62

15. Brasel, J. A. and Boyd, D. B. (1975). Influence of thyroid hormone on fetal brain growth and development. In Fisher, D. A. and Burrow, G. N. (eds.) *Perinatal Thyroid Physiology and Disease.* pp. 59–71. (New York: Raven Press)

16. Eayrs, J. T. (1966). Thyroid and central nervous development. *Sci. Basis Med. Ann. Rev.*, 317–39

17. Eayrs, J. T. (1971). Thyroid and developing brain: anatomical and behavioral effects. In Hamburgh, M. and Barrington, E. J. W. (eds.) *Hormones in Development.* pp. 345–55. (New York: Appleton-Century-Crofts)

18. Smith, D. W., Blizzard, R. M. and Wilkins, L. (1957). The mental prognosis in hypothyroidism of infancy and childhood. *Pediatrics*, **19**, 1011–22

19. Klein, A. H., Meltzer, S. and Kenny, F. M. (1972). Improved prognosis in congenital hypothyroidism treated before the age of three months. *J. Pediatr.*, **81**, 912–15

20. Raiti, S. and Newns, G. H. (1971). Cretinism: early diagnosis and its relation to mental prognosis. *Arch. Dis. Child.*, **46**, 692–4

21. Warne, G. L., Andrews, J. T., McKay, W. J. and Wettenhall, H. N. B. (1978). 99mTc Pertechnetate for detection of ectopic dysgenesis of the thyroid in childhood hypothyroidism. *Aust. Paediatr. J.*, **14**, 11–15

22. Money, J., Clarke, F. C. and Beck, J. (1978). Congenital hypothyroidism and IQ increase: a quarter-century follow-up. *J. Pediatr.*, **93**, 432–4

23. Hulse, J. A. (1982). The place of screening for congenital hypothyroidism in the prevention of handicap. *MD Thesis*, University of Cambridge

24. Mäenpää, J. (1972). Congenital hypothyroidism: aetiological and clinical aspects. *Arch. Dis. Child.*, **47**, 914–23

25. McFaul, R., Dorner, S., Brett, E. M. and Grant, D. B. (1978). Neurological abnormalities in patients treated for hypothyroidism from early life. *Arch. Dis. Child.*, **53**, 611–19

26. Wolter, R., Noel, P., De Cock, P., Craen, M., Ernould, C. H., Malvaux, P., Verstraeten, F., Simons, J., Mertens, S., Van Broeck, N. and Vanderschueren-Lodewyckx, M. (1979). Neuropsychological study in treated thyroid dysgenesis. *Acta Paediatr. Scand. Suppl.*, **277**, 41–6

27. Burt, L. and Kulin, H. E. (1977). Head circumference in children with short stature secondary to primary hypothyroidism. *Pediatrics*, **59**, 628–30

28. Weldon, A. P. and Danks, D. M. (1972). Congenital hypothyroidism and neonatal jaundice. *Arch. Dis. Child.*, **47**, 469–71

29. Larsson, A., Hagenfeldt, L., Blom, L. and Mortensson, W. (1983). Serum alpha-fetoprotein—a biochemical indicator of prenatal hypothyroidism. *Acta Paediatr. Scand.*, **72**, 481–4

30. Klein, A. H., Agustin, A. V. and Foley, T. P. (1974). Successful laboratory screening for congenital hypothyroidism. *Lancet*, **2**, 77–9

31. Dussault, J. H., Coulombe, P., Laberge, C., Letarte, J., Guyda, H. and Khoury, K. (1975). Preliminary report on a mass screening program for neonatal hypothyroidism. *J. Pediatr.*, **86**, 670–4

32. Irie, M., Enomoto, K. and Naruse, H. (1975). Measurement of TSH in dried blood spots. *Lancet*, **2**, 1233–4

33. Fisher, D. A., Dussault, J. H., Foley, T. P., Klein, A. H., LaFrachni, S., Larsen, P. R., Mitchell, M. L., Murphy, W. H. and Walfish, P. G. (1979). Screening for congenital hypothyroidism: results of screening one million North American infants. *J. Pediatr.*, **94**, 704–5

34. Illig, R. (1983). Report on neonatal thyroid screening in Europe. In *Proceedings of the 22nd Annual Meeting of the European Society for Paediatric Endocrinology*, Budapest, 1983

35. Dussault, J. H., Parlow, A., Letarte, J., Guyda, H. and Laberge, C. (1976). TSH measurements from blood spots on filter paper. A confirmatory screening test for congenital hypothyroidism. *J. Pediatr.*, **89**, 550–2

36. Alm, J., Larsson, A. and Zetterström, R. (1978). Congenital hypothyroidism in Sweden: incidence and age at diagnosis. *Acta Paediatr. Scand.*, **67**, 1–3
37. Brock-Jacobsen, B. and Brandt, N. J. (1981). Congenital hypothyroidism in Denmark. *Arch. Dis. Child.*, **56**, 134–6
38. DeJonge, G. A. (1976). Congenital hypothyroidism in the Netherlands. *Lancet*, **2**, 143
39. Hulse, J. A., Grant, D. B., Clayton, B. E., Lilly, P., Jackson, D., Spracklan, A., Edwards, R. W. H. and Nurse, D. (1980). Population screening for congenital hypothyroidism. *Br. Med. J.*, **1**, 675–8
40. New England Congenital Hypothyroidism Collaborative (1982). Pitfalls in screening for neonatal hypothyroidism. *Pediatrics*, **70**, 16–20
41. Hulse, J. A., Grant, D. B., Jackson, D. and Clayton, B. E. (1982). Growth, development and reassessment of hypothyroid infants diagnosed by screening. *Br. Med. J.*, **1**, 1435–7
42. Glorieux, J., Dussault, J. H., Letarte, J., Guyda, M. and Morisette, J. (1983). Preliminary results on the mental development of hypothyroid infants detected by the Quebec Screening Program. *J. Pediatr.*, **102**, 19–22
43. New England Congenital Hypothyroidism Collaborative (1981). Effects of neonatal screening for hypothyroidism: prevention of mental retardation by treatment before clinical manifestations. *Lancet*, **2**, 1095–8

4

CLINICAL ASPECTS OF ACQUIRED THYROID DISEASE IN CHILDHOOD

N. D. BARNES

Thyroid disease may occur at any age and is an important cause of chronic morbidity. The clinical presentation, especially in childhood, is often insidious and atypical presentations surprise even the most experienced clinicians. However, precise diagnostic tests are widely available and treatment is generally straightforward and fully effective. It is therefore necessary to maintain a high index of suspicion for thyroid disease. This brief review of acquired thyroid disease in childhood will not be comprehensive but will attempt to highlight some aspects of practical importance in diagnosis and treatment which seem to the author currently to need emphasis.

Thyroid axis physiology

Thyroid hormones have a profound effect on the rate of oxidative metabolism in most tissues with the notable exception of the CNS. They also have a vital role in the growth and development of organ systems, including the CNS, in late fetal life and throughout childhood.

Prenatal and perinatal development of the structure and function of the thyroid axis has been greatly elucidated by recent work; this has been well reviewed[1] and will not be considered. In the term infant functional maturation is normally complete by about the age of 4 weeks. Although there are changes in total thyroid hormone concentrations until puberty, these reflect changes in binding proteins; at birth, thyroxine-binding globulin (TBG) levels are two to three times higher than adult values and thyroxine-binding pre-albumin (TBPA) levels half adult values[2].

Some data on the thyroid hormones are shown in Table 1[3,4]. The free tri-iodothyronine (T_3) is the key thyroid hormone fraction. Although structurally T_3 is simply thyroxine (T_4) with a single deiodination of the outer ring, it is five times more potent than its parent hormone. Moreover, it circulates less strongly bound to protein and therefore has a greater active component, and it has a shorter half-life and a more rapid turnover. The concentration of free T_3 is closely controlled by central and peripheral mechanisms as well as by the intrinsic secretory capacity of the thyroid gland. The median eminence of the hypothalamus secretes thyrotropin-releasing hormone (TRH) which stimulates production of thyroid-stimulating hormone (TSH) from the pituitary, which in turn stimulates synthesis and release of T_4 and T_3 from the thyroid. Feedback regulation occurs at the pituitary and probably also the hypothalamic level.

However, less than 20% of circulating T_3 is derived from the thyroid. The greater part is generated by peripheral deiodination of T_4, the large pool of which therefore acts as a reservoir of 'prohormone' for T_3. An alternative deiodination affects the inner ring of T_4 and produces the isomer 'reverse T_3' (rT_3) which, in contrast to T_3, has no metabolic action. In addition, rT_3 competes with T_4 for the outer ring deiodinase; this enzyme not only converts T_4 to T_3 but also, more efficiently, rT_3 to di-iodothyronine[5]. These remarkably neat and economical mechanisms permit adjustment of the balance between production of the most active and a totally inactive thyroxine metabolite. They seem to provide a means for sparing the metabolic stimulation of the thyroid in situations in which energy conservation is needed, such as acute illness and starvation, and also in the fetus. How the peripheral deiodinating enzymes are themselves controlled at present remains obscure.

The low T3 (sick euthyroid) syndrome

This state is characterized by low serum T_3 concentrations, high or normal rT_3, variable T_4 and normal TSH[1]. It is now known to be by far the most common alteration of thyroid function in ill adults and is increasingly recognized in children. It seems to represent a secondary hypothyroid state which results from the effects of non-thyroidal illness on several aspects of thyroid hormone metabolism. In teleological terms it may, as indicated above, represent an adaptation to circumstances in which the metabolic stimulation of the thyroid may be harmful. The thyroid status is analogous to that in the fetus during the latter part of pregnancy. Similar alterations in thyroid function may occur in ill preterm infants, in whom the normal postpartum increase in T_4 may be blunted and the T_3 may fall after an initial abrupt rise[1,6]. The relative importance of stress, hypoxia, undernutrition and other factors is not yet clear. Nor is it certain whether in some circumstances, such as the

Table 1 Thyroid hormones

	Thyroxine (T_4)	Tri-iodothyronine (T_3)	Reverse tri-iodothyronine (rT_3)
Structure	HO–⬡–O–⬡–CH_2 CH (NH_2) COOH	HO–⬡–O–⬡–CH_2 CH (NH_2) COOH	HO–⬡–O–⬡–CH_2 CH (NH_2) COOH
Mean serum total concentration (nmol/l)	103	1.8	0.62
Mean serum-free concentration (pmol/l)	27	4.3	3.1
% Free	0.03	0.3	0.5
Relative biological activity	1	5	0
Serum half-life (days)	6.5	1.0	<0.5
Volume of distribution (l)	10.0	38.0	98.0
Body pool (µg)	810.0	46.0	40.0
Metabolic clearance rate (l/day)	1.1	22.0	90.0
Daily production rate (µg/day)	82.0	28.0	28.0

preterm infant in whom lung maturation may be life-saving, adverse effects may outweigh the metabolic benefits of this adaptive mechanism[6]. There is a spontaneous return to normal thyroid function as the patient recovers.

HYPOTHYROIDISM

Causes

Hypothyroidism arising in childhood is most frequently due to disease of the thyroid gland, primary hypothyroidism, but can result from problems affecting the thyroid axis at pituitary or hypothalamic levels, secondary or tertiary hypothyroidism. Apart from the low T_3 syndrome, disorders of peripheral thyroid hormone metabolism are rare. The conditions that may cause hypothyroidism are listed in Table 2. A number of conditions which are strictly congenital rather than acquired are included, since these may present later in childhood. Many such children are now detected in the newborn period by screening while still asymptomatic.

Table 2   Causes of 'acquired' hypothyroidism in childhood

Primary (T_4/T_3 deficiency)
  autoimmune thyroiditis
  iatrogenic (antithyroid drugs, surgery, ^{131}I, iodide)
  dysgenesis
  dyshormonogenesis } with late failure
  subacute thyroiditis
  infiltration (cystinosis, histiocytosis)
  TSH unresponsiveness

Secondary (TSH deficiency)
  pituitary lesions (tumour, trauma, infection, infiltration,
    dysgenesis with late failure)
  isolated TSH deficiency

Tertiary (TRH deficiency)
  hypothalamic lesions (as for pituitary lesions)
  isolated TRH deficiency

Peripheral hormone metabolism
  low T_3 ('sick euthyroid') syndrome
  thyroid hormone unresponsiveness

Chronic lymphocytic thyroiditis

Chronic lymphocytic thyroiditis is by far the most common cause of acquired hypothyroidism in childhood. The underlying autoimmune mechanisms have been investigated extensively and clarified recently[7].

The prevalence of the condition in most populations is not known, but in a 6-year survey of three American states 5179 schoolchildren aged from 11 to 18 were examined and tested to detect thyroid abnormalities after exposure to nuclear fall-out after weapons testing in 1953[8]. Chronic lymphocytic thyroiditis was identified in 62 children, a prevalence of 1.2%. Eighty-five per cent had palpable goitres and girls were affected twice as commonly as boys. Overt clinical hypothyroidism was present in only two children and hyperthyroidism in two children. Most affected children were asymptomatic and clinically euthyroid. Spontaneous resolution of the thyroiditis occurred in 15 of 32 children who received no treatment and 14 of 30 given thyroid hormone supplements. This important study emphasizes that chronic lymphocytic thyroiditis is usually a mild and self-limited disorder and presents a very different picture of the problem from that obtained in referral practice.

Clinical presentation

The onset of hypothyroidism is usually insidious and unless an obvious goitre is present there is often prolonged delay before the diagnosis is made. The major clinical features are summarized in Table 3. The cardinal sign is growth retardation, the process of growth providing a sensitive bioassay for the action of thyroid hormones. Every child with disturbed growth that is not otherwise fully and adequately explained

Table 3 Major clinical and radiological features of hypothyroidism in childhood

Thyroid
  enlarged or atrophic

Skeletal
  growth retardation
  increased upper/lower segment ratio
  retarded bone age
  epiphyseal dysgenesis, slipped femoral capital epiphysis

CNS
  placidity, 'good nature'
  good school progress!
  immobility, lethargy
  delayed tendon reflexes

Other
  facial fullness
  pallor, anaemia, carotinaemia
  muscularity (not obesity)
  dry, coarse skin/hair
  cold intolerance
  constipation
  abnormal sexual development

requires a check on thyroid function. Since the major growth-promoting action of thyroid hormones is on osteogenesis, the retardation of linear growth is associated with marked retardation of the bone age. The growth chart of a child with severe hypothyroidism is shown in Figure 1. With the onset of hypothyroidism the growth curve parts from the previously established channel and falls progressively away as the growth rate drops. The bone age lags increasingly behind the chronological age.

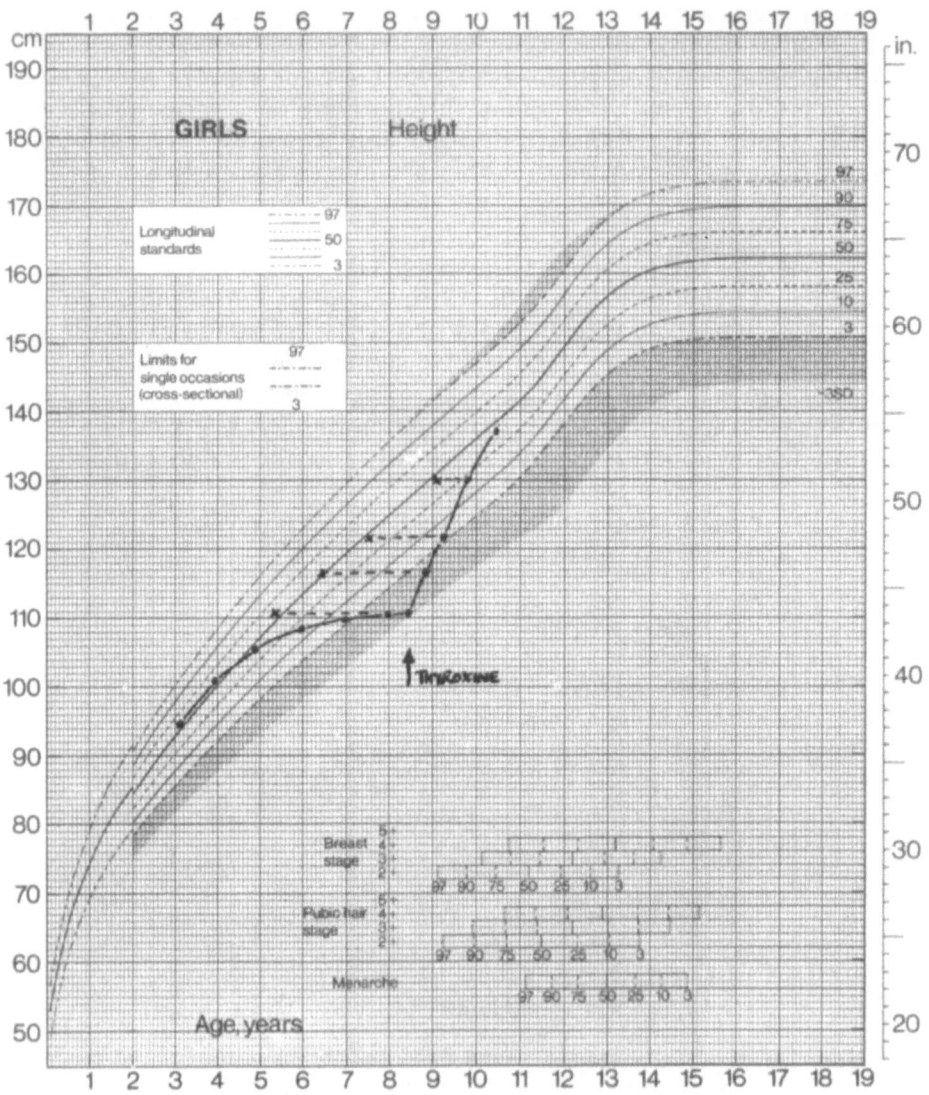

Figure 1 The growth chart of a girl who became hypothyroid and was treated. Bone age estimations are depicted as crosses

Growth may almost cease before the diagnosis is made, but with treatment the catch-up is remarkable. Dental development is also retarded and delayed eruption of the primary or secondary dentition may provide an additional clinical clue to the diagnosis.

Children with hypothyroidism almost invariably show a considerable change in activity and personality, but this is often interpreted as a good rather than a bad sign and, indeed, in many respects it may be. Affected children are quiet, placid and usually good-tempered. Contrary to nearly all accounts of the condition they retain good mental function and alertness and often do remarkably well at school. This sometimes causes diagnostic confusion because the possibility of hypothyroidism, or indeed any illness, may be dismissed in a child apparently functioning so well. The reason for this apparently paradoxical effect of the disease seems to be that, as is well known to parents and teachers, the average child is far too active for her own good. Slowed and calmed a little, her concentration improves, she plods along with her work unaffected by the maelstrom around her and scores especially high marks for endeavour and behaviour. This effect is transient and eventually overt lethargy and mental sluggishness supervene in association with cold intolerance, dry skin and hair, constipation and the full catalogue of symptoms and signs familiar from adult myxoedema. These are, however, late signs and many hypothyroid children continue to make good academic and social progress until diagnosed.

Hypothyroid children are seldom obese and they appear muscular. Excessive muscular development has been described as a rare manifestation of the disease, the Kocher–Debré–Semelaigne syndrome[9], but such children probably represent only the more extreme examples of a change in body composition common to all. This is of practical diagnostic importance because the first impression on seeing a hypothyroid child undressed is often of excess muscularity, sometimes, in boys, even resembling that seen in Duchenne muscular dystrophy and, in girls, superficially resembling the build of Turner's syndrome.

Precocious sexual development has been described as another rare and paradoxical association with juvenile hypothyroidism. Since delay in general development is a cardinal feature of the condition it is indeed remarkable that some children show features of sexual development in advance of their chronological age. However, in a large series of children with long-standing primary hypothyroidism, more than half those of both sexes showed some features of sexual development in advance of their bone age, taken as the best estimate of their physiological or maturational age[10].

Concentration on the relative timing of these aspects of development seems to have diverted attention from their abnormal features, summarized in Table 4. This is also important chiefly because inappropriate investigation may be undertaken before the underlying hypothyroidism

61

is recognized. In both sexes, there is commonly dissociation of unusual degree between pubic hair development, which is sparse or absent, and other secondary sexual characteristics. In girls, remarkable hypertrophy of the labia minora often occurs and may be ascribed inappropriately to local problems. The cystic ovarian hypertrophy may result in an unnecessary laparotomy and the testicular enlargement in an unnecessary biopsy. Enlargement of the sella in association with features of hypothyroidism or galactorrhoea is likely to suggest the presence of a pituitary tumour.

The biochemical correlates of these changes, in addition to the decreased thyroid hormone and increased TSH concentrations, are hyperprolactinaemia with increased immunoreactive FSH and LH levels. In contrast to adults, in children a bolus of TRH does release FSH and, in association with the hyperprolactinaemia and pituitary hyperplasia, suggests that stimulation of hypothalamic TRH secretion may be the primary event. All these manifestations resolve with treatment of the hypothyroidism and normal puberty occurs at an appropriate maturational age.

Table 4 Abnormal sexual development in juvenile hypothyroidism

Girls
    breast development without pubic hair
    hypertrophy of the labia minora
    galactorrhoea
    cystic ovarian enlargement
    globular enlargement of the sella turcica

Boys
    testicular enlargement without pubic hair
    globular enlargement of the sella turcica

Diagnosis

Once suspected, biochemical confirmation of hypothyroidism is usually easily obtained. The serum thyroid hormone levels are low, but the T_3 is often relatively well maintained compared with the T_4. In primary hypothyroidism the TSH is raised, often in children greatly so, whereas in secondary and tertiary hypothyroidism the TSH is characteristically low but may be slightly or moderately raised with hypothalamic disorders. The TRH stimulation test is of the greatest value in investigating borderline primary hypothyroidism and secondary and tertiary problems[11].

Secondary abnormalities of binding proteins are less often seen in childhood than in adult life, but the congenital disorders sometimes cause diagnostic confusion. Screening programmes using primary T_4

estimation have shown that TBG deficiency is surprisingly common with an incidence around 1 in 9000 and X-linked inheritance[12]. X-linked TBG excess is relatively rare, but familial hyperthyroxinaemic states due to other congenital binding abnormalities have recently been recognized[13].

Associated conditions

Autoimmune thyroiditis occurs with increased frequency in a number of conditions which should alert the clinician to maintain extra vigilance. Among the most important of these is insulin-dependent diabetes mellitus. Several surveys have shown a prevalence of thyroid antibodies around 15% and hypothyroidism 5% [14, 15]. Screening of young diabetics is therefore worthwhile.

There is an increased incidence of autoimmune thyroiditis in three genetic conditions associated with severe growth restriction, Down's[16], Turner's[17] and Noonan's[18] syndromes. The expected short stature masks the most important sign of hypothyroidism and in these conditions recognition and treatment of hypothyroidism is rewarding.

Thyroiditis is commonly associated with other autoimmune diseases and several polyglandular syndromes have been defined[19]. These are

Table 5   Polyglandular syndromes

Type I
  hypoparathyroidism
  Addison's
  mucocutaneous moniliasis

Type II
  Addison's
  thyroiditis
  diabetes, type I

Type III
  A diabetes, type I
    thyroiditis
  B thyroiditis
    pernicious anaemia
  C thyroiditis
    other

Other associated conditions
  vitiligo
  alopecia
  keratoconjunctivitis
  Sjogren's syndrome
  malabsorption
  gonadal failure
  chronic active hepatitis
  primary biliary cirrhosis
  myasthenia gravis

summarized in Table 5. It has recently been recognized as being frequently associated with the congenital rubella syndrome[20].

There is an association between primary hypothyroidism and slipped femoral capital epithysis[21].

Infiltration of the thyroid is rare except in cystinosis in which it is invariable and leads eventually to hypothyroidism in survivors, who are more numerous now that the results of renal transplantation have improved[22].

TREATMENT

Thyroid replacement is generally straightforward. Synthetic l-thyroxine is the preparation of choice and giving the prohormone enables the peripheral mechanisms, presumably intact, to make fine adjustment. Except in some infants with congenital hypothyroidism, in whom the set point of the proximal limb of the thyroid axis may be abnormal, the correct dose of thyroxine can be judged by reference to the child's own feedback loop and defined as the smallest dose that suppresses the TSH into the normal range. The serum total thyroxine is then generally in the upper part of the normal range. After the age of 1 year a dose of approximately $4\,\mu g/kg/day$ is needed[23], but great precision of dosage seems to be unnecessary, probably because some excess thyroxine can be rendered inactive by conversion to rT_3. A considerable overdose of thyroxine is therefore necessary to provoke overt hyperthyroid manifestations or unduly rapid advance in growth and maturation, but this is a danger, especially in infants in whom premature craniosynostosis can result[24].

If the hypothyroidism is severe and of long standing, it is wise to start replacement at less than a full dose and increase in one or two increments over a few weeks. It is also important for the child, parents and school-teacher to be warned that the initial effects are not apparent for several days and that transient undesirable side-effects are common. These include emotional and behaviour disturbance, which is occasionally so severe that the treatment is interrupted, aching pain in muscles and joints, and hair loss, which is often worrying but never progresses to a degree sufficient to cause cosmetic problems.

Slipped femoral capital epiphysis may occur soon after, as well as before, treatment is started, perhaps in relation to increased activity. Attention has recently been drawn to the occurrence of pseudotumour cerebri in the early days of treatment, a serious complication which may be more common than has been appreciated[25].

HYPERTHYROIDISM

Neonatal hyperthyroidism

Transient neonatal hyperthyroidism occurs in the infants of mothers who have extremely high titres of thyroid-stimulating immunoglobulins, irrespective of their own current thyroid status. The antibodies cross the placenta and cause a short-lived but sometimes life-threatening hyperthyroid state. This condition has been discussed above and will not be considered further.

A rare persistent form of neonatal hyperthyroidism has also been recognized[26]. This has generally affected children from families in which there is a strong history of Graves', but the mother may not be affected. The onset of hyperthyroidism occurs in the neonatal period and persists for many months or years. Affected children show behaviour disturbance with hyperactivity and emotional lability and some are mentally retarded. In addition, they may have a characteristic skull shape with frontal bossing due to premature synostosis and, after initial acceleration, their growth may be retarded. It seems likely that this disorder represents simply the earliest onset of Graves' disease, but it is not clear whether prompt control of the hyperthyroidism would prevent the sequelae.

Acquired hyperthyroidism

Hyperthyroidism is uncommon in childhood, only about 5% of cases presenting in the first 15 years of life. In addition, the onset of symptoms tends to be more gradual than in adult life and large goitres and obvious opthalmopathy are uncommon. These facts no doubt account for the delay, on average 6–12 months, which occurs before the diagnosis is made.

The great majority of cases are due to Graves' disease, now known to be an autoimmune disorder in which there is generation of thyroid-stimulating immunoglobulins which bind to and stimulate the TSH receptor[7]. There is a high familial incidence, girls are three to five times more frequently affected than boys and there is an increasing incidence through childhood.

Hyperthyroidism in childhood may rarely result from a number of other causes, including excessive administration of thyroid hormones, either iatrogenic or factitious, autonomously functioning adenomas, iodide ingestion (the Jod–Basedow phenomenon), functional thyroid carcinomas, TSH-secreting pituitary adenomas, pituitary resistance to thyroxine and chorionic gonadotrophin-secreting tumours[27]. A transient and usually mild hyperthyroid state may occur in subacute thyroiditis[28] and in patients with co-existing Graves' and Hashimoto's disease[29]; both these conditions may be under-recognized in children.

Clinical features

The clinical features of hyperthyroidism in childhood are summarized in Table 6. In retrospect, parents usually remember that the first symptom in their child was increased nervousness, irritability and emotional lability but, unless enlargement of the thyroid or eye signs lead them to seek medical attention, and especially as the disease often occurs in adolescence, this is almost invariably considered to be psychological in origin. The corollary of the good school progress in hypothyroidism should be poor school progress and this is indeed the case. The handwriting becomes cramped and untidy (this is a remarkably constant early sign), the child is unable to sit still or to concentrate and, combined with the psychological problems, these symptoms form a recipe for disaster. Many affected children are referred first for psychological or psychiatric evaluation. The motor restlessness may be such that it is mistaken for chorea and it persists through sleep so that these children usually sleep fitfully and awake with all their bedclothes thrown on the floor.

Table 6   Major clinical features of hyperthyroidism in childhood

Thyroid
   diffusely enlarged

CNS
   nervousness, irritability, emotional lability
   deterioration in handwriting, school work
   restlessness, hyperactivity, abnormal movements, tremor
   sleeplessness, nightmares

Eyes
   stare, 'bright-eyed' look
   lid retraction, lag
   proptosis

CVS
   tachycardia
   increased pulse pressure

Other
   increased appetite
   weight loss
   diarrhoea
   heat intolerance
   growth acceleration, advanced bone age
   fatigue, weakness, proximal myopathy

Diagnosis

The diagnosis of hyperthyroidism is established by demonstrating raised serum T_3 levels. T_4 levels are usually, but not invariably, raised also.

The diagnosis can be confirmed by demonstrating absent TSH response to TRH stimulation[11]; this test has largely superseded the T_3 suppression test, in which hyperthyroidism was demonstrated by failure of treatment with T_3 for a week to suppress the increased thyroidal radioiodine uptake.

Treatment

Of the three methods of treatment available, medical management with a thionamide compound is generally used initially in children in preference to surgery or radioactive iodine. Carbimazole is the preferred drug in the UK and propylthiouracil in the USA. The main action of these drugs is to prevent thyroid hormone synthesis by blocking the organification of iodine, but there is evidence that carbimazole has an immunosuppressive action[30] and PTU blocks the peripheral conversion of T_4 to T_3[31]. The significance of these effects in the treatment of Graves' is uncertain, but they may explain why euthyroidism can often be maintained with a small twice daily, or even daily, dose in spite of the short plasma half-lives.

Control of the hyperthyroidism is generally easily achieved. A beta blocking agent can be used for symptomatic control until euthyroidism is restored. Side-effects from the thionamide drugs are not infrequently seen in children[32], but they are generally mild, consisting of pruritus, urticaria, a maculopapular rash or arthralgia and they usually respond to a change of drug or a reduction in dosage. Although rare, it is necessary to be alert for more serious problems such as a serum-sickness or systemic lupus-like syndrome, hepatitis or neutropenia. These are reversible but obviously preclude continued use of the drug. Some 2–5% of children are unable to tolerate either drug. If it proves difficult to maintain a stable euthyroid state a higher dose can be given in combination with thyroxine replacement[33]. Compliance often proves a problem.

A 2–3-year course of antithyroid treatment is generally given before withdrawing the drug in the hope that a permanent remission will then occur. At present there is no reliable method of predicting the likelihood of remission, but a short history, mild hyperthyroidism, a small goitre and a low radioiodine uptake are good prognostic factors. Prolonged remission rates varying from 25 to 61% after 2–3 years of medical therapy have been reported in large series[33–35].

Subtotal thyroidectomy is a well tried and effective form of therapy. It is a safe operation in the hands of an experienced surgical team. There have been no deaths in a series of more than 400 children operated on at the Mayo Clinic[36]. However, there is a high incidence, 30–50%, of postoperative hypothyroidism, recurrent hyperthyroidism occasionally occurs and there is a small risk of surgical complications, including hypoparathyroidism, recurrent laryngeal palsy, haemorrhage, infection or keloid formation[33–35].

Radioactive iodine provides a safe and effective form of therapy, well tried in adults. In Europe, this form of treatment has been largely confined to patients past reproductive age for fear of cancer induction, leukaemia and genetic damage. However, a considerable number of children and many young adults have been treated in the United States and, to date, there is no evidence of increased risk to the individual or subsequent progeny[37]. It is a remarkable fact that although external irradiation to the thyroid is strongly carcinogenetic ^{131}I therapy is not. There is a high incidence of hypothyroidism after treatment, but this cannot be avoided and it has been suggested that ablative treatment may further reduce the risk of thyroid carcinoma. At present it seems wise to reserve this form of treatment for children in whom medical therapy has failed and subtotal thyroidectomy is contraindicated. It may, however, be useful in special situations and current evidence suggests that there may have been undue reluctance to use it in childhood.

STRUCTURAL LESIONS OF THE THYROID

Diffuse thyroid enlargement is generally due to autoimmune disease. Asymmetrical enlargement is much less common. The usual finding is a single nodule, but occasionally a multinodular gland may be encountered. Girls are more frequently affected than boys.

Especially in the United States, from which most series have been reported, the incidence of carcinoma has varied according to the use of external irradiation to the cervical area but, in general terms, about one-third of such lesions prove to be carcinomas, one-third adenomas and one-third other lesions, including lymphocytic thyroiditis, subacute thyroiditis, teratoma, abscess, cyst, thyroid dysplasia or dyshormono-genetic goitre[39,40]. The most useful investigation is the thyroid scan, but ultrasound, CT and biopsy may be helpful. Surgical excision is usually needed.

Carcinoma of the thyroid is fortunately not only much less common in childhood than in adult life but also generally less aggressive. It may occur at any age, but the incidence increases throughout life. The close relationship with external irradiation was clearly demonstrated by the remarkable 20-year survey of Winship and Rosvoll in which 878 cases were identified[41]. There was a steep rise in incidence between 1940 and 1950, which reflected increased use of irradiation, and 80% of the children for whom details were available had been exposed; after 1960 there was a rapid decrease in incidence once again. The average interval between irradiation and the diagnosis of cancer was 8.5 years; 71.6% of the tumours were classified histologically as papillary, but most showed follicular elements.

Thyroid carcinoma generally presents as a firm thyroid mass, but metastases to the cervical lymph nodes occur early and may be more impressive and easily felt than the primary in the thyroid. The lymphadenopathy is fortunately unlike the common infective cervical lymphadenopathy of childhood as the glands are lower in the cervical chain and feel firmer.

Medullary carcinoma of the thyroid, a tumour of the calcitonin-secreting C cells, is rarely diagnosed during childhood; it accounted for only 2.6% of the tumours in Winship and Rosvoll's series[41]. Nevertheless, it should be known to paediatricians because of its familial incidence and its association with the mucosal neuroma syndrome or multiple endocrine adenomatosis type III (also known as multiple endocrine neoplasia type IIb). Medullary carcinoma may occur sporadically, but in some families it is inherited as an autosomal dominant trait. In some of these families, affected individuals show a syndrome in which a Marfanoid build and a characteristic facies is associated with multiple neuromas on the tongue, lips and eyelids. There may be ganglioneuromatosis of the gastro-intestinal tract which can present with motility disorders in infancy. Bilateral phaeochromocytomas and parathyroid hyperplasia occur in adult life[42]. The children of families with medullary carcinoma should be screened regularly with calcium infusion or pentagastrin stimulation tests to detect excessive calcitonin production from the C cells which, if detected, is an indication for total thyroidectomy. Metastatic disease has been recorded as young as 3 years and in 12 children aged 10 or less[43]. The opportunity to detect this genetic disease as early as possible must therefore not be missed.

References

1. Fisher, D. A. and Klein, A. H. (1981). Thyroid development and disorders of thyroid function in the newborn. *N. Engl. J. Med.*, **304**, 702–12
2. Braverman, L. E., Dawber, N. A. and Ingbar, S. H. (1966). Observations concerning the binding of thyroid hormones in sera of normal subjects of varying ages. *J. Clin. Invest.*, **45**, 1273–9
3. Oppenheimer, J. H. and Surks, M. I. (1974). Quantitative aspects of hormone production, distribution, metabolism and activity. In *Handbook of Physiology. Section 7, Vol. 3, Endocrinology*, pp. 197–214. (Washington: American Physiological Society)
4. Pittman, C. S. (1979). Hormone metabolism. In De Groot, L. J., Cahill, G. F. and Odell, W. D. (eds.) *Endocrinology*. Vol. 1, pp. 365–72. (New York: Grune and Stratton)
5. Pittman, J. A., Tingley, J. O., Nickerson, J. F. and Hill, S. R. (1960). Antimetabolic activity of 3,3′,5′-triiodo-DL-thyronine in man. *Metabolism*, **9**, 293–5
6. Erenberg, A. (1982). Thyroid function in the preterm infant. *Pediatr. Clin. N. Am.*, **29**, 1205–11
7. Strakosch, C. R., Wenzel, B. E., Row, V. V. and Volpe, R. (1982). Immunology of autoimmune thyroid diseases. *N. Engl. J. Med.*, **307**, 1499–1505

8. Rallinson, M., Dobyns, B. M., Keating, F. R., Rall, J. E. and Tyler, F. H. (1975). Occurrence and natural history of chronic lymphocytic thyroiditis in childhood. *J. Pediatr.*, **86**, 675–82

9. Najjar, S. S. (1974). Muscular hypertrophy in hypothyroid children: the Kocher–Debré–Semelaigne syndrome. *J. Pediatr.*, **85**, 236–9

10. Barnes, N. D., Hayles, A. B. and Ryan, R. J. (1973). Sexual maturation in juvenile hypothyroidism. *Mayo Clin. Proc.*, **48**, 849–56

11. Barnes, N. D. (1975). Serum T.S.H. measurement in children with thyroid disorders. *Arch. Dis. Child.*, **50**, 497–9

12. Fisher, D. A., Dussault, J. H., Foley, T. P., Klein, A. H., Lafranchi, S., Reed Larsen, P., Mitchell, M. L., Murphey, W. H. and Walfish, P. G. (1979). Screening for congenital hypothyroidism: results of screening one million North American infants. *J. Pediatr.*, **94**, 700–5

13. Stockigt, J. R., White, E. L. and Barlow, J. N. (1982). Differences between familial hyperthyroxinaemic syndromes. *N. Engl. J. Med.*, **307**, 824–5

14. Riley, W. J., Maclaren, N. K., Lezotte, D. C., Spillar, R. P. and Rosenbloom, A. L. (1981). Thyroid autoimmunity in insulin-dependent diabetes mellitus: the case for routine screening. *J. Pediatr.*, **98**, 350–4

15. Court, S. and Parkin, J. M. (1982). Hypothyroidism and growth failure in diabetes mellitus. *Arch. Dis. Child.*, **57**, 622–4

16. Lobo, E. de H., Khan, M. and Tew, J. (1980). Community study of hypothyroidism in Down's syndrome. *Br. Med. J.*, **280**, 1253

17. Pai, G. S., Leach, D. C., Weiss, L., Wolf, L. and Van Dyke, D. L. (1977). Thyroid abnormalities in 20 children with Turner's syndrome. *J. Pediatr.*, **91**, 267–9

18. Vesterhus, P. and Aarskog, D. (1973). Noonan's syndrome and autoimmune thyroiditis. *J. Pediatr.*, **83**, 237–40

19. Neufeld, M., Maclaren, N. and Blizzard, R. (1980). Autoimmune polyglandular syndromes. *Pediatr. Ann.*, **9**, 154–62

20. Avruskin, T. W., Brakin, M. and Juan, C. (1982). Congenital rubella and myxedema. *Pediatrics*, **69**, 495–6

21. Hirano, T., Stamelos, S., Harris, V. and Dumbovic, N. (1978). Association of primary hypothyroidism and slipped capital femoral epiphysis. *J. Pediatr.*, **93**, 262–4

22. Burke, J. R., El-Bishti, M. M., Maisey, M. N. and Chantler, C. (1978). Hypothyroidism in children with cystinosis. *Arch. Dis. Child.*, **53**, 947–51

23. Resvani, I. and DiGeorge, A. M. (1977). Reassessment of the daily dose of oral thyroxine for replacement therapy in hypothyroid children. *J. Pediatr.*, **90**, 291–7

24. Penfold, J. L. and Simpson, D. A. (1975). Premature craniosynostosis—a complication of thyroid replacement therapy. *J. Pediatr.*, **86**, 360–3

25. Van Dop, C., Conte, F. A., Koch, T. K., Clark, S. J., Wilson-Davis, S. L. and Grumbach, M. M. (1983). Pseudotumor cerebri associated with initiation of levothyroxine therapy for juvenile hypothyroidism. *N. Engl. J. Med.*, **308**, 1076–80

26. Hollingsworth, D. R. and Mabry, C. C. (1976). Congenital Graves' disease. *Am. J. Dis. Child.*, **130**, 148–55

27. Reiter, E. C., Root, A. N., Rettig, K. and Vargas, A. (1981). Childhood thyromegaly: recent developments. *J. Pediatr.*, **99**, 507–18

28. Hurley, J. R. (1977). Thyroiditis. *Disease-a-Month*, **24**, 1–68

29. Kidd, A., Okita, N., Row, V. V. and Volpe, R. (1980). Immunologic aspects of Graves' and Hashimoto's diseases. *Metabolism*, **29**, 80

30. McGregor, A. M., Rees Smith, B., Hall, R., Collins, P. N., Botazzo, G. F. and Petersen, M. M. (1982). Specificity of the immunosuppressive action of carbimazole in Graves' disease. *Br. Med. J.*, **284**, 1250–1

31. Saberi, M., Sterling, F. H. and Utiger, R. G. (1975). Reduction in extrathyroidal triiodothyronine production by propylthiouracil in man. *J. Clin. Invest.*, **55**, 218–23

32. Armhein, J. A., Kenny, F. N. and Ross, D. (1970). Granulocytopenia, lupus-like syndrome and other complications of propylthiouracil therapy. *J. Pediatr.*, **76**, 54–63

33. Barnes, H. V. and Blizzard, R. M. (1977). Antithyroid drug therapy for toxic diffuse goitre (Graves' disease): 30 years experience in children and adolescents. *J. Pediatr.*, **91**, 313–20

34. Buckingham, B. A., Costin, G., Roe, T. F., Weitzman, J. J. and Kogut, M. A. (1981). Hyperthyroidism in children: a re-evaluation of treatment. *Am. J. Dis. Child.*, **135**, 112–17

35. Hothem, A. L., Thomas, C. G. and Van Wyk, J. J. (1978). Selective treatment in the management of thyrotoxicosis in children. *Ann. Surg.*, **187**, 593–8

36. Howard, C. P. and Hayles, A. B. (1978). Hyperthyroidism in childhood. *Clin. Endocrinol. Metab.*, **7**, 127–43

37. Safa, A. M., Schumacher, O. P. and Rodriguez-Antunez, A. (1975). Long-term follow-up in children and adolescents treated with radioactive iodine (^{131}I) for hyperthyroidism. *N. Engl. J. Med.*, **292**, 167–71

38. Freitas, J. E., Swanson, D. P., Gross, M. D. and Sisson, J. C. (1979). Iodine-131: optimal therapy for hyperthyroidism in children and adolescents? *J. Nucl. Med.*, **20**, 847–50

39. Kirkland, R. T., Kirkland, J. L., Rosenberg, H. S., Harberg, F. J., Librik, L. and Clayton, G. W. (1973). Solitary thyroid nodules in 30 children and report of a child with a thyroid abscess. *Pediatrics*, **51**, 85–90

40. Scott, M. D. and Crawford, J. D. (1976). Solitary thyroid nodules in childhood: is the incidence of thyroid carcinoma declining? *Pediatrics*, **58**, 521–5

41. Winship, T. and Rosvoll, R. V. (1970). Thyroid carcinoma in childhood: final report on a 20-year study. *Clin. Proc. Child. Hosp. Natl. Med. Ctr.*, **26**, 327

42. Dyck, P. J., Carney, J. A., Sizemore, G. W., Okazaki, H., Brimisoin, W. S. and Lambert, E. H. (1979). Multiple endocrine neoplasia, type 2b: phenotypic recognition, neurological features and their pathological basis. *Ann. Neurol.*, **6**, 302–14

43. Kaufman, F. R., Roe, T. F., Isaacs, H. and Weitzman, J. J. (1982). Metastatic medullary thyroid carcinoma in young children with mucosal neuroma syndrome. *Pediatrics*, **70**, 263–7

SECTION 3

Disorders of
Sexual Development

Chairman: D. A. PRICE

5

PATHOGENESIS AND INVESTIGATION OF AMBIGUOUS GENITALIA

M. O. SAVAGE

Disorders of sexual differentiation were originally classified according to their clinical features and descriptive terms such as the adrenogenital syndrome and testicular feminization were adopted. In recent years, however, and particularly during the past decade, many of the basic biochemical abnormalities in these syndromes have been defined which has led to a change from a clinical to an aetiological approach in the investigation and management of patients with intersex disorders.

In order to adopt an aetiological approach, however, it is necessary to have some knowledge of the normal physiology of human fetal sexual differentiation.

NORMAL FETAL SEXUAL DIFFERENTIATION

It was the classical experiments of Jost[1] in the 1940s and 1950s which established two fundamental principles of mammalian sexual differentiation. The first is that the natural tendency of the fetus is to develop as a female, and the second is that hormones secreted by the fetal testis play an essential role in the formation of the male phenotype. During the first 8 weeks of fetal life the gonads and internal and external structures are sexually undifferentiated, preserving the potential for both male and female development. In the female, internal structures and external genitalia develop spontaneously. In the male, however, it is the Y chromosome which plays a limited but nevertheless pivotal role in the differentiation in the development of the testis.

Male genital development occurs during a critical period from the 10th to the 16th week of fetal life. The fetal testis is stimulated by placental human chorionic gonadotrophin to secrete testosterone which has two main functions. First, by local diffusion from the adjacent testis, the Wolffian ducts are virilized to become the epididymis, vas deferens and seminal vesicle. Secondly, by circulating peripherally, testosterone reaches the androgen target cell where it is converted by the microsomal enzyme 5α-reductase to its metabolite dihydrotestosterone which is responsible for virilization of the urogenital sinus and external genitalia.

At the same time, the Sertoli cell of the testis secretes a glycoprotein known as anti-müllerian hormone or müllerian-inhibiting factor[2]. This substance, by an active process and also probably by local diffusion, inhibits the formation of the müllerian ducts which would otherwise develop into the female internal structures.

The whole process is more complicated than female development and therefore more vulnerable, and any abnormality in the chain of events from testicular differentiation to secretion and peripheral action of these hormones will lead to incomplete virilization of the male fetus.

CLASSIFICATION OF PATIENTS WITH AMBIGUOUS GENITALIA (Table 1)

Despite current preoccupation with biochemical mechanisms, the original classification of Klebs based on the identification of gonadal sex is still in current usage. There are essentially three types of intersexuality: female pseudohermaphroditism, where there is virilization of the female fetus; male pseudohermaphroditism, where there is incomplete virilization of the male fetus; and thirdly, a group, somewhat heterogeneous, in which there is abnormal differentiation of the gonads.

THE FEMALE PSEUDOHERMAPHRODITE (Table 2)

Virilization of the normal female fetus is usually confined to the external genitalia and is due to the inappropriate production of either fetal or maternal androgens. By far the most important cause is congenital adrenal hyperplasia and each of these enzyme deficiencies may cause fetal virilization. The remaining causes are unimportant. Of the enzyme defects, 21-hydroxylase deficiency is by far the most common. Deficiency of this enzyme, inherited as an autosomal recessive trait, leads to accumulation of the precursor immediately before the enzyme which is 17-hydroxyprogesterone. This is converted to androstenedione, a weak androgen, and then to testosterone, a potent androgen which is responsible for virilization of the fetus. Lack of circulating cortisol stimulates the negative feedback loop resulting in excess ACTH production. Salt-loss due to lack of aldosterone secretion and virilization are the two predominant clinical features of the affected infant.

Table 1   Classification of patients with ambiguous genitalia

Identification of gonadal sex (Klebs, 1876)

(1) Female pseudohermaphroditism, virilization of genetic female with normal ovaries

(2) Male pseudohermaphroditism, incomplete virilization of genetic male with differentiated testes

(3) Abnormal gonadal differentiation, e.g. true hermaphrodite, XX male, mixed gonadal dysgenesis

Table 2   Female pseudohermaphrodite

Features	Aetiology
46 XX	congenital adrenal hyperplasia deficiency of
Normal ovaries	(1) 21-hydroxylase
	(2) 11β-hydroxylase
Normal uterus and fallopian tubes	(3) 3β-hydroxysteroid dehydrogenase
Virilization of *external* genitalia	maternal virilizing tumour
	maternal progestagens
	idiopathic

THE MALE PSEUDOHERMAPHRODITE (Table 3)

The male pseudohermaphrodite has a normal male karyotype, two differentiated testes, and may have a wide clinical spectrum of impaired virilization. There are essentially two aetiological categories[3]. In the first the defect is in the testis and in the second it is in the peripheral action of androgens.

Table 3   Male pseudohermaphrodite

Features	Aetiology
46 XY	(1) impaired testicular function
Two differentiated testes	inborn errors of testosterone biosynthesis
Wide clinical spectrum of impaired virilization	(2) impaired peripheral androgen metabolism 5α-reductase deficiency androgen receptor defects

DEFICIENT TESTOSTERONE BIOSYNTHESIS

Deficient testosterone biosynthesis due to an inherited enzyme deficiency is the most important testicular cause. If any of the enzymes in the biosynthetic pathway are deficient, testosterone cannot be synthesized in sufficient quantities during the critical period of embryogenesis when male differentiation is taking place. The result is that certainly the external genitalia, and possibly the internal genitalia, will be incompletely virilized. If an enzyme is deficient early in the pathway, both cortisol and aldosterone synthesis may be affected in addition to testosterone.

DEFICIENT PERIPHERAL ANDROGEN ACTION

The most important disorders causing male pseudohermaphroditism are those due to impaired peripheral androgen metabolism. Peripheral androgen action may be disturbed in three principal ways. Deficiency of 5α-reductase[4] leads to impaired conversion of testosterone to dihydrotestosterone. Abnormality of the cytoplasmic receptor will lead to impaired binding of the androgen, either testosterone or dihydrotestosterone, to this receptor, and thirdly, some patients with apparently normal receptor binding may have postreceptor resistance.

In 5α-reductase deficiency there is a selective lack of virilization of the external genitalia due to deficiency of dihydrotestosterone, and the prepubertal phenotype is essentially female, most patients being brought up as girls. This enzyme deficiency is inherited as an autosomal recessive trait and most cases hitherto described have been identified in communities with a high incidence of consanguinity.

At puberty, due to the normal testosterone levels, virilization occurs, resulting in the formation of a male body habitus and male psychosexual orientation which leads to conversion from a female to a male gender identity. The external genitalia, however, remain poorly virilized. The pathognomonic biochemical finding in 5α-reductase deficiency is an elevation in the ratio of plasma testosterone to dihydrotestosterone concentrations.

Androgen receptor defects[5] can be extremely variable in their clinical expression. There are essentially four phenotypes, two female and two male. At either end of this spectrum there is no genital ambiguity. In complete testicular feminization the phenotype is entirely female. Also, the adult male with infertility has no ambiguity. It is the two middle groups, incomplete testicular feminization and so-called Reifenstein syndrome, which present as paediatric problems. These patients have partial androgen insensitivity and provide perhaps the most difficult management problem in all disorders of sexual differentiation.

At puberty after many urological procedures, a reasonable cosmetic result can be achieved. However, the phallus always remains small, being resistant both to endogenous and exogenous androgens. In addition, there is often pubertal gynaecomastia due to a combination of androgen resistance and excess oestrogen secretion by the testes.

ABNORMAL GONADAL DIFFERENTIATION (Table 4)

The final aetiological category includes patients with abnormal differentiation of the testes resulting in deficient secretion of both testosterone and anti-müllerian hormone during fetal life[6]. In mixed gonadal dysgenesis there is usually a testis on one side and a streak gonad on the other. Most patients are raised as female but may have short stature.

Table 4 Abnormal gonadal differentiation causing ambiguous external genitalia

Mixed gonadal dysgenesis (XO/XY mosaicism)
True hermaphroditism (60% 46 XX)
Syndrome of rudimentary testes
Dysmorphic syndromes associated with hypogonadism
XX male

I would like to describe the approach in terms of clinical assessment and investigation of the infant who is born with genital ambiguity.

CLINICAL ASSESSMENT (Table 5)

Many disorders of sexual differentiation are genetically determined and a careful family history may therefore be helpful. In addition, examination of the baby for features such as widely spaced nipples indicating possible XO cell line is also important. Examination of the external genitalia, however, is likely to provide the most helpful clues to the possible aetiology, and the patients are divided into those with no palpable gonads, those with one palpable gonad and those with two palpable gonads. Despite this over-simplification, a patient with no palpable gonads is likely to be a female pseudohermaphrodite and therefore to have the 21-hydroxylase form of congenital adrenal hyperplasia. The patient with either one or asymmetrical gonads is likely to have abnormal gonadal differentiation due either to mixed gonadal dysgenesis or to true hermaphroditism, and the patient with two palpable gonads is likely to be a male pseudohermaphrodite who has either a receptor defect, 5α-reductase deficiency, or impaired testosterone synthesis.

The possibility of true hermaphroditism with bilateral ovotestes should also be considered.

Table 5   Infant with ambiguous genitalia

Clinical assessment
Family history, general examination for dysmorphic features

Examination of external genitalia
(1) No gonads
        female pseudohermaphrodite CAH (21-OH def.)
        (male pseudohermaphrodite)
(2) One gonad
        abnormal gonadal differentiation
           mixed gonadal dysgenesis (XO/XY)
           true hermaphroditism
(3) Two gonads
        male pseudohermaphrodite receptor defect
                          5α-reductase deficiency
                          impaired T synthesis
        true hermaphroditism

LABORATORY ASSESSMENT (Table 6)

The laboratory assessment can also be approached from the same standpoint and in each group a karyotype is mandatory. Plasma 17-hydroxy-progesterone or 11-deoxycortisol measurement should exclude congenital adrenal hyperplasia. The patient with asymmetrical gonadal development may need a gonadal biopsy to exclude the presence of ovarian tissue and possibly a laparotomy to define the intra-abdominal genital structures. In the patient with two gonads, i.e. the probable male pseudohermaphrodite, an HCG test[5] to stimulate androgen secretion should distinguish between the three aetiological categories. There are many regimens and 1000 units daily for 3 days is one that is effective and of which we have experience. Plasma concentrations of testosterone, dihydrotestosterone, dehydroepiandrosterone and androstenedione should be measured basally and 24 hours after the third injection.

Table 6   Infant with ambiguous genitalia

Laboratory assessment
(1) No gonads
        karyotype, plasma 17 OH-progesterone, 11-deoxycortisol
(2) One gonad
        karyotype, HCG test, gonadal biopsy laparotomy
(3) Two gonads
        karyotype, HCG test (HCG 1000 U daily × 3), plasma T,
           DHT, DHEA, Δ_4 A on days 0 and 3
        in vitro androgen-binding studies
        sinogram

In vitro androgen-binding studies may provide information about quantitative or qualitative defects of the androgen receptor. These studies are now becoming highly sophisticated and cannot be described in detail. Finally, a sinogram is important to exclude a vaginal remnant.

In conclusion, I have emphasized the importance of defining the primary biochemical defect in patients with ambiguous genitalia. It is also right, however, to admit that, in terms of management, endocrinology has, with the notable exception of congenital adrenal hyperplasia, a relatively limited role in the management of these disorders at the present time. It is only, however, by the detailed investigation of these patients that our knowledge of this complex field can grow and this must ultimately be to the benefit of future patients with genital ambiguity.

References

1. Jost, A. (1953). Problems of foetal endocrinology: the gonadal and hypophyseal hormones. *Recent Prog. Horm. Res.*, **VIII**, 379–421
2. Josso, N., Picard, J. Y. and Tran, D. (1977). The antimüllerian hormone. *Recent Prog. Horm. Res.*, **33**, 117–60
3. Imperato-McGinley, J. and Peterson, R. E. (1976). Male pseudohermaphroditism: the complexities of male phenotype development. *Am. J. Med.*, **61**, 251–72
4. Peterson, R. E., Imperato-McGinley, J., Gautier, T. and Sturla, E. (1977). Male pseudohermaphroditism due to steroid 5x-reductase deficiency. *Am. J. Med.*, **62**, 170–91
5. Griffin, J. E. and Wilson, J. D. (1980). The syndromes of androgen resistance. *N. Engl. J. Med.*, **302**, 198–209
6. Savage, M. O. (1982). Ambiguous genitalia, small genitalia and undescended testes. In *Clinics in Endocrinology and Metabolism*. Vol. II (1), pp. 127–58. (Philadelphia: W. B. Saunders)
7. Grant, D. B. and Savage, M. O. (1981). Clinical aspects of intersex. In Brook, C. G. D. (ed.) *Clinical Paediatric Endocrinology*. pp. 40–60. (Oxford: Blackwell Scientific Publications)
8. Grant, D. B., Laurance, B. M., Atherden, S. M. and Ryness, J. (1976). HCG stimulation test in children with abnormal sexual development. *Arch. Dis. Child.*, **51**, 596–601

References

6

MEDICAL AND PSYCHO-LOGICAL MANAGEMENT OF CONGENITAL ADRENAL HYPERPLASIA

I. A. HUGHES

INTRODUCTION

Congenital adrenal hyperplasia (CAH) or the adrenogenital syndrome is an autosomal recessive disorder of cortisol biosynthesis[1]. A certain knowledge of the pathways of adrenal steroid biosynthesis is required to interpret the clinical and biochemical features of CAH due to various enzyme deficiencies. These pathways, together with the enzymes involved, are shown schematically in Figure 1. More than 90% of cases are due to 21-hydroxylase deficiency. Consequently, the review will emphasize this variant of CAH, while other much rarer enzyme deficiencies will only be mentioned briefly. Table 1 summarizes the main clinical features of CAH in relation to the specific enzyme defect. Much of the clinical and biochemical data to be described has been obtained through management of 25 children with CAH currently attending the Paediatric Endocrine Clinic of the University Hospital of Wales.

Pathophysiology

Whichever enzyme is absent, the net result is cortisol deficiency. The consequence of decreased cortisol synthesis due to 21-hydroxylase deficiency is shown in simple outline in Figure 2. The response, as in many endocrine disorders, is an increased trophic hormone secretion, in this case adrenocorticotrophin (ACTH). This leads to increased production of 17OH-progesterone (17OHP), the immediate precursor steroid of the

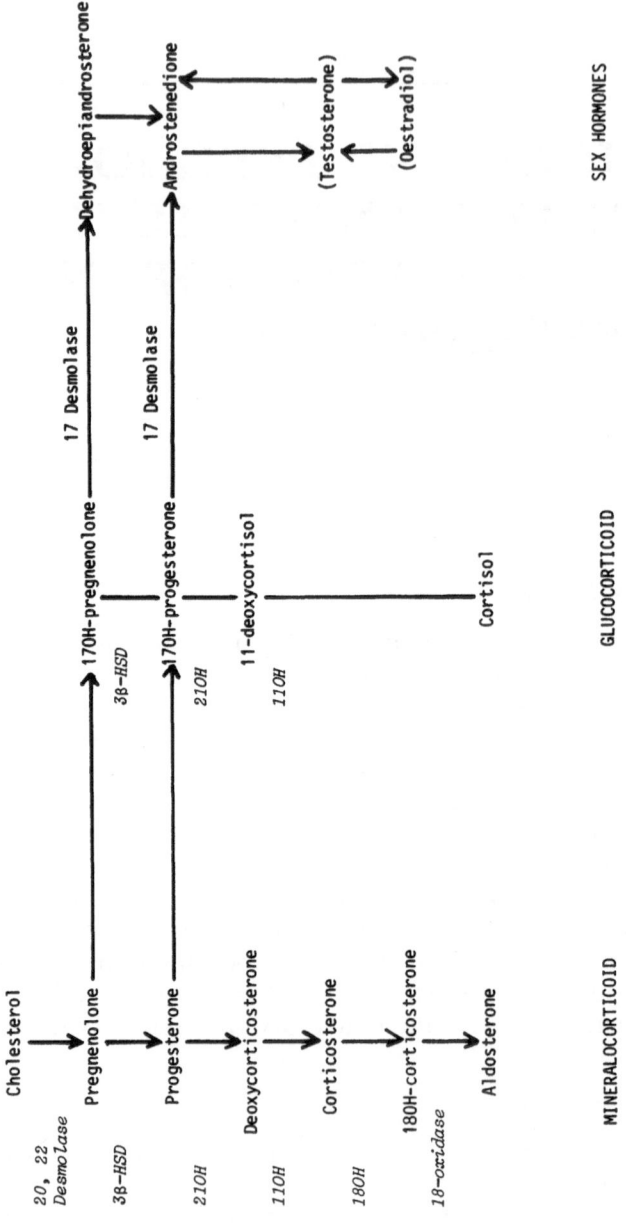

Figure 1 Scheme of adrenal steroid biosynthesis

enzyme block[2]. Following steroid side-chain cleavage, there is conversion to androstenedione, a weak androgen; this in turn is converted mainly in the liver to the potent androgen, testosterone[3]. Androgens produce the clinical hallmark of CAH—virilization.

Table 1 Summary of main clinical features of CAH according to type of enzyme defect

Enzyme defect	
20,22-Desmolase	Incomplete masculinization in male. Normal external genitalia in female. Severe salt-wasting. Rarely survive
3β-Hydroxysteroid dehydrogenase	Inadequate masculinization in male and mildly virilized external genitalia in female. Severe salt-wasting
17α-Hydroxylase	Usually presents with delayed sexual development in both sexes. Hypertension. Hypokalaemic alkalosis
21-Hydroxylase	Virilization of external genitalia in female, of varying severity. Genitalia usually normal in male at birth. Salt-wasting in 50% of cases. Occasional hypoglycaemia. Pseudoprecocious puberty in non-salt-losing males. Late onset cases can present as delayed menarche, hirsutism, infertility
11β-Hydroxylase	Virilization of external genitalia in female. Hypertension, but onset may be delayed. Late-onset cases as in 21-hydroxylase deficiency

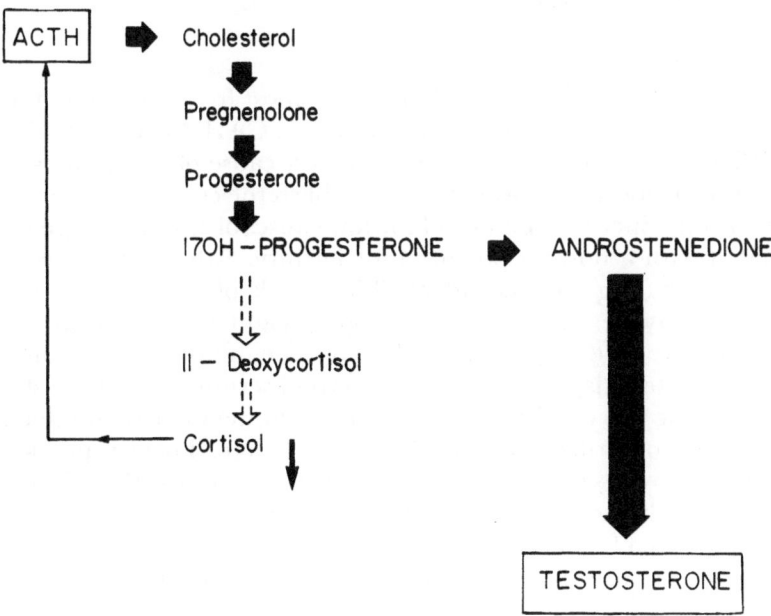

Figure 2 Consequences of 21-hydroxylase deficiency. Androstenedione conversion to testosterone is mainly extra-adrenal

Since 21-hydroxylation is also required for aldosterone biosynthesis, salt-wasting is an additional feature of CAH. Recent studies indicate that two-thirds of cases are salt-losers[4]. The explanation for the difference between the two types continues to be a subject of debate[5,6]. Recent studies by New et al.[6] postulate that in salt-losers, 21-hydroxylation is defective in both the zona fasciculata and glomerulosa, whereas in the non-salt-losers the defect is confined only to the zona fasciculata. The accumulation of steroid precursors such as 17OHP, progesterone and 16OH-progesterone in the plasma also contributes to salt-loss, since these act as natiuretic hormones by competitive inhibition of aldosterone binding to its receptor in the renal tubule[7].

Salt-loss does not usually occur in CAH due to 11β-hydroxylase deficiency because of increased secretion of deoxycorticosterone, a potent mineralocorticoid (see Figure 1). This leads to hypertension, characteristic of 11β-hydroxylase deficiency; the onset, however, may be delayed by several years. In a large group of cases, all with documented 11β-hydroxylase deficiency, recently described by Zachmann et al.[8], two infants developed salt-wasting in the neonatal period. Both patients excreted large quantities of urinary tetrahydrodeoxycorticosterone; no explanation could be found for the salt-loss.

DIAGNOSIS OF CAH

Clinical

Ambiguous genitalia of the newborn is the most frequent presentation. This has been discussed in detail in Chapter 5. CAH due to 21-hydroxylase deficiency in a female is the commonest cause of ambiguous genitalia of the newborn. It is essential to establish the correct diagnosis and sex of rearing, since CAH is one of the few causes of ambiguous genitalia associated with a normal potential for fertility. Salt-losing crises typically occur during the second or third week of life, but an earlier indication may be static or falling body weight despite an adequate sodium intake. The diagnosis in affected male infants can be confused with pyloric stenosis, although the pattern of serum electrolytes should distinguish the two conditions. The non-salt-losing male infant does not develop signs of virilization until 2–4 years of age. There is penile and pubic hair growth, but normal prepubertal size testes. Rapid somatic growth and advanced skeletal maturation are accompanying features. Even an affected female may only develop signs of mild clitoromegaly, labial fusion or pubic hair growth in later childhood. The reason for this late onset is unclear.

21-Hydroxylase deficiency occurring in the postpubertal age group is increasingly recognized as the underlying cause for hirsutism, mild degrees of virilization, oligo- or primary amenorrhoea and both male and female infertility[9-13]. Increased awareness of the condition has resulted from the development of sensitive and specific immunoassays for steroids, and their application in dynamic studies of adrenal function. The demonstration of a close genetic linkage between the HLA-B and 21-hydroxylase loci has also led to the detection of cases hitherto unrecognized[14].

Biochemical

The diagnosis is confirmed using one or more of the investigations listed in Table 2. Traditionally, the 24-hour urinary excretion of 17-oxo-steroids and pregnanetriol is measured. The results are not reliable because of the changing pattern in urinary steroid excretion characteristic of early neonatal life[15,16]. Furthermore, an accurate 24-hour urine collection is seldom achieved from an infant; only a random urine sample is needed to determine the 11-oxygenation index[17]. Measurement of plasma 17OHP concentration is currently the most reliable test for 21-hydroxylase deficiency. Concentrations are markedly elevated in untreated infants[18-20]. Levels in normal infants can be elevated within hours of birth due to placental production of 17OHP[21,22], but mean concentrations fall to below 10 nmol/l by 36 hours of age (Figure 3). Data illustrated in Figure 4 indicate that concentrations of 17OH-progesterone may also be elevated in preterm ill infants without adrenal disease[23], although the concentrations seldom reach levels observed in untreated CAH infants.

Table 2   Diagnostic tests in CAH due to 21-hydroxylase deficiency

Urinary
    17-oxosteroids
    pregnanetriol
    11-oxygenation index
    electrolytes

Plasma
    electrolytes
    17OH-progesterone
    androgens
    plasma renin activity
    ACTH

The concentrations of androgens—androstenedione, dehydroepiandrosterone sulphate and testosterone[24,25]—are also elevated in untreated CAH, due to both 21- and 11β-hydroxylase deficiencies. Specific confirmation of 11β-hydroxylase deficiency requires measurements of

11-deoxycortisol in plasma[26] and the 24-hour urinary excretion of tetra-hydro-11-deoxycortisol (THS) and its 6-hydroxylated metabolite, 6α-THS which appears to be excreted in large quantities in the urine of affected infants[27]. Measurement of plasma ACTH concentration is of no value in specifying the precise enzyme defect, and may occasionally be normal in untreated infants[28]. Other steroid concentrations shown to be elevated in untreated 21-hydroxylase deficiency include progesterone[29], 17OH-pregnenolone[30] and 21-deoxycortisol[31].

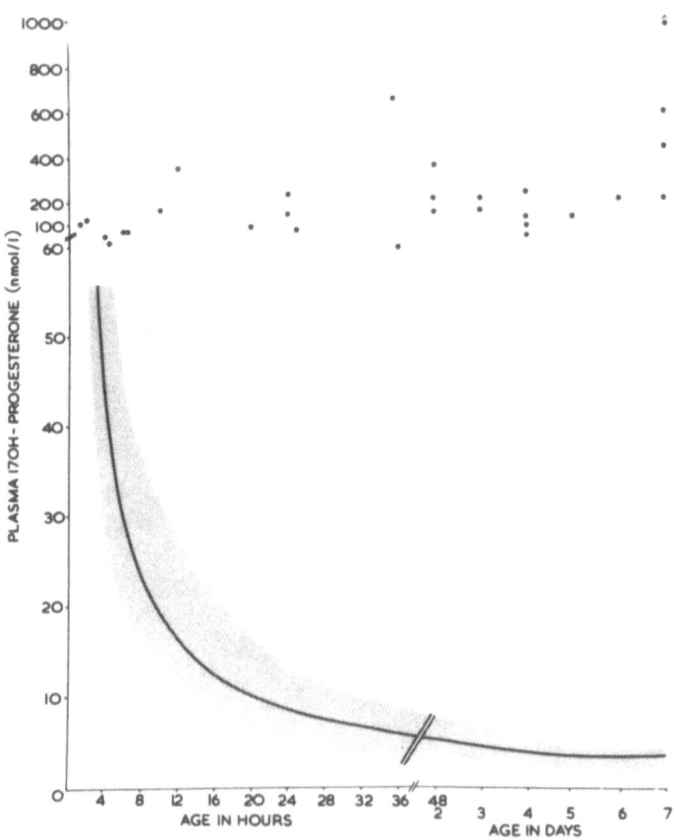

Figure 3 Plasma 17OH-progesterone concentrations in normal term and CAH (●) infants during the first 7 days of life. The line represents the mean and the shaded area encompasses the range in normal infants. Reproduced with permission of the editor of *Archives of Disease in Childhood*

Salt-losing infants typically have hyponatraemia, hyperkalaemia, azotaemia and early metabolic acidosis. Hypoglycaemia occurs occasionally. Plasma renin activity is markedly elevated in response to the hyponatraemia and decreased extracellular fluid volume[32, 33].

MEDICAL MANAGEMENT

Early

Intravenous saline is required initially for the infant who has a salt-losing crisis. This is given as normal saline, the amount calculated based on the sodium deficit and the degree of dehydration. Dextrose (5%) should also be infused because of the risk of hypoglycaemia. Unless there is peripheral circulatory collapse, glucocorticoids can be withheld until blood samples for steroid analyses have been collected. Initially, mineralocorticoid therapy is given as deoxycorticosterone acetate (DOCA), 1–2 mg every 12 hours by intramuscular injection. However, this preparation is no longer widely available in the UK. If necessary, an intravenous infusion of aldosterone, 500 μg every 4–6 hours, can be substituted, although this is seldom necessary. Deoxycortone glucoside (Percorten) is another mineralocorticoid preparation, available as a

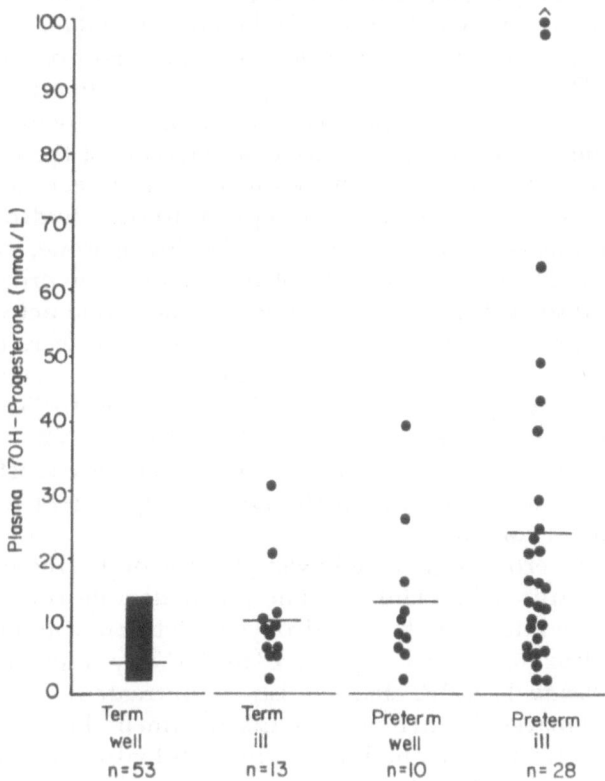

Figure 4 Plasma 17OH-progesterone concentrations in term and preterm infants in relation to illness. The data represent the mean and range of values in each group of infants. Repeat blood samples were collected from some infants; 'n' refers to the number of 17OHP measurements in each group. (Reproduced with permission of the Editor of *Archives of Diseases in Childhood*)

water-soluble injection in a concentration of 50 mg per 5 ml. Once the infant is rehydrated and the sodium deficit has been partially corrected, oral mineralocorticoid therapy using 9α-fludrocortisone (Florinef) can be started. The usual dose is 0.1–0.2 mg daily, but occasionally higher doses are required. The blood pressure must be monitored regularly. Supplementation of oral feeds with 2–3 g of salt daily in divided doses is sometimes necessary until semi-solid feeding is established. The rare patient in whom there is a problem with treatment compliance can be given a long-acting mineralocorticoid, deoxycorticosterone pivalate (DOCP) 25 mg each month by intramuscular injection. The earlier practice of using subcutaneous implants of DOCA pellets (125 mg) which provided mineralocorticoid replacement for about 6 months has now been largely discontinued.

Glucocorticoid replacement therapy is required to suppress increased ACTH secretion, even though there is evidence of endogenous cortisol secretion (Hughes, personal observation). Only a *replacement* dose is required from initiation of therapy and should be based on surface area. It is unnecessary to start with a large glucocorticoid dose to suppress increased ACTH secretion, followed by a reduction to a maintenance dose later in infancy. This protocol invariably produces some suppression of the rapid growth velocity characteristic of the first year of life. Consequently, based on the known cortisol secretion rate of 12 ± 3 mg/m²/day[34], the author's practice is to start hydrocortisone, 20–25 mg/m²/day, in three divided doses. Hydrocortisone, rather than cortisone, is used because about 50% of an oral dose of hydrocortisone is consistently absorbed, it is the physiological hormone active in man (cortisone is metabolically inactive) and the cortisol secretion rate is standardized for surface area. The average surface area of a newborn infant is 0.25 m². A replacement hydrocortisone dose of 20–25 mg/m²/day amounts to about 5 mg per day given in divided doses as 2, 1 and 2 mg. There is also a significant glucocorticoid effect from the use of 9α-fludrocortisone in salt-losers; 0.1 mg of the latter is equivalent to approximately 1.5 mg of cortisol.

The plasma steroid response following the use of this regime in early infancy is illustrated in Figure 5. The mean starting dose of hydrocortisone in five infants with 21-hydroxylase deficiency and one infant with 11β-hydroxylase deficiency was 23 mg/m²/day. Elevated concentrations of plasma 17OHP, characteristic of untreated 21-hydroxylase deficiency, fell markedly after only 2 weeks' treatment. Plasma 11-deoxycortisol concentrations in the infant with 11β-hydroxylase deficiency decreased from more than 2000 nmol/l to 240 nmol/l within 2 months of starting treatment. Twelve months (in three infants) and 18 months (in two infants) after initiating therapy, concentrations of plasma 17OHP remained adequately suppressed; the mean hydrocortisone dose was 18.0 and 16.0 mg/m²/day, respectively. The infant with 11β-hydroxylase

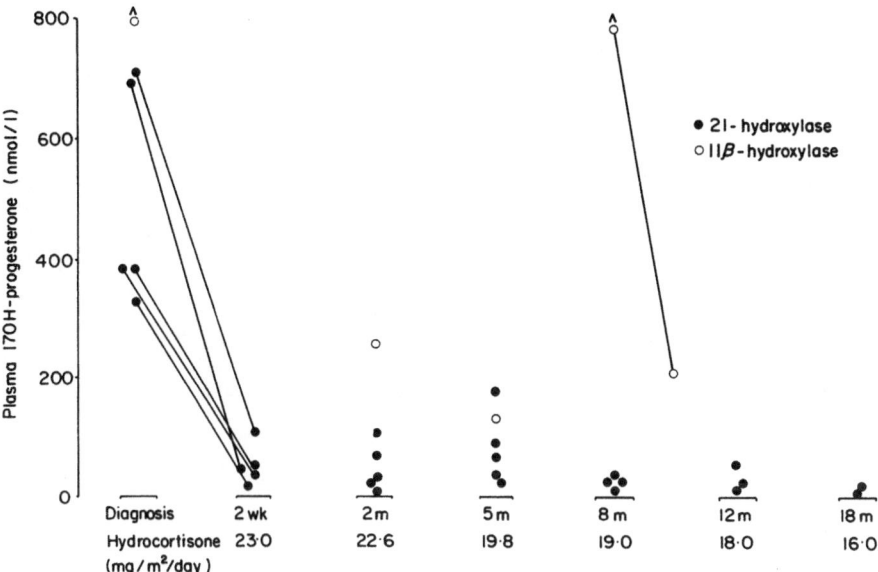

Figure 5 Plasma 17OH-progesterone concentrations (●) before and after starting hydrocortisone treatment in five infants with 21-hydroxylase deficiency. Also shown are values for plasma 11-deoxycortisol (○) in an infant with 11β-hydroxylase deficiency. Ô indicates values greater than 2000 nmol/l

deficiency again showed an elevated plasma concentration of 11-deoxy-cortisol 8 months after the start of treatment. This was the result of poor treatment compliance. However, within 2 months of re-instituting appropriate glucocorticoid replacement, the plasma 11-deoxycortisol concentration had decreased markedly. Figure 6 shows the course of concomitant plasma 17OHP and testosterone concentrations in two male infants with 21-hydroxylase deficiency following hydrocortisone therapy. Plasma levels of both steroids initially fell rapidly, but while 17OHP levels continued to decrease, there was a transient rise in plasma testosterone concentrations at about 3 months of age. This coincided with the surge in plasma testosterone concentration observed in normal male infants at this age caused by increased gonadotrophin secretion and Leydig cell testosterone production[35,36]. By 3–4 months of age, plasma testosterone concentrations in the infants with CAH had decreased to prepubertal levels (less than 1 nmol/l), indicating adequate glucocorticoid replacement therapy. Although the purpose of a transient increase in pituitary–gonadal activity in the male infant is unknown, it is possible that abolishing this response with excessive glucocorticoid replacement in an infant with CAH may predispose to some pituitary–gonadal dysfunction in later life.

The most rapid period of growth in postnatal life occurs during the first year. The normal infant grows at the rate of approximately

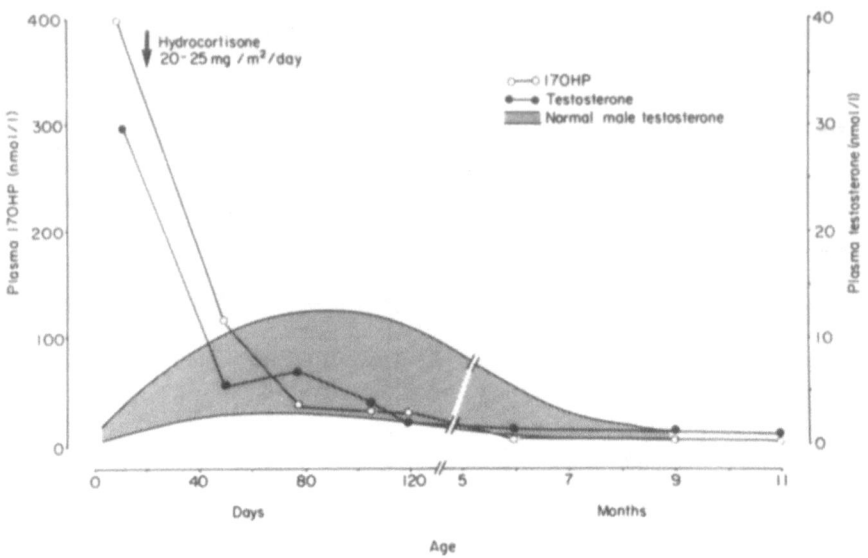

Figure 6 Plasma 17OH-progesterone (○) and testosterone (●) concentrations in two male infants with 21-hydroxylase deficiency before and after starting treatment with hydrocortisone. The shaded area represents the range of values for plasma testosterone in normal males during the first 9 months of age

24 cm/year during the first 6 months, and at 16–18 cm/year over the entire first postnatal year[37]. An analysis of growth velocity in the same five infants during the first 6 and 12 months' treatment with maintenance glucocorticoid therapy showed no suppression of linear growth (Figure 7). Two male infants had an increased growth velocity compared to normals; whether this adversely affects skeletal maturation is not possible to assess yet because of the inconsistencies in bone age determination at this age.

In summary, based on preliminary results in a small number of infants, the recommended treatment for an infant with CAH should be hydrocortisone given as a maintenance dose from the outset. This amounts to 20–25 mg/m²/day given in three divided doses. Salt-losers, in addition, should be given 0.1–0.2 mg 9α-fludrocortisone daily. The response to treatment can closely be monitored with serial measurements of plasma 17OHP and testosterone concentrations.

Longer-term management

The aim of long-term therapy in CAH is to ensure normal growth in infancy and childhood, development of puberty at the appropriate age, followed by the acquisition of adult reproductive potential. To attain this goal, it is necessary to strike a delicate balance between achieving adequate suppression of adrenal androgen secretion in order to prevent rapid growth and advanced skeletal maturation, but also ensure that normal linear growth is not suppressed with excessive glucocorticoid

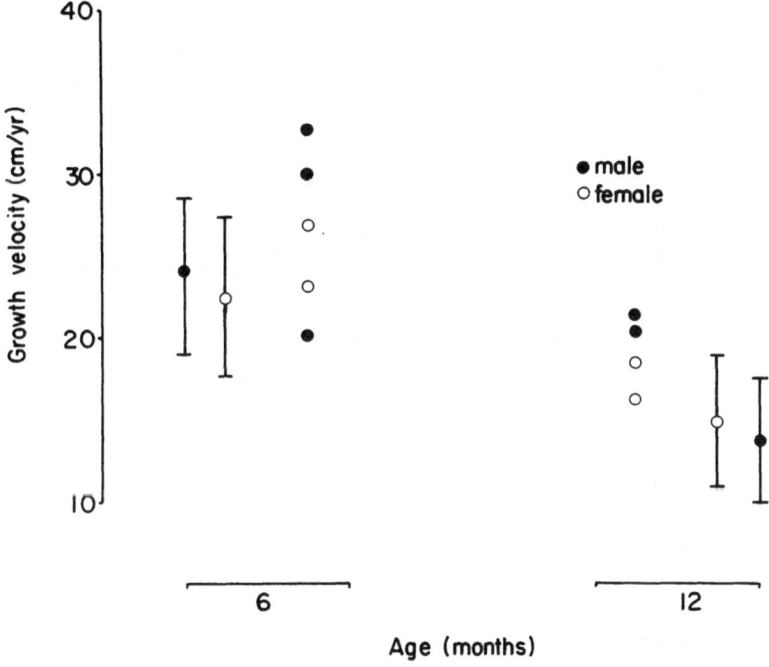

Figure 7   Growth velocity during the first 6 and 12 months of age in infants with CAH. The bar lines represent the mean ± 2 SD growth velocity in normal male (●) and female (○) infants, respectively, at each age

replacement. If this balance is not achieved, the outcome for adult height can be extremely poor (see Figure 8). The diagnosis in this girl with non-salt-losing CAH was delayed until 4 years of age. By that time, her height was on the 97th centile and skeletal age was advanced to 9.5 years. Treatment was started with prednisone in a dose sufficient to cause marked growth suppression in addition to inhibiting adrenal androgen secretion. At 9 years of age, she had a growth spurt coincident with the onset of puberty (skeletal age 12.0 years); at this time treatment was changed to hydrocortisone given in a maintenance dose. Although a further modest growth spurt was achieved, menarche occurred soon afterwards and subsequently linear growth ceased due to epiphyseal fusion. Final height was 4.3 SD below the mean adult height for females. The example illustrates the additive effect of advanced skeletal maturation (and hence a significant reduction in the number of 'growth years') and the potent growth-inhibiting action of excessive glucocorticoid therapy in causing a marked reduction in final height in patients with CAH.

In order to achieve normal growth and reproductive potential, treatment in CAH requires careful monitoring using both clinical and biochemical parameters. How this can be achieved is described separately for prepubertal and postpubertal patients.

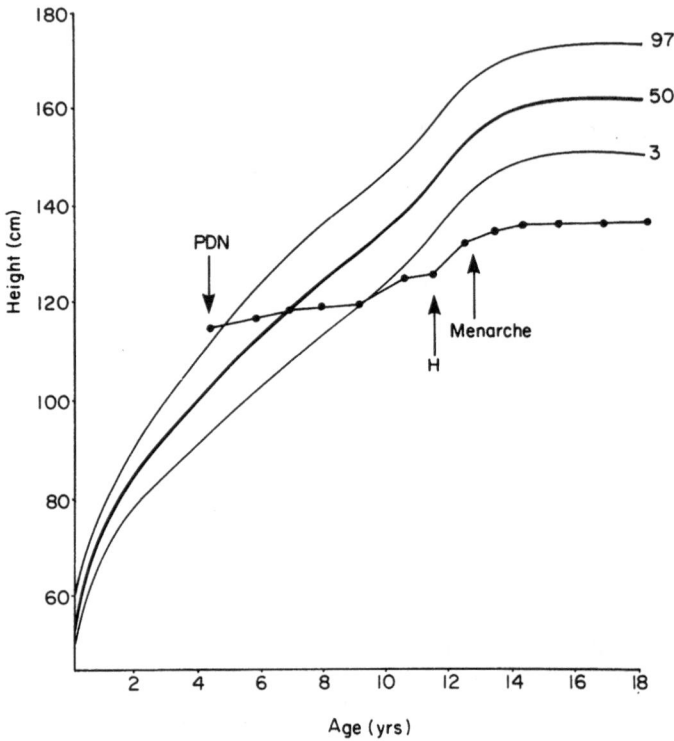

Figure 8   Longitudinal growth in a girl with late-treated CAH. PDN and H indicate treatment with prednisone and hydrocortisone, respectively

Prepubertal

The regimen of oral hydrocortisone given in three divided doses is continued throughout childhood. Whether the largest dose of hydrocortisone should be given in the morning or at night has not been satisfactorily resolved[38, 39]. The author normally gives 50% of the total daily dose at bedtime, and the remainder divided equally at 08.00 and 16.00 hours. Treatment can be monitored using serial measurements of plasma 17OHP and testosterone concentrations[24, 30]. A single estimation of the plasma 17OHP concentration is an unreliable index of therapeutic control[40]. The value can be influenced by factors such as diurnal rhythm, episodic secretion, time and dose of previous steroid medication, and the stress of venepuncture on plasma adrenal steroid concentrations[20].

However, because of the close correlation between plasma 17OHP and testosterone concentrations in treated CAH patients[24], simultaneous measurement of both these steroids at 09.00 hours before the morning hydrocortisone dose is taken, is a useful index of control[41]. The development of sensitive immunoassays for 17OHP in capillary blood collected on to filter paper[42,43] offers an attractive method to measure serial plasma 17OHP concentrations, particularly in treated infants.

The recent development of sensitive immunoassays to measure steroid concentrations in saliva[44] has obvious practical benefits to monitor treatment, particularly in children. Previous studies show that saliva 17OHP measurements accurately reflect levels of the steroid in plasma, over a wide range of concentrations[45]. Using frequent saliva sample collection performed by children at home, it has been possible to monitor 17OHP concentrations in relation to diurnal rhythm, different

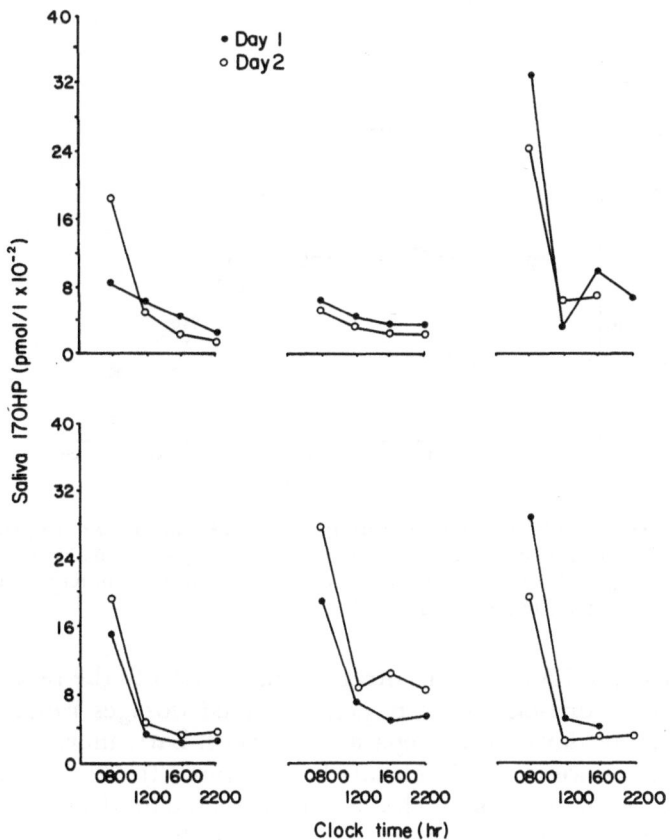

Figure 9 Two-day consecutive saliva 17OH-progesterone profiles determined at 2-monthly intervals over a 12-month period in a girl with treated CAH. Reproduced with permission of the editor of *Hormone Research*

95

glucocorticoid preparations and variable dose regimens of hydrocortisone[46]. The pronounced 17OHP diurnal rhythm present in CAH is illustrated in Figure 9. A 16-year-old patient, treated with a single daily dose of dexamethasone, collected weekend saliva samples on six separate occasions during a 1-year period. A normal 17OHP diurnal rhythm was maintained on this treatment, and the pattern was reproducible from day to day and from month to month. Figures 10 and 11 show 24-hour

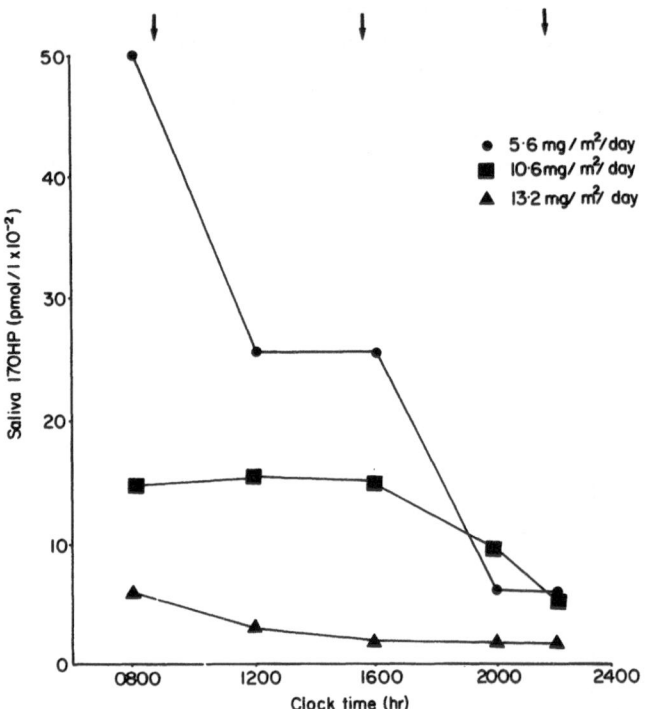

Figure 10   Saliva 17OH-progesterone profiles over a 24-hour period in a patient with CAH treated with three different dose regimens of hydrocortisone as indicated by the symbols (●, ■, ▲). The arrows indicate the times of administration. Reproduced with permission of the editor of *Hormone Research*

profiles of saliva 17OHP concentrations in relation to the replacement dose of hydrocortisone. One patient received dosages ranging from 5.6–13.2 mg/m²/day on three separate occasions. Early morning 17OHP concentrations were clearly elevated (5000 pmol/l) during treatment with the lowest dose, although levels had decreased to within the normal range by the evening. A maintenance dose of only 13.2 mg/m²/day was sufficient to suppress 17OHP concentrations throughout most of the day in this particular patient; the optimal daily dose appeared to be 10.6 mg/m². In three different patients receiving varying doses of hydrocortisone and studied in the same manner (Figure 11), the optimal daily hydrocortisone dose appeared to be 9–10 mg/m²; there was some evidence of over-suppression when the dose exceeded 12 mg/m²/day. In prepubertal children with CAH, the maintenance dose of hydrocortisone can usually be reduced to 10–15 mg/m²/day. However, there is considerable individual variation in the effectiveness of a given maintenance dose in suppressing adrenal steroid secretion.

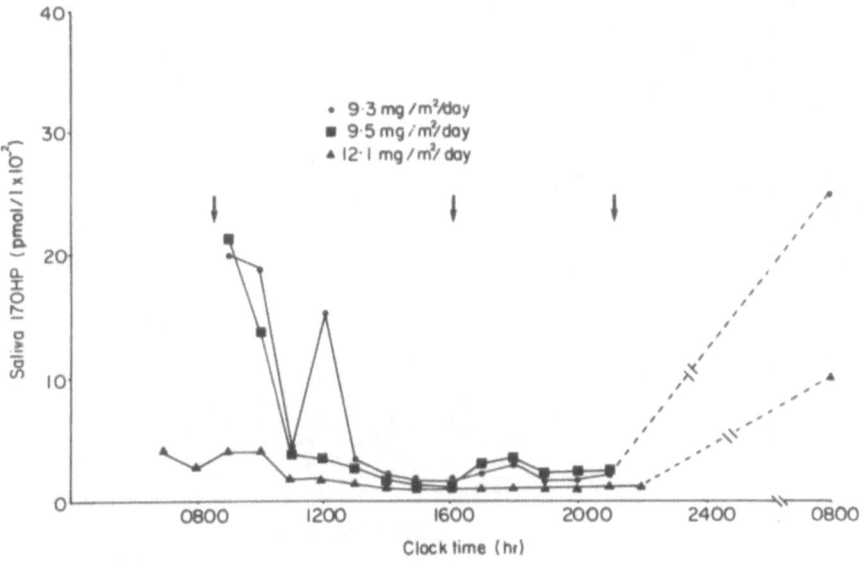

Figure 11   Saliva 17OH-progesterone profiles over a 24-hour period in three patients with CAH treated with different doses of hydrocortisone as indicated by the symbols (●, ■, ▲). Reproduced with permission of the editor of *Hormone Research*

The half-life of hydrocortisone is only 80–100 minutes. Thus, for maintenance therapy it needs to be administered daily in three divided doses. As the bedtime dose is rarely given later than 22.00 hours in prepubertal children, at least 10 hours elapse before the next dose of hydrocortisone is due. Early morning 17OHP concentrations, therefore, are invariably elevated (see Figures 10 and 11). Longer-acting glucocorticoid preparations will suppress adrenal steroid secretion throughout the 24-hour period, but they also produced significant growth retardation[47,48]. Figure 12 illustrates the effect of substituting prednisolone (in equivalent dosage) for the bedtime hydrocortisone dose in two prepubertal patients with CAH. Comparison of the daily saliva 17OHP profiles before and 2 weeks after the change in therapy showed a marked reduction in early morning concentrations of 17OHP, although a diurnal rhythm had been maintained. Other workers have shown that adequate adrenal suppression can be obtained by using prednisone administered twice daily in dosages as low as 4.2 mg/m^2/day[49,50]. The value of serial saliva 17OHP measurements in monitoring treatment in CAH is summarized in Figure 13. Weekend saliva 17OHP profiles in patients treated with hydrocortisone were analysed in relation to the degree of therapeutic control based on clinical criteria. Typical profiles of the three categories of control, i.e. under-, adequately- and over-treated, could be derived, as shown in Table 3.

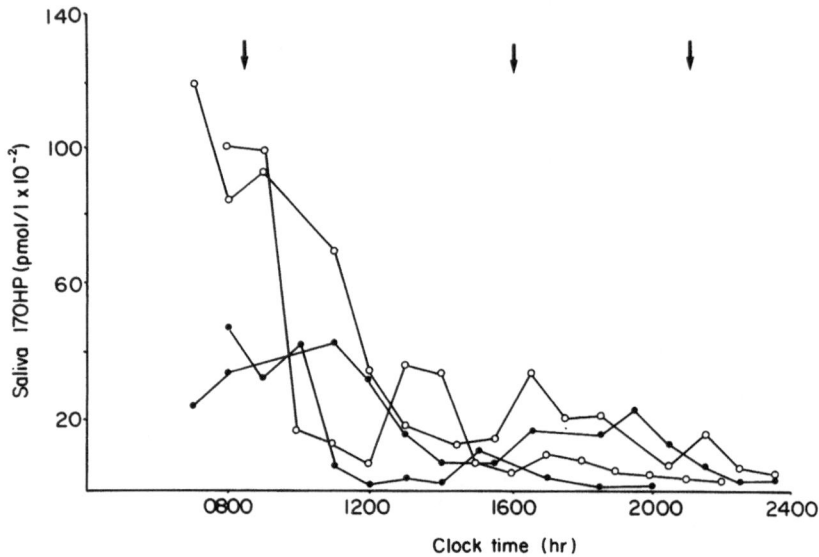

Figure 12 Saliva 17OH-progesterone profiles over a 24-hour period in two pre-pubertal patients with CAH during treatment with hydrocortisone alone (O———O) and after treatment with hydrocortisone and prednisolone at night (●———●). Reproduced with permission of the editor of *Hormone Research*

Salt-losing patients appear to become less dependent on mineralo-corticoid therapy in later childhood. Until recently, it was recommended that mineralocorticoid replacement could be discontinued by

Table 3 Typical saliva 17OHP profiles in relation to degree of control in CAH

| Time | Saliva 17OHP (pmol/l) | | |
	Under-treated	Adequately-treated	Over-treated
08.00	6000	1500	500
12.00	4000	1000	<150
16.00	2500	600	<150
22.00	2000	400	<150

about 4 years of age[51]. However, with the use of assays for plasma renin activity (PRA) as an index of salt-repletion, it has been recognized that salt-losers do not 'grow out' of the need for mineralocorticoid replacement[52,53]. Increased dietary salt-intake is the main compensatory mechanism, but such patients are liable to develop a salt-losing crisis if the

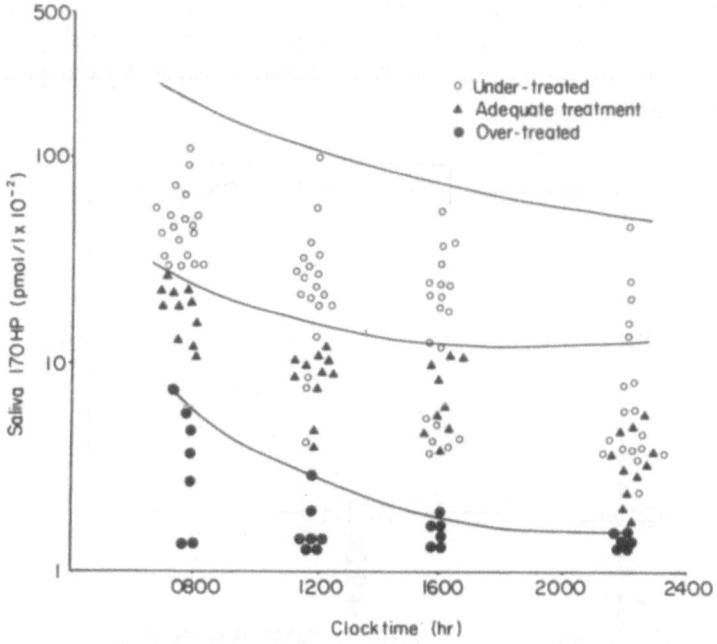

Figure 13 Two-day consecutive saliva 17OH-progesterone profiles in a group of prepubertal patients with CAH treated with hydrocortisone in three divided doses. The results are classified according to the degree of therapeutic control as defined by clinical criteria. Saliva 17OHP concentrations are plotted on a logarithmic scale. Reproduced with permission of the editor of *Hormone Research*

salt intake is curtailed[53]. Plasma 17OHP concentrations (or urinary pregnanetriol and 17-oxosteroid excretion) are increased, suggesting inadequate glucocorticoid replacement therapy. The postulated mechanism is schematically represented in Figure 14. Salt-depletion (unrecognized other than by elevated PRA) acts as a stress-mediated stimulus for increased ACTH-dependent adrenal precursor steroid secretion. These steroids are also natiuretic. Glucocorticoid replacement is increased inappropriately, rather than instituting mineralocorticoid therapy to promote salt-repletion. There is evidence that increased activity of the renin–angiotensin system has a direct stimulatory effect on ACTH secretion[54], although angiotensin II infused in a surgically castrate XX adult patient with CAH failed to increase plasma ACTH concentrations[55]. In a recent study, reinstituting fludrocortisone therapy reduced PRA to normal, caused a significant reduction in glucocorticoid requirements, which in turn led to improved linear growth[56]. Even patients with no clinical evidence of salt-wasting may show elevated PRA[57]; they should also be given sufficient mineralocorticoid replacement to reduce PRA to normal. The adequacy of mineralocorticoid replacement is monitored by serial measurements of PRA. Biochemical parameters of control complement information obtained using clinical criteria of control, such as signs of hypercortisolism, skeletal maturation and linear growth.

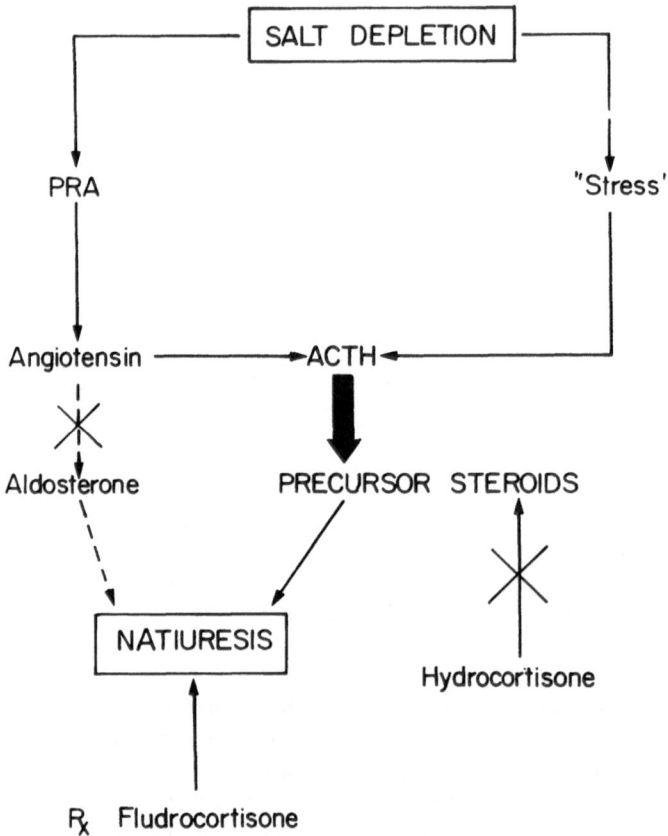

Figure 14 Renin–angiotensin system in CAH and its effect on plasma steroid levels in salt-depleted patients

Growth in CAH—prepubertal

Long-term follow-up in treated patients shows that final adult height in both males and females is significantly lower than expected when compared with the normal population[58,59]. Most studies refer to patients whose treatment was monitored before sensitive immunoassays for steroids in blood (and recently in saliva) became available. The data shown in Figure 15 indicate that there is a close correlation between serial plasma 17OHP measurements and height velocity expressed as a

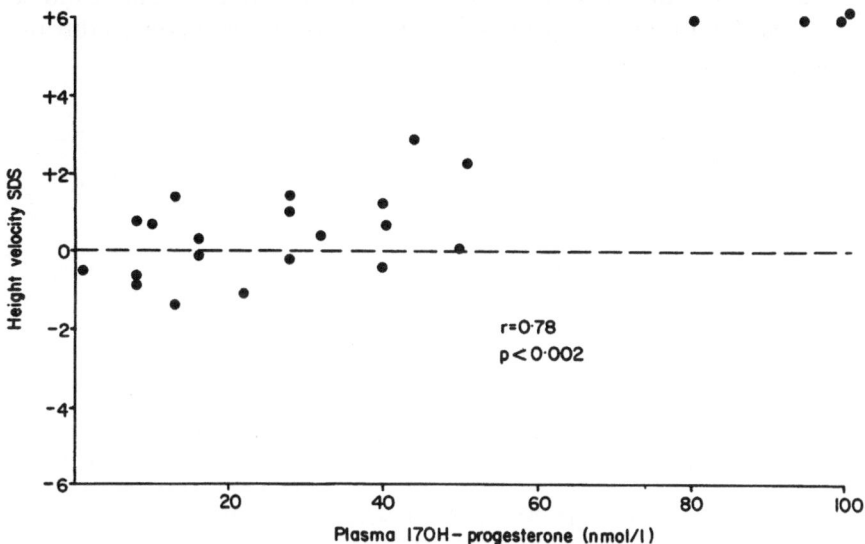

Figure 15 Relationship between height velocity and serial plasma 17OH-progesterone concentrations in treated prepubertal CAH patients. Velocity scores for chronological age were calculated from height velocities based on standing height measurements performed at 6-month intervals. The mean concentration of 17OHP during each 6-month period was used to analyse the correlation. Reproduced with permission of the editor of *Hormone Research*

standard deviation score. Similar results were obtained when growth was analysed in relation to serial plasma testosterone and saliva 17OHP measurements[41]. The growth curves in two children with 21-hydroxylase deficiency whose treatment has been monitored regularly, as previously discussed, are shown in Figure 16. Figure 17 summarizes the present height of all prepubertal patients (excluding infants less than 1 year of age previously described) who currently attend clinic. The data is expressed as a standard deviation score (SDS), where the normal for chronological or bone age is 0 ± 1 SD. Height is within normal limits for chronological age in all but two patients; when height is related to bone age, however, several patients are short due to advanced skeletal maturation. Ultimate adult height may be slightly reduced in some of these children.

Longer-term management (postpubertal)

Puberty should occur at the appropriate age in patients with CAH if treatment has been carefully monitored throughout infancy and childhood. When skeletal maturation is significantly advanced, puberty occurs early when androgen concentrations are adequately suppressed. Plasma testosterone concentrations in boys are no longer a reliable index of control, due to the increasing testicular testosterone secretion during puberty.

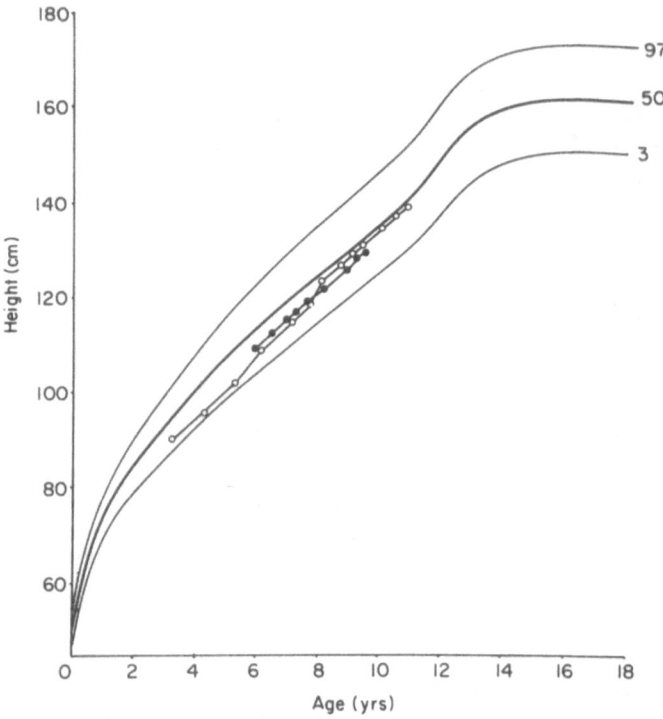

Figure 16 Longitudinal growth in two prepubertal children with CAH treated with hydrocortisone in three divided doses

Inadequately-treated girls with elevated plasma testosterone levels have delayed onset of menarche or later menstrual irregularities[58,60]. This may occur despite adequate daily hydrocortisone replacement. However, when therapy was changed to a longer-acting preparation such as dexamethasone given in equivalent dosage, plasma testosterone concentrations decreased to normal with the subsequent onset of menarche and regular menses[61,62]. Based on the dose of dexamethasone required to reduce plasma testosterone concentrations to normal, the potency ratio of dexamethasone to cortisol was approximately 80:1

rather than 30:1 usually quoted in standard texts[62, 63]. A single dose of dexamethasone, 0.25–0.75 mg/day will provide sufficient glucocorticoid replacement to maintain normal plasma 17OHP and testosterone concentrations throughout the day. A recent study in adult patients with CAH also concludes that dexamethasone, used in similar dosages, was better than either hydrocortisone or cortisone acetate in suppressing precursor steroid levels[64].

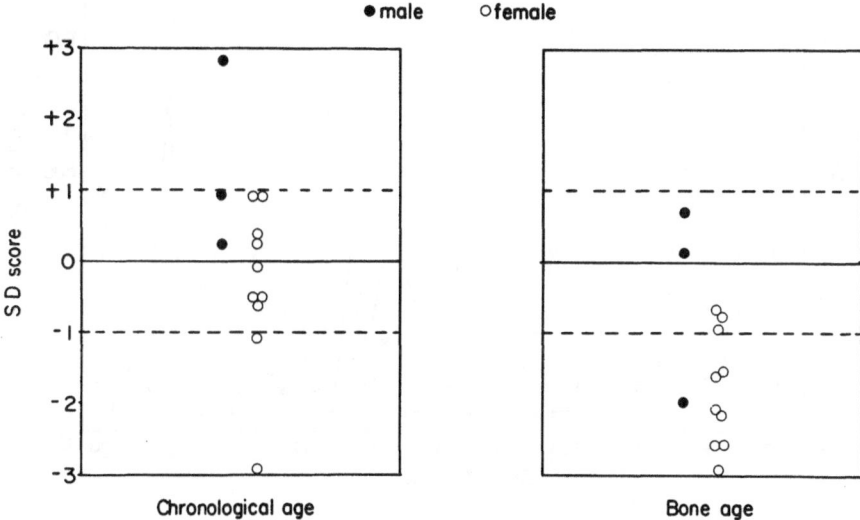

Figure 17 Height expressed as a standard deviation score (SDS) in relation to chronological and bone age in a group of prepubertal children with CAH. A mean ± 1 SD height SDS of 0 ± 1 represents the limits for normal children

Once menses are established, treatment in the female is directed towards the development and maintenance of regular ovulatory cycles. Approximately 50% of cycles in normal girls are anovulatory for up to 3 years after menarche[65, 66]. Saliva steroid measurements provide an extremely useful monitor of ovarian function in postmenarchal girls with CAH. Figures 18 and 19 show the patterns of saliva 17OHP and progesterone concentrations throughout the menstrual cycle before and after therapy was changed to dexamethasone in a female with CAH. Initially, plasma testosterone concentrations exceeded 5 nmol/l, vaginal bleeding was episodic and steroid profiles showed no consistent pattern. Following dexamethasone therapy, there was a consistent increase in 17OHP and progesterone concentrations during the second half of the cycle, indicating that this was probably ovulatory, even though basal body temperature was monophasic. Glucocorticoid replacement with daily dexamethasone appears to be a satisfactory treatment regimen in older children whose statural growth is almost complete. Normal reproductive potential can be ensured for the adult female who, in the long-term, is more likely to comply with a once-daily dose treatment regimen.

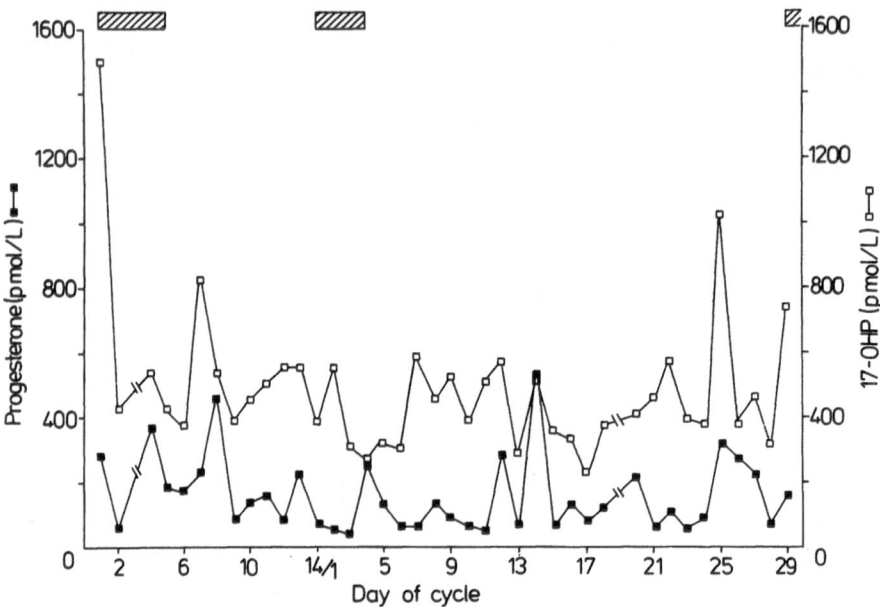

Figure 18 Daily saliva progesterone (●) and 17OH-progesterone (○) levels throughout a menstrual cycle in a postmenarchal female with poorly controlled CAH. Episodes of vaginal bleeding are indicated by the hatched areas. Reproduced with permission of the editor of *Hormone Research*

Long-term treatment for the adult male with CAH is less clear-cut. Salt-losers should continue glucocorticoid and mineralocorticoid for life. Non-salt-losers, however, appear to experience no ill effects when they stop glucocorticoid replacement. Studies of testicular size and spermatogenesis in adults who had stopped treatment or had not even started treatment have, in general, shown no abnormalities[59, 67]. Several of these patients have fathered children. However, in a recent case report[13], an untreated infertile male with small testes and oligospermia developed normal sized testes and sperm count on treatment and was subsequently fertile. Non-salt-losing adult males with CAH should be persuaded to continue regular maintenance glucocorticoid therapy long-term. Furthermore, an adrenocortical tumour developing in a 60-year-old woman with CAH who had never been treated has recently been reported[68]. Adequate long-term replacement therapy is essential for the patient with 11β-hydroxylase deficiency in order to prevent the development of irreversible hypertension, which can be malignant[8, 69].

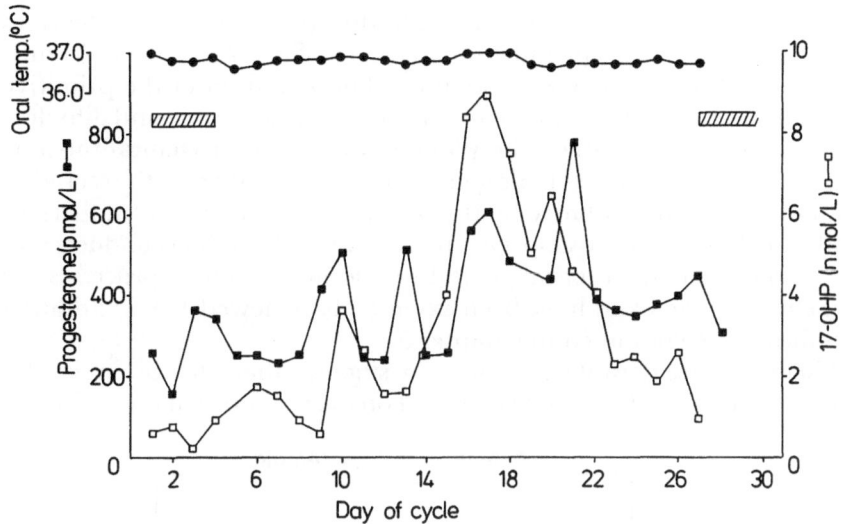

Figure 19 Daily saliva progesterone (●) and 17OH-progesterone (○) levels throughout a menstrual cycle in a postmenarchal female with CAH repeated after adequate therapeutic control was achieved. Also shown is the basal body temperature chart. Reproduced with permission of the editor of *Hormone Research*

As discussed previously, final adult height for both males and females is significantly lower than the mean adult height for the normal population. Analysis of the small number of patients in this clinic who had completed their growth gave similar results (Figure 20). There is a marked female predominance in this age group, probably reflecting the number of unexplained infant male deaths which occurred in previous years[70]. These analyses of adult stature reflect the results of treatment given to a generation of patients with CAH who were monitored by insensitive methods of steroid analyses. Hopefully, there will be an improvement in the outcome for adult stature and reproductive potential for those patients currently in their childhood years.

PSYCHOLOGICAL MANAGEMENT

A mother asks two pertinent questions after the birth of her baby. What is the sex? Is he/she all right? When the first question cannot be answered immediately, the effect on the parents can be devastating. To understand some of the psychological problems that may arise, both for the parents and later for the girl with CAH, it is necessary to briefly discuss some of the concepts of physiological and psychosexual differentiation in the human.

(1) *Physiological sexual differentiation.* This is inherently female. Male development requires the presence of 'inducers', active at critical times in organogenesis. This includes the presence of a cell-surface H-Y antigen, and a Y chromosome to organize differentiation of the primitive gonad into a testis; the subsequent synthesis of testosterone and dihydrotestosterone to differentiate the Wolffian ducts and urogenital tubercle into internal and external male genitalia, respectively; and the secretion of a non-steroidal substance by the sertoli cells of the testis (müllerian-inhibiting factor) to cause specific regression of the müllerian ducts and inhibition of female internal genital development. These processes are well characterized and have been extensively reviewed[71, 72], in addition to information contained in Chapter 5.

There is considerable evidence to suggest that the brain is also inherently female. This has been based on observations made in animal

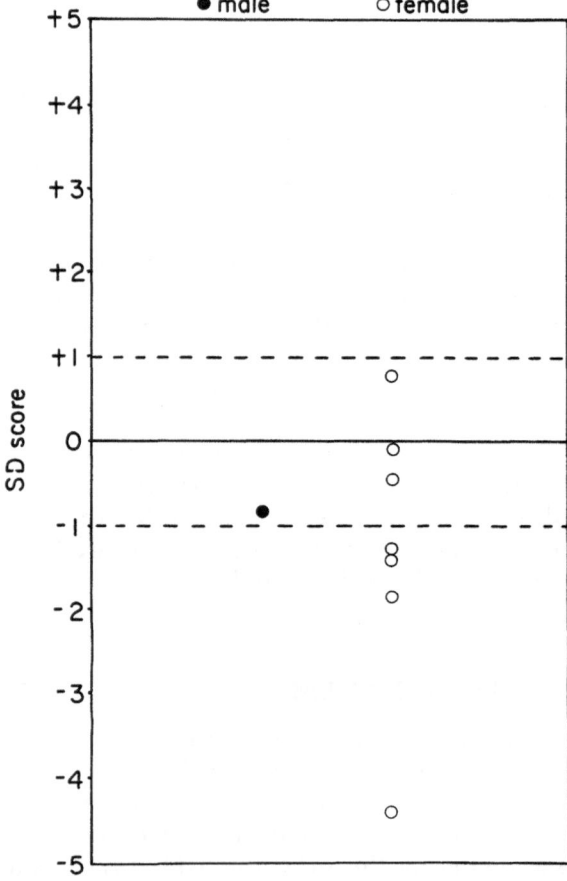

Figure 20   Adult height in patients with CAH expressed as a standard deviation score (SDS). A mean ± SD height SDS of 0 ± 1 represents the limits of normality

models, particularly the rat brain[73]. The same conclusion may not necessarily apply in the human. Masculinization of the male brain depends on testosterone being converted to oestradiol by aromatization. Differentiation of the female brain is also steroid-dependent; it is currently thought that sexual differentiation of the brain depends on the degree of exposure to gonadal steroids. This is controlled in the rat by binding of oestradiol to α-fetoprotein, whereas testosterone, which is not bound, enters neurons and by aromatization results in a high intra-neuronal concentration of oestradiol.

There are also sex differences in the structure of the central nervous system. The preoptic area of the rat brain contains an intensely staining region of increased neuronal density which is much larger in the male than in the female. This region has been termed the sexually dimorphic nucleus of the preoptic area[74]. Castration of the newborn male rat leads to a reduction, whereas androgens given to the female cause a significant increase in size of the nucleus. Clearly, sex steroids play an important role in sexual differentiation of the brain, at least in rodents and other laboratory animals.

(2) *Gender identity*. This refers to how an individual perceives self as being male, female, or even ambivalent. It is not determined by the nature of chromosomes, gonads or prenatal hormones. Gender identity is entirely dependent on the sex of assignment and subsequent rearing practice. This is derived through a process of learning which is usually firmly embedded in the child by 18 months–2 years of age. Gender identity has a profound influence when making decisions on sex re-assignment later than in the newborn period.

(3) *Gender role or sex-dimorphic behaviour*. This is defined as the actions, activities and behaviour of an individual which indicates to him/her and others the degree to which that person is male, female or ambivalent. In his extensive writings on the subject, Money has stated that gender role is the public expression of gender identity, whereas the latter is the private experience of gender role[75]. There is considerable data to suggest that gender role is at least influenced by the prenatal hormone environment.

(4) *Sexual orientation*. This can be considered as an extension of gender role and refers to the development in adulthood of erotic responsiveness to one sex or the other. The choice of sexual partner in addition to sexual fantasies and dreams may be heterosexual, homosexual or bisexual. There has been considerable debate concerning the influence of pre-natal hormones on the development of sexual orientation but, in general, it appears to be predominantly affected by the sex of rearing.

There are several disorders of sexual differentiation in the human which are suitable for the study of psychosexual behaviour. They include chromosomal abnormalities such as Klinefelter's and Turner's syndromes, anorchia, the androgen insensitivity syndromes, defects in androgen biosynthesis, including 5α-reductase deficiency, and variants of CAH. Recent papers have summarized the extensive literature written during the past 25 years about the influence of fetal androgens on psychosexual development in CAH[76,77]. Briefly, females with CAH exhibit a normal gender identity, i.e. conforming with the sex of rearing. This occurs, whatever the degree of virilization of the external genitalia, provided the infant has been assigned female before 2 years of age. If parents and doctors prevaricate about the assignment beyond this age, then the child may later be ambiguous in gender identity. The sex of rearing in a female infant born with ambiguous genitalia due to CAH should unquestionably be female, even though the degree of virilization may suggest otherwise.

There appears to be an effect of prenatal androgens on gender role or sex-dimorphic behaviour in females with CAH. When Ehrhardt et al.[78,79] compared a group of early-treated female CAH patients with both matched normal controls and unaffected siblings, there were significant differences in behaviour patterns. For example, girls with CAH showed a higher energy expenditure in play and sports and preferred boys to girls as playmates. They were less interested in dressing-up and playing with dolls, and were less inclined to display signs of parenting, such as playing with infants, play rehearsals for weddings and marriage and for being pregnant. The label of 'tomboy' was used both by themselves and by others. Male infants with CAH also showed greater energy expenditure in play and athletics compared with controls.

Data on sexual orientation is not so complete. Nevertheless, the information available indicated a heterosexual orientation in the majority of females with CAH, although some were bisexual; none were exclusively homosexual in their orientation. The evidence, so far, indicates that prenatal androgens affect only some aspects of gender role in the postnatal development of females with CAH.

Psychological management of the patient with CAH starts at birth when precise diagnosis must be established without delay (Figure 21). There is no place for making guesses of the infant's sex. The parents should be kept informed that the results of confirmatory tests will be available as soon as possible. Fortunately, a diagnosis of 21-hydroxylase deficiency, the commonest cause of ambiguous genitalia of the newborn, can now be confirmed within a few days of birth, based on plasma 17OHP determination and 48-hour lymphocyte culture to analyse the peripheral karyotype[80]. It should be emphasized to the parents that despite masculinized external genitalia, the internal genitalia (including ovaries) are female, and she will be able to have children. No doubt must be expressed in any way about the sex of rearing being female. The author has had the experience of trying to persuade the parents and extended family of a virilized Indian infant with 11β-hydroxylase deficiency that the appearance of the genitalia did not dictate that the

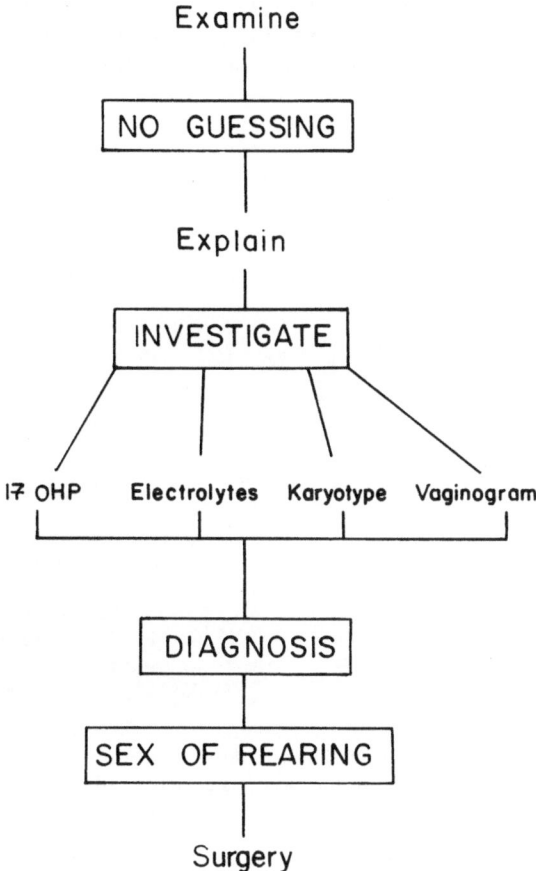

Figure 21 Plan of management at birth in the infant with ambiguous genitalia due to 21-hydroxylase deficiency

sex of rearing be male. They accepted the decision to rear as female more readily when shown radiographs from a perineal sinogram (Figure 22) which clearly demonstrated a uterine cavity. Parents must be discouraged from choosing a name appropriate for either sex, since this would reinforce any continuing doubts about the sex assignment.

Genital surgery should be performed early, between 6 and 12 months of age. This aspect is discussed fully in Chapter 7. The cosmetic result of surgery is an enormous relief to the parents. Until then, they are often social recluses, unwilling to have friends, relatives and baby-sitters care for the infant. In the early days, it is useful to show photographs taken of other infants before and after surgery to emphasize the normal-looking appearance of the genitalia following surgery. Further surgery is usually required at the time of puberty in order to enlarge the vaginal introitus, particularly if a vaginoplasty procedure was not performed in infancy. It must be appreciated that further surgery on the genital area at this time coincides with heightened sexual awareness and erotosexual behaviour[76].

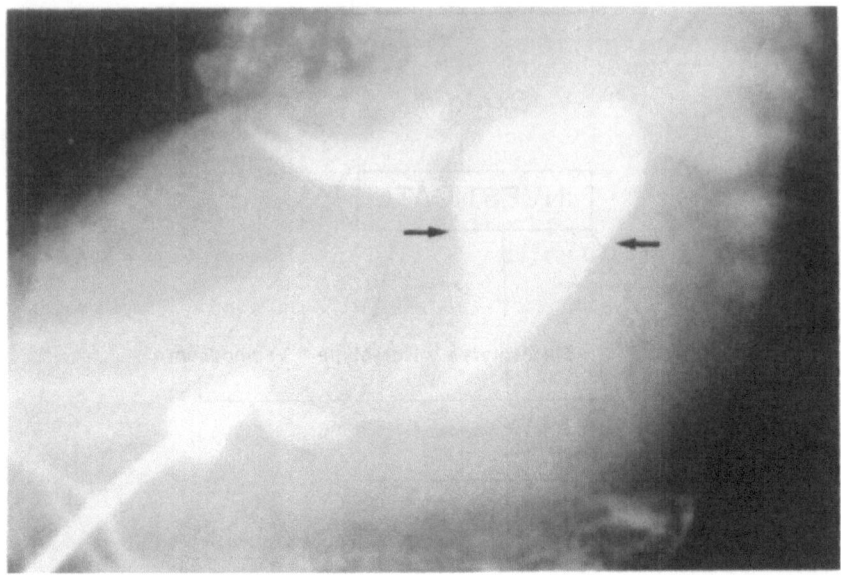

Figure 22 Perineal sinogram in a female infant with ambiguous genitalia due to 11β-hydroxylase deficiency. The uterine cavity is clearly outlined (arrowed)

CONCLUSIONS

(1) 21-Hydroxylase deficiency accounts for more than 90% of cases of CAH; ambiguous genitalia in the newborn is the commonest presentation. Two-thirds are salt-losers.

(2) Maintenance glucocorticoid treatment is required from the outset (20–25 mg/m²/day). 9α-Fludrocortisone, 0.1–0.2 mg daily, is adequate mineralocorticoid replacement; this should be continued for life. Clinical non-salt-losers with elevated PRA require mineralocorticoid replacement.

(3) Treatment is monitored clinically by measurement of growth velocity, skeletal maturation and signs of hypercortisolism. Biochemical indices include serial measurements of plasma 17OHP, testosterone, PRA and, if available, saliva 17OHP.

(4) A long-acting glucocorticoid preparation, such as dexamethasone, is suitable replacement for the patient who has completed statural

growth. Daily hydrocortisone (10–$15\,mg/m^2/day$) in three divided doses is required for children with CAH; some patients may achieve improved control with substituting a small dose of prednisolone at bedtime.

(5) Detailed, regular monitoring of treatment should ensure normal growth and adult reproductive potential in patients with CAH. There is no evidence for a marked disturbance in psychosexual behaviour in older patients, provided the diagnosis and sex of assignment was established correctly in early life.

ACKNOWLEDGEMENTS

The collaboration of Dr Riad-Fahmy, Dr R. F. Walker, Dr G. F. Read, Mr J. Dyas and many technical staff at the Tenovus Institute is gratefully appreciated. Part of this work was supported by the Welsh Scheme for Health and Social Research.

References

1. Hughes, I. A. (1982). Congenital and acquired disorders of the adrenal cortex. *Clin. Endocrinol. (Oxf.)*, **11**, 89–125
2. Strott, C. A., Yoshimi, T. and Lipsett, M. B. (1969). Plasma progesterone and 17-hydroxyprogesterone in normal men and children with congenital adrenal hyperplasia. *J. Clin. Invest.*, **48**, 930–9
3. Horton, R. and Frasier, S. D. (1967). Androstenedione and its conversion to plasma testosterone in congenital adrenal hyperplasia. *J. Clin. Invest.*, **46**, 1003–9
4. Fife, D. and Rappaport, E. B. (1983). Prevalence of salt-losing among congenital adrenal hyperplasia patients. *Clin. Endocrinol. (Oxf.)*, **19**, 259–64
5. Ulick, S., Eberlin, W. R., Bliffeld, A. R., Chu, M. D. and Bongiovanni, A. M. (1980). Evidence for an aldosterone biosynthetic defect in congenital adrenal hyperplasia. *J. Clin. Endocrinol. Metab.*, **51**, 1346–53
6. New, M. I., Dupont, B., Pang, S., Pollack, M. and Levine, L. S. (1981). An update of congenital adrenal hyperplasia. *Recent Prog. Horm. Res.*, **37**, 105–81
7. Keenan, B. S., Holcombe, J. H., Kirkland, R. T., Potts, V. E. and Clayton, G. W. (1979). Sodium homeostasis and aldosterone secretion in salt-losing congenital adrenal hyperplasia. *J. Clin. Endocrinol. Metab.*, **48**, 430–6
8. Zachmann, M., Tassinari, D. and Prader, A. (1983). Clinical and biochemical variability of congenital adrenal hyperplasia due to 11β-hydroxylase deficiency. A study of 25 patients. *J. Clin. Endocrinol. Metab.*, **56**, 222–9
9. Riddick, D. H. and Hammond, C. B. (1975). Adrenal virilism due to 21-hydroxylase deficiency in postmenarchal female. *Obstet. Gynecol.*, **45**, 21–4
10. Newmark, S., Dluhy, R. G., Williams, G. H., Pochi, P. and Rose, L. I. (1977). Partial 11- and 21-hydroxylase deficiencies in hirsute women. *Am. J. Obstet. Gynecol.*, **127**, 594–8
11. Sarris, S., Swyer, G. I. M., Ward, R. H. T., Laurence, D. M., McGarrigle, H. H. and Little, V. (1978). The treatment of mild adrenal hyperplasia and associated infertility with prednisone. *Br. J. Obstet. Gynaecol.*, **85**, 251–3

12. Blankstein, J., Faiman, C., Reyes, F. I., Schroeder, M. L. and Winter, J. S. D. (1980). Adult-onset familial 21-hydroxylase deficiency. *Am. J. Med.*, **68**, 441–8

13. Wischusen, J., Baker, H. W. G. and Hudson, B. (1981). Reversible male infertility due to congenital adrenal hyperplasia. *Clin. Endocrinol. (Oxf.)*, **14**, 571–7

14. Levine, L. S., Dupont, B., Lorenzen, F., Pang, S., Pollack, M., Oberfield, S., Kohn, B., Lerner, A., Cacciari, E., Mantero, F., Cassio, A., Scaroni, C., Chiumello, G., Rondanini, G. F., Gargantini, L., Giovanelli, G., Virdis, R., Bartolotta, E., Migliori, C., Pintor, C., Tato, L., Barboni, F. and New, M. I. (1980). Cryptic 21-hydroxylase deficiency in families of patients with classical congenital adrenal hyperplasia. *J. Clin. Endocrinol. Metab.*, **51**, 1316–24

15. Shackleton, C. H. L., Mitchell, F. L. and Farquhar, J. W. (1972). Difficulties in the diagnosis of the adrenogenital syndrome in infancy. *Pediatrics*, **49**, 198–205

16. Shackleton, C. H. L. (1976). Congenital adrenal hyperplasia caused by defect in steroid 21-hydroxylase. Establishment of definitive urinary steroid excretion pattern during first weeks of life. *Clin. Chim. Acta*, **67**, 287–98

17. Edwards, R. W. H., Matkins, H. L. J. and Barratt, T. M. (1964). The steroid 11-oxygenation index: a rapid method for use in the diagnosis of congenital adrenal hyperplasia. *J. Endocrinol.*, **30**, 181–94

18. Barnes, N. D. and Atherden, S. M. (1972). Diagnosis of congenital adrenal hyperplasia by measurement of plasma 17-hydroxyprogesterone. *Arch. Dis. Child.*, **47**, 62–5

19. Youssefnejadian, E. and David, R. (1975). Early diagnosis of congenital adrenal hyperplasia by measurement of 17α-hydroxyprogesterone. *Clin. Endocrinol.*, **4**, 451–4

20. Hughes, I. A. and Winter, J. S. D. (1976). The application of a serum 17OH-progesterone radioimmunoassay to the diagnosis and management of congenital adrenal hyperplasia. *J. Pediatr.*, **88**, 766–73

21. Sippell, W. G., Becker, H., Versmold, H. T., Bidlingmaier, F. and Knorr, D. (1978). Longitudinal studies of plasma aldosterone, corticosterone, deoxycorticosterone, progesterone, 17-hydroxyprogesterone, cortisol and cortisone determined simultaneously in mother and child at birth and during the early neonatal period. I. Spontaneous delivery. *J. Clin. Endocrinol. Metab.*, **46**, 971–85

22. Hughes, I. A., Riad-Fahmy, D. and Griffiths, K. (1979). Plasma 17OH-progesterone concentrations in newborn infants. *Arch. Dis. Child.*, **54**, 347–9

23. Murphy, J. R., Joyce, B. G., Dyas, J. and Hughes, I. A. (1983). Plasma 17OH-progesterone concentrations in ill newborn infants. *Arch. Dis. Child.*, **58**, 532–4

24. Hughes, I. A. and Winter, J. S. D. (1978). The relationships between serum concentrations of 17OH-progesterone and other serum and urinary steroids in patients with congenital adrenal hyperplasia. *J. Clin. Endocrinol. Metab.*, **46**, 98–104

25. Pang, S., Levine, L. S., Chow, D. M., Faiman, C. and New, M. I. (1979). Serum androgen concentrations in neonates and young infants with congenital adrenal hyperplasia due to 21-hydroxylase deficiency. *Clin. Endocrinol. (Oxf.)*, **48**, 228–34

26. Hughes, I. A., Arisaka, O., Perry, L. A. and Honour, J. W. Early diagnosis of 11β-hydroxylase deficiency in an infant with ambiguous genitalia using specific plasma and urinary steroid analyses. (Submitted for publication)

27. Honour, J. W., Anderson, J. M. and Shackleton, C. H. L. (1983). Difficulties in the diagnosis of congenital adrenal hyperplasia in early infancy: the 11β-hydroxylase defect. *Acta Endocrinol.*, **103**, 101–9

28. Fukishima, D. K., Finkelstein, J. W., Yoshida, K., Boyar, R. M. and Hellman, L. (1975). Pituitary adrenal activity in untreated congenital adrenal hyperplasia. *J. Clin. Endocrinol. Metab.*, **40**, 1–12

29. Lippe, B. M., LaFranchi, S. H., Lavin, N., Parlow, A., Coyotupa, J. and Kaplan, S. A. (1974). Serum 17α-hydroxyprogesterone, progesterone, estradiol and testosterone in the diagnosis and management of congenital adrenal hyperplasia. *J. Pediatr.*, **85**, 782–7

30. McKenna, T. J., Jennings, A. S., Liddle, G. W. and Burr, I. M. (1976). Pregnenolone, 17OH-pregnenolone and testosterone in plasma of patients with congenital adrenal hyperplasia. *J. Clin. Endocrinol. Metab.*, **42**, 918–25
31. Fukushima, D. K., Nishina, T., Wu, R. H. K., Hellman, L. and Finkelstein, J. W. (1979). Rapid assay of plasma 21-deoxycortisol and 11-deoxycortisol in congenital adrenal hyperplasia. *Clin. Endocrinol. (Oxf.)*, **10**, 367–75
32. Hughes, I. A. and Winter, J. S. D. (1977). Early diagnosis of salt-losing congenital adrenal hyperplasia in a newborn boy. *Can. Med. Assoc. J.*, **117**, 363–5
33. Koshimizu, T. (1979). Plasma renin activity and aldosterone concentration in normal subjects and patients with salt-losing type of congenital adrenal hyperplasia during infancy. *Clin. Endocrinol. (Oxf.)*, **10**, 515–22
34. Kenny, F. M., Preeyasombat, C. and Migeon, C. J. (1966). Cortisol production rate. II. Normal infants, children, and adults. *Pediatrics*, **37**, 34–42
35. Forest, M. G., Sizonenko, P. C., Cathiard, A. M. and Bertrand, J. (1974). Hypophysogonadal function in humans during the first year of life. I. Evidence for testicular activity in early infancy. *J. Clin. Invest.*, **53**, 819–28
36. Winter, J. S. D., Hughes, I. A., Reyes, F. I. and Faiman, C. (1976). Pituitary–gonadal relations in infancy. 2. Patterns of serum gonadal steroid concentrations in man from birth to 2 years of age. *J. Clin. Endocrinol. Metab.*, **42**, 679–86
37. Smith, D. W. (1977). Growth and its disorders. In *Major Problems in Clinical Pediatrics.*. Vol. 15. (Philadelphia: W. B. Saunders)
38. Brook, C. G. D., Zachmann, M., Prader, A. and Mürset, G. (1974). Experience with long-term therapy in congenital adrenal hyperplasia. *J. Pediatr.*, **85**, 12–19
39. Winter, J. S. D. (1980). Marginal comment: current approaches to the treatment of congenital adrenal hyperplasia. *J. Pediatr.*, **97**, 81–2
40. Frisch, H., Parth, K., Schober, E. and Swoboda, W. (1981). Circadian patterns of plasma cortisol, 17-hydroxyprogesterone, and testosterone in congenital adrenal hyperplasia. *Arch. Dis. Child.*, **56**, 208–13
41. Hughes, I. A. and Read, G. F. (1982). Simultaneous plasma and saliva steroid measurements as an index of control in congenital adrenal hyperplasia (CAH): a longitudinal study. *Horm. Res.*, **16**, 142–50
42. Pang, S., Hotchkiss, J., Drash, A. L., Levine, L. S. and New, M. I. (1977). Microfilter paper method for 17α-hydroxyprogesterone radioimmunoassay: its application for rapid screening for congenital adrenal hyperplasia. *J. Clin. Endocrinol. Metab.*, **45**, 1003–8
43. Sólyom, J. (1981). Blood-spot 17α-hydroxyprogesterone radioimmunoassay in the follow-up of congenital adrenal hyperplasia. *Clin. Endocrinol. (Oxf.)*, **14**, 547–53
44. Riad-Fahmy, D., Read, G. F., Walker, R. F. and Griffiths, K. (1982). Steroids in saliva for assessing endocrine function. *Endocr. Rev.*, **3**, 367–95
45. Walker, R. F., Hughes, I. A. and Riad-Fahmy, D. (1979). Salivary 17α-hydroxyprogesterone in congenital adrenal hyperplasia. *Clin. Endocrinol. (Oxf.)*, **11**, 631–7
46. Hughes, I. A. and Read, G. F. (1984). Control in congenital adrenal hyperplasia monitored by frequent saliva 17OH-progesterone concentrations. *Horm. Res.*, **19**, 77–85
47. Laron, Z. and Pertzelan, A. (1968). The comparative effect of 6α-fluoroprednisolone, 6α-methylprednisolone, and hydrocortisone on linear growth of children with congenital adrenal virilism and Addison's disease. *J. Pediatr.*, **73**, 774–82
48. Rappaport, R., Bouthreuil, E., Marti Henneberg, C. and Basmaciogullari, A. (1973). Linear growth, bone maturation and growth hormone secretion in prepubertal children with congenital adrenal hyperplasia. *Acta Paediatr. Scand.*, **62**, 513–19
49. Huseman, C. A., Varma, M. M., Blizzard, R. B. and Johanson, A. (1977). Treatment of congenital virilizing adrenal hyperplasia patients with single and multiple daily doses of prednisone. *J. Pediatr.*, **90**, 538–42

50. Bacon, G. E. and Kelch, R. P. (1979). Congenital adrenal hyperplasia due to 21-hydroxylase deficiency: a review of current knowledge. *J. Endocrinol. Invest.*, **2**, 93–100
51. Raiti, S. and Newns, G. H. (1970). The management of congenital adrenal hyperplasia. *Br. J. Hosp. Med.*, **3**, 509–12
52. Grant, D. B., Dillon, M. J., Atherden, S. M. and Levinsky, R. J. (1977). Congenital adrenal hyperplasia: renin and steroid values during treatment. *Eur. J. Pediatr.*, **126**, 89–96
53. Hughes, I. A., Wilton, A., Lole, C. A. and Gray, O. P. (1979). Continuing need for mineralocorticoid therapy in salt-losing congenital adrenal hyperplasia. *Arch. Dis. Child.*, **54**, 350–5
54. Rayyis, S. S. and Horton, R. (1971). Effect of angiotensin II on adrenal and pituitary function in man. *J. Clin. Endocrinol. Metab.*, **32**, 539–46
55. Wigerhof, M., Mellinger, R. C. and Zafer, M. S. (1983). Failure of angiotensin II to stimulate increases in concentrations of adrenal androgens, 17-hydroxyprogesterone, or adrenocorticotropin in congenital 21-hydroxylase deficiency. *J. Clin. Endocrinol. Metab.*, **56**, 627–31
56. Jansen, M., Wit, J. M. and Van Den Brande, J. L. (1981). Reinstitution of mineralocorticoid therapy in congenital adrenal hyperplasia. Effects on control and growth. *Acta Paediatr. Scand.*, **70**, 229–33
57. Rösler, A., Levine, L. S., Schneider, B., Novogroder, M. and New, M. I. (1977). The interrelationship of sodium balance, plasma renin activity and ACTH in congenital adrenal hyperplasia. *J. Clin. Endocrinol. Metab.*, **45**, 500–12
58. Klingensmith, G. J., Garcia, S. C., Jones, H. W., Jr, Migeon, C. J. and Blizzard, R. M. (1977). Glucocorticoid treatment of girls with congenital adrenal hyperplasia: effects on height, sexual maturation, and fertility. *J. Pediatr.*, **90**, 996–1004
59. Urban, M. D., Lee, P. A. and Migeon, C. J. (1978). Adult height and fertility in men with congenital virilizing adrenal hyperplasia. *N. Engl. J. Med.*, **299**, 1392–6
60. Jones, H. W., Jr and Verkauf, B. S. (1971). Congenital adrenal hyperplasia: age at menarche and related events at puberty. *Am. J. Obstet. Gynecol.*, **109**, 292–8
61. Richards, G. E., Grumbach, M. M., Kaplan, S. L. and Conte, F. A. (1978). The effect of long acting glucocorticoids on menstrual abnormalities in patients with virilizing congenital adrenal hyperplasia. *J. Clin. Endocrinol. Metab.*, **47**, 1208–15
62. Hughes, I. A. and Read, G. F. (1982). Menarche and subsequent ovarian function in girls with congenital adrenal hyperplasia. *Horm. Res.*, **16**, 100–6
63. Meikle, A. W. and Tyler, F. H. (1977). Potency and duration of action of glucocorticoids. Effects of hydrocortisone, prednisone and dexamethasone on human pituitary–adrenal function. *Am. J. Med.*, **63**, 200–7
64. Horrocks, P. M. and London, D. R. (1982). A comparison of three glucocorticoid suppressive regimes in adults with congenital adrenal hyperplasia. *Clin. Endocrinol. (Oxf.)*, **17**, 547–56
65. Apter, D. (1980). Serum steroids and pituitary hormones in female puberty: a partly longitudinal study. *Clin. Endocrinol. (Oxf.)*, **12**, 107–20
66. Hughes, I. A., Read, G. F., Wilson, D. W. and Griffiths, K. (1983). Development of ovarian function in adolescent girls. Presented at the *2nd Joint Meeting of British Endocrine Societies*, April 5–8, York (abstract no. 42)
67. Prader, A., Zachmann, M. and Illig, R. (1977). Normal spermatogenesis in adult males with congenital adrenal hyperplasia after discontinuation of therapy. In Lee, P. A., Plotnick, L. P., Kowarski, A. A. and Migeon, C. J. (eds.) *Congenital Adrenal Hyperplasia.* pp. 397–401. (Baltimore: University Park Press)
68. Van Seters, A. P., Van Aalderen, W., Moolenaar, A. J., Gorsiro, M. C. B., Van Roon, F. and Backer, E. T. (1981). Adrenocorticoid tumour in untreated congenital adrenocortical hyperplasia associated with inadequate ACTH suppressibility. *Clin. Endocrinol. (Oxf.)*, **14**, 325–34

69. Hague, W. M. and Honour, J. W. (1983). Malignant hypertension in congenital adrenal hyperplasia due to 11β-hydroxylase deficiency. *Clin. Endocrinol. (Oxf.)*, **18**, 505–9

70. Murtaza, L., Sibert, J., Hughes, I. A. and Balfour, I. C. (1980). Congenital adrenal hyperplasia—a clinical and genetic survey. Are we detecting male salt-losers? *Arch. Dis. Child.*, **55**, 622–5

71. Haseltine, F. and Ohno, S. (1981). Mechanisms of gonadal differentiation. *Science*, **211**, 1272–7

72. Wilson, J. D., Griffin, J. E., George, F. W. and Leshin, M. (1981). The role of gonadal steroids in sexual differentiation. *Recent Prog. Horm. Res.*, **37**, 1–39

73. Gorski, R. A. (1982). Effects of androgen exposure on the perinatal animal brain. *Ann. Intern. Med.*, **94**, 488–93

74. Gorski, R. A., Harlan, R. E., Jacobson, C. D., Shryne, J. E. and Southam, A. M. (1980). Evidence for the existence of a sexually dimorphic nucleus in the preoptic area of the rat. *J. Comp. Neurol.*, **193**, 529–40

75. Money, J. (1981). The development of sexuality and eroticism in humankind. *Q. Rev. Biol.*, **56**, 379–403

76. Baker, S. W. (1980). Psychosexual differentiation in the human. *Biol. Reprod.*, **22**, 61–72

77. Ehrhardt, A. A. and Meyer-Bahlburg, H. F. L. (1981). Effects of prenatal sex hormones on gender-related behaviour. *Science*, **211**, 1312–24

78. Ehrhardt, A. A., Epstein, R. and Money, J. (1968). Fetal androgens and female gender identity in the early-treated adrenogenital syndrome. *Johns Hopkins Med. J.*, **122**, 160–7

79. Ehrhardt, A. A. and Baker, S. W. (1974). Fetal androgen, human CNS differentiation and behaviour sex differences. In Friedman, R. C., Richart, R. M. and Vande Wiele, R. L. (eds.) *Sex Differences in Behaviour*. pp. 53–76. (New York: Wiley)

80. Hughes, I. A. and Davies, P. A. (1980). Neonatal endocrine and metabolic emergencies. *Clin. Endocrinol. Metab.*, **9**, 583–604

7

SURGICAL MANAGEMENT OF INTERSEX IN CHILDHOOD

J. DEWHURST

This paper concerns only the surgical management of intersex patients who are to be reared as female. It will deal predominantly with the management of the genetic female with congenital adrenal hyperplasia, but what will be said about the surgery required for this category of patient is appropriate with some modification for other intersex patients whose gender role is to be female.

Genetic female patients with congenital adrenal hyperplasia have a twofold external genital anomaly—enlargement of the clitoris and excessive fusion of the genital folds which come together in front of the vagina and urethra, thus creating an artificial urogenital sinus with a single opening which lies usually in the region of the base of the clitoris. Figure 1 illustrates these abnormalities in a child with congenital adrenal hyperplasia; Figure 2 shows in diagrammatic form that the fused genital folds may be thin, somewhat thicker or very thick indeed with narrowing of the lower vagina as well. It must be stressed, however, that the internal genital organs are always present and that the vagina is always patent at some point, although this point may be difficult to identify.

The necessary surgery, therefore, includes reduction in the size of the phallus and the opening of the vagina.

The reduction in the size of the phallus is not invariably required. If it is small enough not to be a cause of embarrassment later, it may be left alone. This, however, is, in my experience, the exception and not the rule. In congenital adrenal hyperplasia phallic reduction is usually necessary.

For many years I used to amputate the phallus in this fashion. A circular incision is made around the base of the organ and the loose connective tissue stripped from its shaft. During this procedure the restraining bands that are holding the clitoris down on its ventral surface in a position of chordee are divided and the organ is seen to be larger than was previously believed. The base is then clamped and ligated and the organ removed.

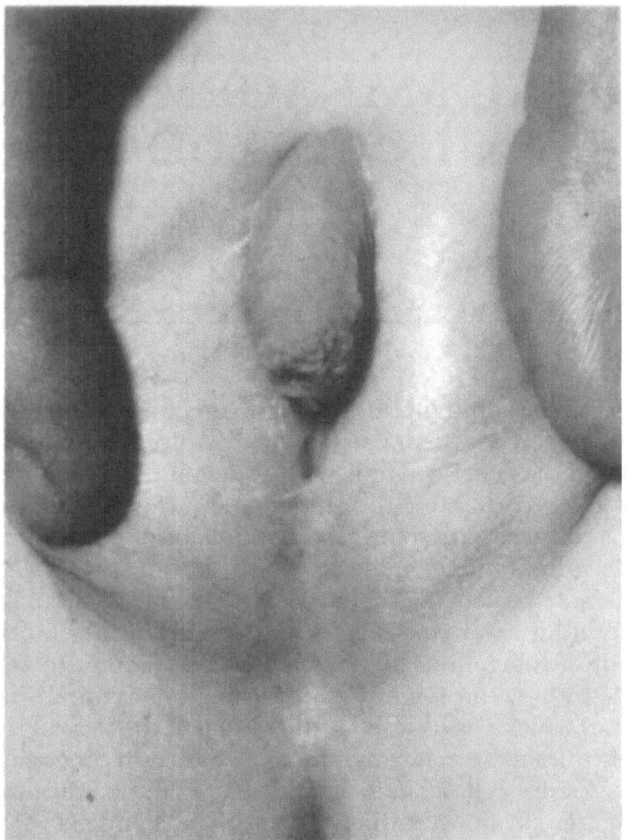

Figure 1   A 4-year-old female child with congenital adrenal hyperplasia

I think it probable that there are few real disadvantages to this procedure since, in my experience, patients so treated later have satisfactory intercourse and some achieve orgasm. The suggestion that the sensitive glans may be removed, however, sometimes causes concern to parents who fear that their daughter may not be able to have normal intercourse when she grows up; accordingly I have, for several years now, adopted a method devised by Dr Hugh Allen of London, Ontario.

In this technique the corpora cavernosa are stripped clean in the same fashion as before; the blood supply to the glans is preserved on the ventral side of the organ; the nerve supply is more difficult to preserve, since the nerves run in the sheath of the corpora cavernosa which must be incised to allow them to be reflected laterally and to preserve them.

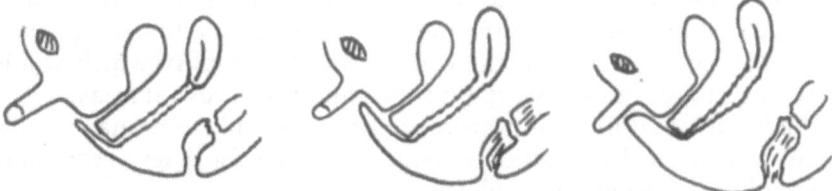

Figure 2 Diagrammatic representation of the external genital abnormalities present in congenital adrenal hyperplasia. In each figure there is similar enlargement of the clitoris, although the fused labial folds which come together beneath the vagina and urethra become increasingly thicker from left to right

The corpora cavernosa are then excised and the glans stitched back in place (Figure 3). The redundant skin can be fashioned into the appearance of labia minora and a good functional result can be achieved.

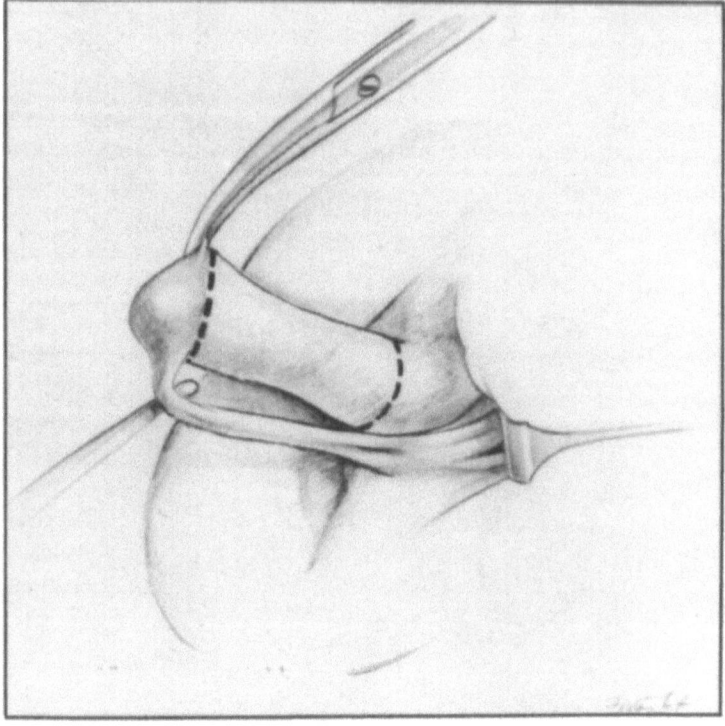

Figure 3 Diagrammatic illustration of the part of the enlarged clitoris to be removed once the blood supply and the nerve supply have been preserved. Following excision of the corpora cavernosa the glans is stitched back in place

119

This procedure can, of course, be undertaken at any time in childhood but, in my view, is best done in the neonatal period. The advantages of this are that the congenital adrenal hyperplasia will be well controlled and the child can be discharged from hospital without any visible evidence of maleness so that the parents can more readily accept their child as female and no one else can see an abnormality which would allow them to spread the story that the child was a sexual freak.

The fused labial folds, however, are more difficult to manage in the infant and surgical correction is best postponed for a few years and, preferably, until soon after puberty.

The procedure for dividing the fused labial folds is, in principle, simple (Figure 4). A vertical incision is made through them to expose

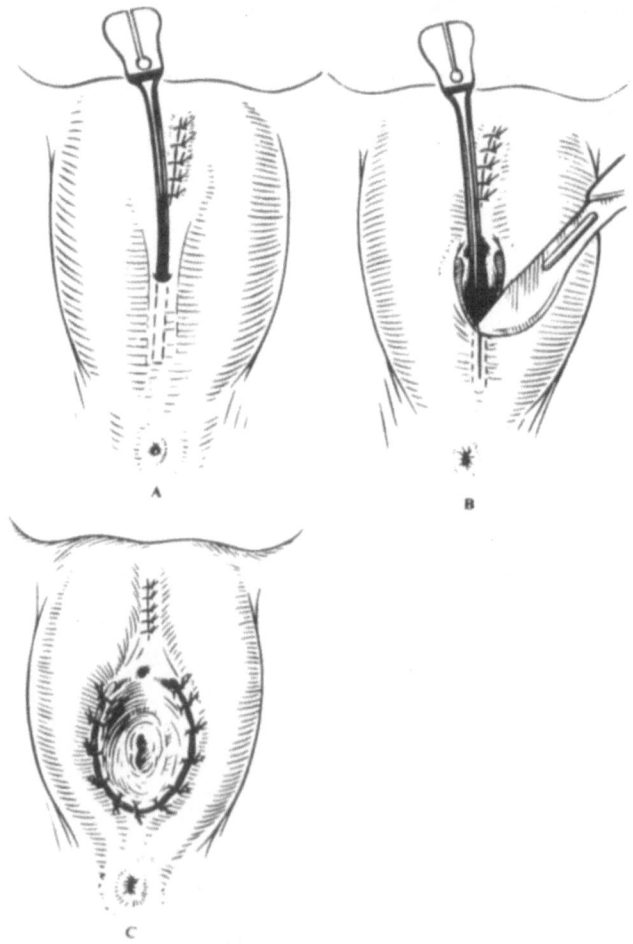

Figure 4 Diagrammatic representation of division of thin fused labial folds in congenital adrenal hyperplasia

the vagina beneath. A few stitches then unite the cut edges together and the child is left with a comparatively normal vulva. This is shown in Figure 4 in diagrammatic form and in Figure 5 on an actual patient.

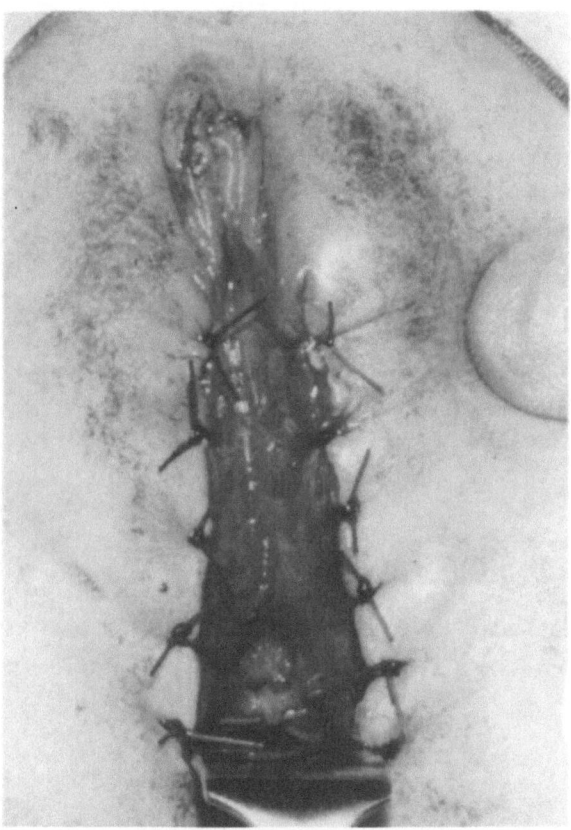

Figure 5 A case of drug-induced masculinization in a genetic female child. The labial folds have become fused so far forward that a lengthy incision backwards is necessary before the vagina is reached, into which a small speculum has now been inserted

If the folds are thicker and longer, more difficulty may be experienced in identifying the vagina and exteriorizing it properly. The incision may require to be extended well posteriorly before the vagina is reached (Figure 5). If the folds are very thick it is necessary to bring further skin into the vulval ring to enlarge it adequately. This may be undertaken in several ways, but the one illustrated in Figure 6 concerns the raising of two triangular flaps of skin on each side of the vagina; these flaps are so constructed that their height from base to apex is not greater than one-and-a-half times the base in order to preserve the blood supply. A mid-line incision is then made through the narrowed part of the vagina and

121

the flaps swung into place to enlarge the vulval ring. There are other plastic techniques which can be employed to give a similar result.

I have said that in my view it is better to leave division of the fused labial folds until soon after puberty; if they are thin, of course, the

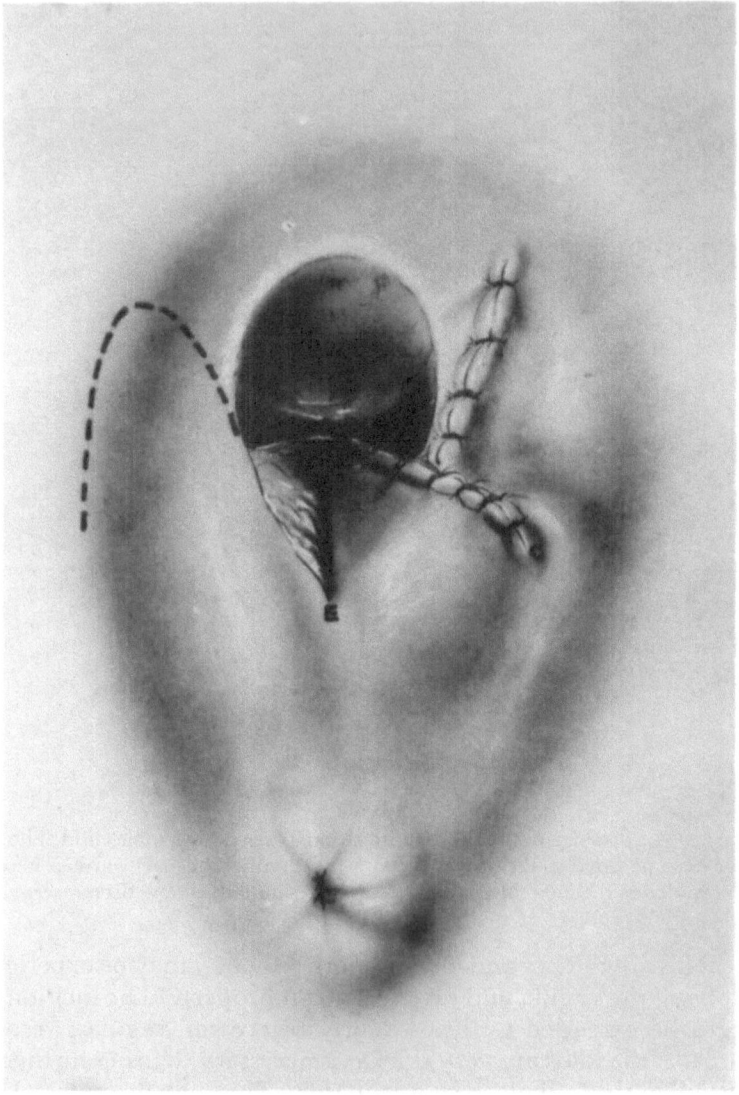

Figure 6 Diagrammatic illustration of one technique which may be used to enlarge the vagina in a patient with congenital adrenal hyperplasia when very thick fusion of the labial folds is present. A midline incision is first made through the narrow portion of the vagina; a triangular flap of skin, the dotted outline of which is seen on the left of the picture, is then raised; this flap is then folded into the defect in the vagina, as shown on the right, and the donor site is closed

122

procedure may be undertaken earlier, but it is always difficult in the newborn, since the tissues are vascular, the organs very tiny, and bleeding deep in the opening one is trying to enlarge can be difficult to stop properly. If the folds are thick, of course, it is imperative that the procedure is postponed until soon after puberty.

Other procedures that may need to be considered in different forms of intersex are the removal of a testis present in the labia or scrotum on one or both sides which seldom presents a problem (Figure 7). In certain genetic males who are to be reared as females the vagina may be very short and limited only to that which has been formed from the urogenital sinus. If this is so some form of enlargement may later be required. This can be accomplished by various surgical procedures, but in my view the best initial step is to attempt graduated dilatation by the patient herself using dilators such as are illustrated in Figure 8. With sufficiently motivated patients a good result is possible, as illustrated in Figure 8.

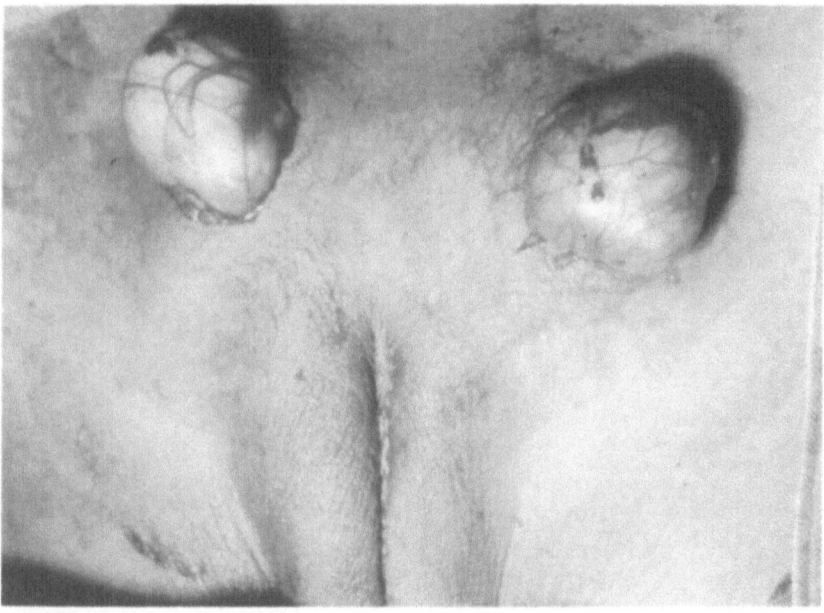

Figure 7 Simple display of testes in the groins of a genetic male child with 5α-reductase deficiency

Other procedures to which reference may be made concern the removal of an unwanted testis within the abdomen if the child is to be brought up in the female role, or the removal of a uterus from, for example, a true hermaphrodite who is to be brought up in the male role. The removal of such a uterus presents no great difficulty, but since the relationship of the organ to the bladder base is more difficult to identify than in the normal patient, it may be prudent not to carry the dissection too far downwards and risk bladder injury. It is better to leave a small amount of the lower portion of the uterus behind and not risk injury in this way.

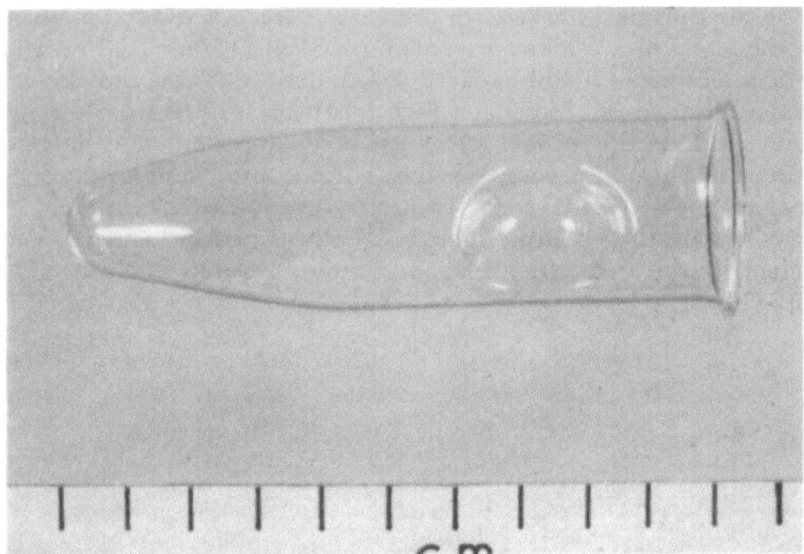

Figure 8 Dilator suitable for vaginal elongation by graduated dilatation

8

FETAL GROWTH CONTROL: THE ROLE OF INSULIN AND RELATED PEPTIDES

R. D. G. MILNER

INTRODUCTION

Sir Francis Teale, in whose memory this lecture is held, was a bacteriologist with wide-ranging interests. In taking as my theme 'Fetal growth control' I would be flattered to imagine that his curiosity as a biologist would be aroused were he with us today, for I shall endeavour in this review to focus on mechanisms that may be of relevance to the general control of cellular growth.

The regulation of fetal growth involves the mother and the placenta as well as the fetus, and Gluckman and Liggins have recently published an authoritative general review of this subject[1]. By focussing on insulin and related peptides which are growth factors I am keeping faith with a long-standing preoccupation that insulin might be important in fetal growth because of the prenatal development of the infant of a diabetic mother (IDM).

In the course of 9 months the human fetus passes from a fertilized egg to become a 3 kg baby. In doing so the equivalent of 44 cellular divisions take place and the control of growth at different stages of intra-uterine development obviously differs widely. During embryogenesis the control of normal cellular division and differentiation lies within the genome. We may contrast with this the third trimester when the fetus behaves in some respects like an individual receiving total parenteral nutrition via the umbilical cord and who is able to make appropriate endocrine and metabolic responses to perturbations of food supply by that route.

It is worth reflecting that the first 1.5 of the 3.0 kg takes two-thirds of pregnancy to develop. In the first 1.5 kg there is about 50 g of fat, whereas the second 1.5 kg acquired in the last 12 weeks of gestation includes 500 g fat. This multiplication and filling of fetal adipocytes in late pregnancy has an obvious clinical manifestation in the chubby IDM whose excess adipose tissue is mainly responsible for its overweight. In clinical practice the glucoregulatory action of insulin is readily perceived, but in biological terms the anabolic actions of this hormone give it a high priority for being important in growth control. Such speculation is reinforced by the appreciation that, among the family of growth-promoting peptides, there are two insulin-like growth factors, -I and -II, which derive their names from the fact that they share some of the metabolic actions of insulin.

INSULIN

The morphological and functional development of the B cell has been the subject of intense and sustained study, and in recent reviews I have summarized much of the current literature[2-5]. Interest in this topic has come from those who consider insulin to play an important part in fetal development, and latterly from investigators who consider that fetal islets or B cells may be suitable for transplantation and the treatment of diabetes.

Points which are relevant to our theme of the control of fetal growth are as follows. The human B cell is recognizable from the 10th week of gestation. Insulin is found in fetal blood from the earliest specimens collected at weeks 12 to 14. Insulin secretion from human fetal pancreas is glucose insensitive until approximately week 28 of gestation. In other species the point at which glucose sensitivity occurs varies; in the rabbit it is 27 days (term is 31 days), in the rat 21 days (term is 22 days). In all three examples the development of glucose sensitivity by the B cell precedes and heralds the storage of subcutaneous and deep tissue fat and it is tempting to link the two events causally. Alternatively, it is possible that as the B cell becomes able to recognize glucose the preadipocyte develops receptors which permit insulin-stimulated lipogenesis to occur. Other circumstantial evidence of an anabolic role for insulin in the last trimester of human pregnancy comes from the change in pattern of cellular growth in many organs at this time[6]. From weeks 12 to 24 growth is mainly by increase in cell number with little increase in cell size. Thereafter the rate of cell division slows, whereas there is a rapid increase of cell size (Figure 1). This is compatible with glucose-stimulated insulin secretion playing an important part in protein synthesis as well as lipogenesis.

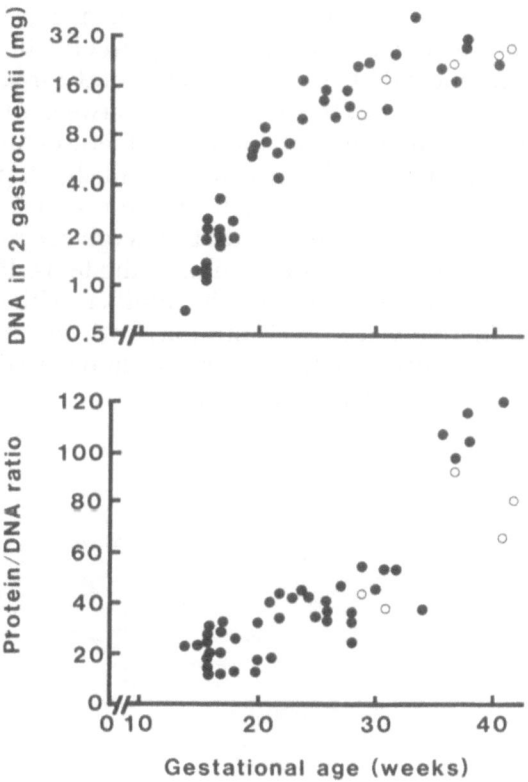

Figure 1 Total DNA and protein/DNA ratio in the gastrocnemii of human fetuses and newborn of 13–42 weeks' gestational age. Small-for-dates infants are shown by open circles. From Widdowson *et al.* (1972) with permission

A direct association between plasma insulin levels and fetal body weight was first noted by Girard *et al.*[7], but the best experimental demonstration of this phenomenon came from Fletcher *et al.*[8], who showed that body weight and log insulin concentrations were significantly correlated in 30-day rabbit fetuses and that after experimental reduction of the litter size to improve growth of the survivors the same relationship was preserved (Figure 2).

The classical clinical models illustrating the effects of insulin on fetal growth are the IDM and the infant born with transient diabetes mellitus. Although most of the overweight of the IDM is adipose, Naeye[9] has argued that the size of other cells may be increased by 10%. This observation has been confirmed using a hyperinsulinaemic fetal rhesus monkey model where the administration of insulin via a minipump for

21 days at the end of pregnancy resulted in a 34% increase in body weight but no significant increase in length[10]. Examination of individual organs showed a significant increase in the weight of the placenta, heart, liver and spleen, but not the lungs, kidneys or brain. The increased liver weight was shown to be due to cellular hyperplasia by the measurement of hepatic protein and DNA. Unfortunately, total carcass analysis for lipid was not carried out, but the discrepancy between the difference in total body weight of experimental and control fetuses and that explicable by the organs measured make it very likely that most of the difference was due to fat accumulation by the insulin-infused fetuses. Recently Picon *et al.* have confirmed that hyperglycaemia in the pregnant rat results in increased fat deposition in the fetus. Pregnancy was extended to 23.5 days by injecting the mother with progesterone. Experimental animals given glucose infusions from day 20.5 to 23.5 had heavier fetuses than control animals. Increased lipogenesis in the experimental fetuses was demonstrated using tritium.

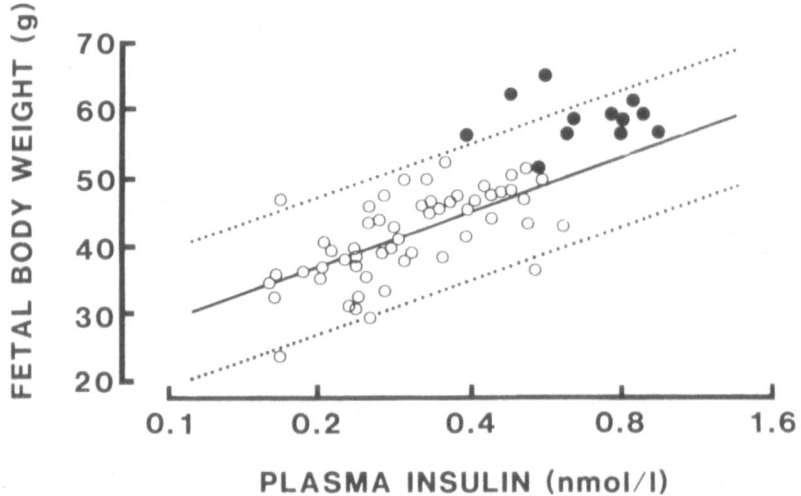

Figure 2 Plasma insulin and body weight at 30 days' gestation of litter-reduced fetal rabbits (closed circles) after surgical reduction of litter size to two at 9 days' gestation compared with that of normal 30-day fetal rabbits (open circles). From Fletcher *et al.* (1982) with permission

The larger effect of insulin on adipocyte development in late gestation than on the lean body mass is explicable if we make the hypothesis that somatic cellular growth in the normal fetus is taking place closer to its maximum than is the development of adipose storage tissue. Fatty growth could be by increase in adipocyte size or number or both. This facet of fetal growth is of more than theoretical interest; it may have a bearing on disease patterns in adult life. For example, if fetal hyper-insulinaemia causes fetal adiposity by an increase in adipocyte number the outcome may be a newborn infant who has a lifelong tendency to obesity and the complications thereof. The conundrum of the obese child has no start or end[12], but a recent epidemiological study of Pima Indians has shown that the offspring of women who had diabetes during pregnancy were two to three times more likely to become obese adults than those born to normal women or women who developed diabetes in later life[13]. This is important evidence because it shows how something going wrong before birth may have lifelong consequences and even be a mechanism for the transmission of acquired disease from one generation to the next.

The fetal deposition of both structural and storage lipid under insulin control may also have subtle but long-lasting consequences. Widdowson *et al.*[14] have shown that infants born to Dutch mothers have significantly more unsaturated tissue fat (palmitoleic and linoleic acids) than those born to British mothers and this reflects maternal dietary habits. Whilst most such fat is storage material, if the same is true for structural lipid, it is possible that degenerative disease of middle and old age may have its origin partly in the nutritional experience of the fetus. These two examples illustrate ways in which fetal growth control may have long-term sequelae: by a control mechanism (insulin) being over- or under-active and by nutrient supply being abnormal in quantity or quality.

PEPTIDE GROWTH FACTORS

There are a number of peptides which share the property of stimulating cellular growth. Some have been characterized physicochemically and of these a number share a broadly similar tertiary structure[15]. There are other growth factors which are as well, or better, defined in physico-chemical terms such as epidermal growth factor[16] and platelet-derived growth factor[17] which have contrasting structures. All growth factors share the property of stimulating a positive pleiotypic response in cells and they may be classified with respect to the type of cell or tissue on which they act and whether in addition to causing cellular proliferation they induce differentiation or dedifferentiation (see Table 1). All the peptide growth factors are of potential relevance to fetal growth control, but attention is focussed here on two which have particularly close ties with insulin.

Since the discovery that growth hormone stimulates cartilage growth via another peptide or peptides, originally referred to as sulphation factor, the results of research in this field have often been confused and confusing. Sulphation factor is a term used to describe a biological ac-tivity: the incorporation of radioactive sulphur into glycosaminoglycans that form part of the extracellular matrix of cartilage. It was not until the much more recent purification of two growth factors, insulin-like growth factors -I and -II (IGF-I and -II), that it has been possible to dissect the mass of previously published information and discriminate between biological fact and artefact. Growth factors have been measured by bioassay, radioimmunoassay and radioreceptor assay, and confusion has been generated usually by the use of heterologous assay systems. Our own work has employed mainly bioassay systems in which the property of plasma to stimulate sulphate or thymidine incorporation into cartilage has been referred to as somatomedin-like activity (SLA). We have been purists in attempting, whenever possible, to use cartilage of the same species and same stage of development as the test system for the plasma under investigation. By taking these precautions it has been possible to demonstrate a close association between SLA and growth rate before and after birth in the rat, and that cartilage responded to different growth factors before and after birth[22].

Table 1   Growth factors and their actions

Growth factor(s)	Target tissue	Differentiation	Dedifferentiation
Somatomedins[18]	Ectoderm Mesoderm Endoderm	Maturation of cartilage and muscle Hepatic glycogen synthesis	None known
Epidermal growth factor[16]	Ectoderm Mesoderm Endoderm	Maturation of epithelial structures, e.g. lung, skin, intestine	Cartilage, thyroid, secondary palate
Fibroblast growth factor[19]	Mesoderm	None known	Muscle, endothelium
Platelet-derived growth factor[17]	Mesoderm	Maturation of cartilage	Bone resorption
Nerve growth factor[20]	Ectoderm	Sympathetic nervous system	Cartilage
Erythropoietin[21]	Mesoderm	Erythroid maturation	None known

From the literature it seems reasonable to equate IGF-I with somato-medin C and IGF-II with multiplication-stimulating activity (MSA) (for review see references 23 and 24) and this usage is followed here. The history of the insulin-like growth factors is a fascinating story in its own right in which the convergence of several avenues of research resulted in the characterization of the peptides. On the one hand, there was the starting-point of sulphation factors and the somatomedins, peptides believed to be under the control of growth hormone that were responsible for skeletal growth. On the other, there was the property of plasma that resembled insulin biologically but which could not be suppressed by insulin antibody: non-suppressible insulin-like activity (NSILA). Independently, a fibroblast growth-promoting polypeptide released from cultured rat liver cells was identified[25]. Finally, with the characterization of IGF-I and -II, it became clear that both the skeletal growth-promoting and non-suppressible insulin-like properties of plasma resided in the same peptides and MSA and IGF-II were closely related. The purification of IGF-I and -II, the raising of antibodies and the development of immunoassay systems for these peptides have made possible rapid advances that have done much to clarify our ideas on the part played by insulin and the insulin-like growth factors in fetal growth control.

IGF-I AND -II IN THE FETAL CIRCULATION

Confusing results came from the use of inappropriate bioassay and heterologous immunoassay systems in the measurement of somatomedins in the fetal circulation. More recently these technical deficiencies have been overcome and a clearer picture of the circulating levels of IGF-I and -II during growth before and after birth has emerged in both man and experimental species. IGF-I but not IGF-II has been shown by Merimee et al.[26], among others, to be the factor essential for normal postnatal growth. Growth hormone-deficient patients have low circulating IGF-I and -II levels and both rise in response to treatment. Pygmies have normal IGF-II levels but low IGF-I levels and these do not increase in response to growth hormone treatment, indicating that dwarfism in the pygmy is due to a failure of IGF-I synthesis and release.

Changes in plasma IGF-I and -II before and after birth have been described in the sheep[27]. The normal gestation of a sheep fetus is 145–150 days. Early in pregnancy (50–80 days) fetal lamb plasma IGF-I-like levels are about one-third those found in the adult. The mean value rises from 0.29 U/ml at 50–80 days to 0.7 U/ml at 140–150 days. In the immediate perinatal period there is no change, but 3–7 days after birth IGF-I peaks at a mean value of 2.4 U/ml, returning to levels characteristic of the adult by the age of 60 days. In contrast IGF-II levels are higher in the fetus than in the adult at all stages of gestation and fall to characteristic adult values 12 hours postpartum (Figure 3). In the same laboratory a cross-sectional study was performed using cord blood from 206 human infants[28]. Cord IGF-I levels were lower than those found in the adult, rose with gestational age and correlated positively with birth weight at a given gestational age. The concentration of IGF-II, on the other hand, did not change with gestational age and was similar to the value found in the adult. Cord IGF-II levels did not correlate with birth weight, gestational age or IGF-I levels. It would be easy to infer from these results that IGF-I was closely related to fetal growth and that IGF-II was not, mimicking what is seen postnatally. However, it must be remembered that only IGF-I was measured by radioimmunoassay and that IGF-II was measured by radioreceptor assay using rat placental membrane as the ligand. This is important because conflicting results have been published by Bennett et al.[29]. These workers used radio-immunoassays for IGF-I and -II and found the plasma concentration of both peptides to increase with gestational age but to be lower than the characteristic adult concentration at term. Birth weight was strongly correlated with both IGF-I and IGF-II in the cord blood.

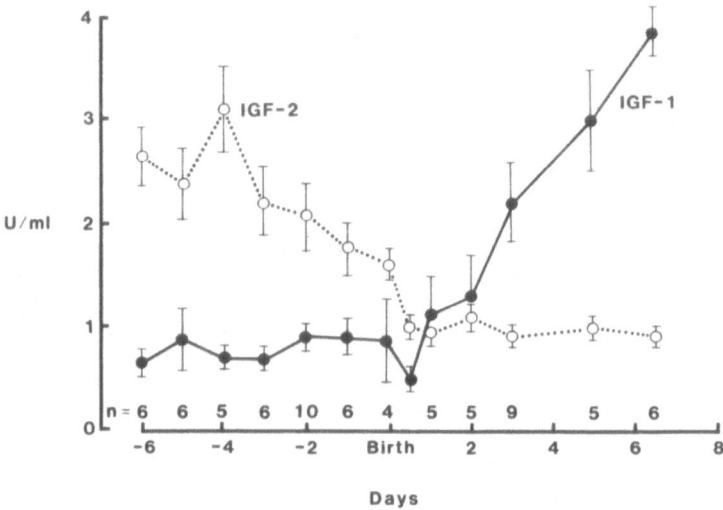

Figure 3 IGF-I (closed circles) and IGF-II (open circles) concentrations in 17 sheep fetuses and lambs in which the time of birth was known and hormone values are expressed in relation to the day of birth. The observations are mixed cross-sectional and longitudinal and the number is shown above the abscissa. From Gluckman and Butler (1983) with permission

IGF-I and -II share with some other growth factors the property of being bound to a carrier protein or proteins in the circulation[30]. In the adult, IGF-I bound to its carrier protein elutes from serum during gel-filtration with an approximate molecular weight of 150000 daltons. Cord blood serum from neonates of more than 30 weeks' gestation behaves similarly, whereas that from fetuses of less than 27 weeks' gestation elutes with a molecular weight of 40000 daltons. Between 27 and 30 weeks there is a bimodal pattern of elution (Figure 4)[31]. In this context it is noteworthy that in the hypophysectomized rat the 150000 dalton binding protein disappears whilst the 40000 dalton protein persists. Treatment with growth hormone restores both IGF and the 150000 dalton binding protein in the circulation.

These observations lead me to speculate that the rise in circulating levels of IGF-I seen towards the end of pregnancy reflect the maturation of hepatic growth hormone receptors and the preparation of the fetus for the pattern of growth factor synthesis and release that will operate after birth. They do little to clarify the apparent paradox of rapid fetal growth in the presence of low circulating levels of IGF-I and -II.

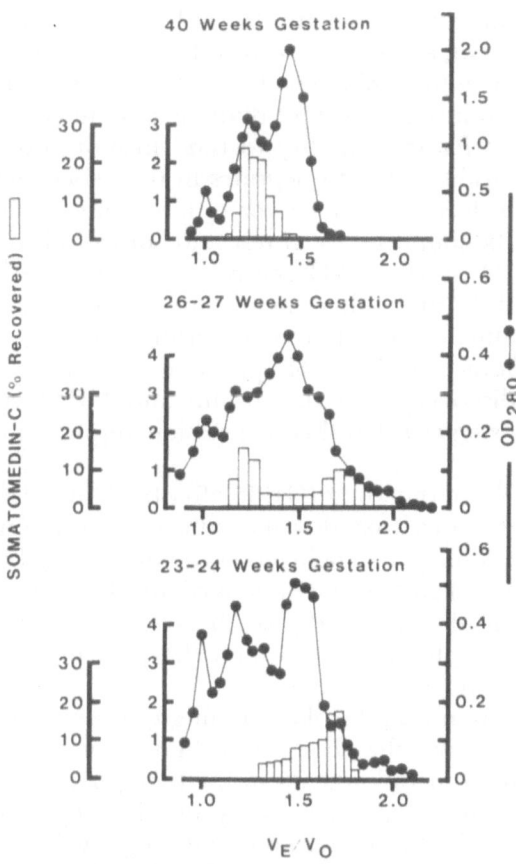

Figure 4 Sephacryl 200 chromatography of cord sera from three infants of different gestational ages. The bars represent immunoreactive Sm-C calculated as a percentage of the total measured in all fractions and illustrate the change in molecular weight of protein-bound Sm-C with increasing gestational age. Redrawn from D'Ercole *et al.* (1980) with permission

INSULIN, IGF-I AND -II AND THE PLACENTA

The gradual increase of circulating IGF-I levels during fetal life co-incides with increased activity of the fetal B cell, particularly with respect to glucose-stimulated insulin secretion. Such an association would be too weak to count as even circumstantial evidence of an effect of insulin upon IGF-I generation, but other evidence linking the two is strong. Anecdotal reports of clinical problems may occasionally be of profound importance in unravelling a biological tangle. The observation that an infant born with transient diabetes mellitus had low cord blood levels of insulin and IGF-I, but a normal IGF-II, is such a case[32]. Insulin therapy starting on the 4th day of life was followed by prompt clinical improvement, a delayed rise in IGF-I, but no change in IGF-II. Other results of a totally different kind also link insulin and IGF-I; fibroblasts from an insulin-resistant diabetic patient were compared to control fibroblasts for their ability to bind insulin and IGF-I[33]. The intensity of the binding of both peptides in the experimental cells was reduced due to a decrease in receptor number but not in affinity. No difference could be found between test and control fibroblasts in their binding of IGF-II. The IGF-II receptor is a single polypeptide not disulphide-linked to any other membrane component, whereas the receptors for insulin and IGF-I are structurally homologous disulphide-linked multi-subunit complexes of apparent molecular weight 350 000 daltons[34]. The discovery that the insulin and IGF-I receptors were affected together suggests that their expression might be under common genetic control.

The abrupt fall of circulating IGF-II after birth in the sheep immediately provokes the idea that the placenta may play some part in its genesis. The role of the placenta in fetal growth is undoubtedly complex and in the context of this review it is particularly relevant to consider ways in which insulin and the growth factors may affect placental metabolism and mechanisms by which the placenta could influence peptide growth factor biosynthesis.

The first suggestion that the placenta might have a trophic action on fetal growth came from the observation that ovine placental lactogen could induce somatomedin activity in the hypophysectomized rat[35]. It was then shown that hypophysectomy of the pregnant rat at mid-gestation had no effect on maternal circulating levels of somatomedin determined by bioassay, but that this fell sharply once delivery had occurred[36]. The idea that a placental hormone released into the maternal circulation can replace pituitary growth hormone as the trophic agent for somatomedin synthesis received further support[37]: a growth hormone-deficient woman became pregnant. At 35 weeks' gestation she had normal levels of IGF-I and -II in the circulation. These fell abruptly, together with circulating placental lactogen, following delivery of her baby.

The effect of placental hormones on fetal tissues is less clear. The gradient from mother to fetus for peptides such as placental lactogen is manifold, making it less likely, but not impossible, that a similar mechanism operates on the fetal side of the placental barrier.

Since the discovery that human placental membranes specifically bind insulin, but not growth hormone, prolactin or glucagon[38], the binding characteristics of insulin, IGF-I and -II to placental membranes have been compared. The receptor for insulin is specific and has high affinity and low capacity. Binding is maximum by 28 weeks gestational age, but placentas from small-for-gestational-age infants have fewer receptors than those from appropriately grown preterm or term infants[39]. There are specific binding sites for IGF-I and -II on human placental membranes, but rat placenta studied in the same way showed specific binding of IGF-II but very little binding of IGF-I[40]. The significance of these observations is unclear at present apart from the facile, but probably correct, inference that placental growth, and thereby fetal nutrition, is sensitive to the anabolic actions of insulin.

RECEPTORS FOR INSULIN AND THE GROWTH FACTORS

Despite the differences that have already been described between the receptor for IGF-II and those for IGF-I and insulin which resemble each other, cross-reactivity between the three hormones and their receptors has been documented in a variety of cells *in vitro*[23]. A novel approach to the analysis of how the different peptides exert their metabolic and growth-promoting actions has been the use of a specific antagonist to the insulin receptor: namely a Fab fragment derived from naturally occurring antibodies. In this way King *et al.*[41] were able to show that the metabolic actions of insulin and IGF-II (MSA) in rat adipocytes were both mediated via the insulin receptor. Contrariwise, the stimulation of thymidine incorporation into DNA in cultured human fibroblasts by insulin or IGF-II was unaffected by insulin receptor blockade, indicating that this action was the result of IGF receptor stimulation.

The possibility of interaction between the peptides and their receptors in the fetus *in utero* is plausible and must be considered in the account of receptor ontogeny that follows. The development of insulin receptors has received most attention. Insulin-binding by human liver membranes has been studied in fetuses of 15–18 weeks, 19–25 weeks and 26–31 weeks[42]. Receptor number increased from 15 to 25 weeks, but not thereafter, whereas the affinity of binding was markedly greater in membranes from 26–31-week fetuses when compared to the earlier stages. When rat liver membranes were studied by the same techniques, binding capacity and affinity also increased with gestational age and at term both were greater than in the adult. At the same stage of development in the rat there is also maturation of insulin metabolism by the hepatocyte[43]. In another study the puzzling observation was made that human fetal liver membranes possessed receptors for insulin and IGF-II but not for IGF-I[44]. This is contrary to the majority of the evidence and requires confirmation. Several types of cell have been shown to possess both IGF-I and -II receptors: rat fibroblast and liver cell membranes, human skin fibroblasts and placental membranes[45].

Muscle cells also develop an increasing density of insulin receptors during embryonic life. Sandra and Przybylski[46] have demonstrated specific insulin receptors on chick skeletal muscle cells in culture. These increase from 500 per proliferating myoblast to 3000 per cell equivalent in the mature myotube.

Monocytes harvested from cord blood have five times as much insulin-binding activity as those from adult blood[47] and cord blood monocytes from IDMs have a higher concentration of insulin receptors than those of normal infants[48]. Strict control of maternal diabetes during pregnancy resulted in the fetal monocyte insulin receptor concentration returning to normal.

Finally, receptors for the growth factors have been demonstrated indirectly in human fetal cartilage which responds to the growth-stimulating action of plasma by increased sulphate and thymidine incorporation from early in gestation[49].

THE RELEASE AND EFFECTS OF GROWTH FACTORS IN THE FETUS

After birth the liver is the principal site for somatomedin synthesis and this takes place under growth hormone control[24]. Fetal growth had long been thought to be independent of pituitary growth hormone because of the survival of anencephalic monsters *in utero*. Using the decapitated rabbit fetus as a model we showed that although bodily growth occurred it was abnormal when the cellular composition of different organs was examined[50]. We then demonstrated that although fetal decapitation abolished growth hormone from the fetal circulation it had no effect on circulating somatomedin-like activity[51]. Initially the site of fetal somatomedin synthesis was thought to be the liver, but when nephrectomized fetal lambs grew poorly *in utero* it seemed possible that the kidney might be a second site of synthesis[52].

The concept of somatomedin being produced in a specific organ in the fetus and of it behaving as a hormone was overturned in 1980 when D'Ercole *et al.* reported that somatomedin C could be recovered from tissue culture medium in which a variety of tissues from 17-day mouse fetuses had been grown[53]. These included liver, intestine, brain, kidney, heart and lung but not placenta. Even more interesting was the observation that 11-day embryonic limb bud micromass cultures also released somatomedin C-like peptide into the medium in excess of the tissue content. The synthesis and release of a particular growth factor does not appear to be a property of all the cells in an organ or tissue. For example, we have separated and cultured myoblasts and fibroblasts from 21-day fetal rat muscle and have shown that the myoblasts release IGF-I (SMC) into the culture medium whereas the fibroblasts do not[54]. It seems that the synthesis and release of peptide growth factors might be the property of most, if not all, embryonic and fetal cells, that the factors act locally and not distantly: they are autocrine or paracrine, but not endocrine signals. It follows that circulating levels do not necessarily reflect biologic activity.

The points in the cell cycle at which different factors act has been worked out in BALB/c 3T3 mouse fibroblasts[55,56]. Platelet-derived growth factor and fibroblast growth factor are 'competence' factors which act in the G_0 phase. The somatomedins, insulin and epidermal growth factor act subsequently in the G_1 phase as 'progression' factors. Subsequent phases (S, G_2 and M) are regulated by the cell intrinsically. If all fetal cells possess receptors for insulin and peptide growth factors and most or all cells synthesize growth factors it is not surprising that experiments to determine the effects of such factors on fetal cellular growth may produce complicated results. We have shown that fetal rat cartilage responds to a variety of peptide growth factors: somatomedin C, mouse epidermal growth factor and platelet-derived growth factor by increasing thymidine incorporation and that the actions of somatomedin and diluted human plasma were synergistic[57]. When Kaplowitz et al.[58] grew 11-day mouse embryo limb buds in low density as monolayer cultures in medium containing 0.2% serum, none of the following peptides stimulated cellular growth: epidermal growth factor, fibroblast growth factor, multiplication-stimulating activity, insulin or somatomedin C. When the cells were grown in high density micromass cultures all of these growth factors had a significant effect on the rate of cellular proliferation. Maximum effect was achieved by a combination of insulin or somatomedin C, epidermal growth factor, fibroblast growth factor and medium in which fetal liver had been grown. The authors surmised that, in addition to the known growth factors, the active component of liver medium represents a previously unrecognized growth factor. Adams et al. have extended and complemented these results in an elegant study[59] of IGF-I and -II synthesis by fetal and postnatal rat fibroblasts. They observed that from 2 to 50 days postnatal age fibroblasts switch from IGF-II to IGF-I biosynthesis. Sheep placental lactogen, but not growth hormone, was able to stimulate IGF-II production by fetal fibroblasts. In contrast, fibroblasts from postnatal animals responded to both placental lactogen and growth hormone by increasing the production of IGF-I. The results are compatible with a mechanism in which the fetal fibroblast has a placental lactogen receptor and responds to stimulation by IGF-II biosynthesis. As development proceeds the placental lactogen receptor disappears, to be replaced by a growth hormone receptor, stimulation of which results in the release of IGF-I. The growth hormone receptor recognizes placental lactogen as a messenger under experimental conditions which, of course, are not pertinent to what happens *in vivo*.

INSULIN, NUTRITION AND THE GROWTH FACTORS

Growth of the skeleton is accompanied by growth of lean body mass and for this to occur the individual must be anabolic. Anabolism requires a satisfactory supply of nutrient and the appropriate hormonal milieu. Overall, undernutrition is a commoner and more important clinical problem than overnutrition and there has been a sustained interest in the endocrine response to starvation and malnutrition[60]. Both marasmus and kwashiorkor are characterized by hypoinsulinaemia, but somewhat surprisingly by high plasma growth hormone levels[61]. Somatomedin measured by bioassay is consistently low in both clinical and experimental undernutrition and this is due partly to the presence of inhibitors in the plasma and partly to a true reduction of somatomedin levels[18, 62]. We have shown that undernutrition of the rat fetus or neonate is always accompanied by reduced cartilage metabolic activity, low plasma insulin, low somatomedin-like activity and high plasma growth hormone levels[63–65].

The general association of undernutrition, hypoinsulinaemia and low somatomedin led to a study of hepatocyte growth hormone receptors in rats at different planes of nutrition[62]. The authors had earlier proposed that growth hormone-binding by the liver was under insulin control[66] and when they found that growth hormone-binding by the liver fell in parallel with insulin and somatomedin, they deduced that insulin could control hepatic somatomedin generation by its action on the growth hormone receptor.

We have extended this concept by proposing that the generation of peptide growth factors in the fetus is dependent on the level of anabolism which, in its turn, is the product of adequate nutrient supply and the prevailing level of insulin in the circulation. Small-for-gestational-age infants have high cord plasma growth hormone levels but low somatomedin activity[67]. The converse proof comes from a study of the effects of endogenous or exogenous fetal hyperinsulinaemia. We injected rabbit fetuses with long-acting insulin on day 27 and found that they had raised cartilage metabolic activity and circulating somatomedin activity when harvested on day 29[68]. If pregnant rats receive a chronic glucose infusion that produces fetal hyperglycaemia and fetal hyperinsulinaemia the plasma somatomedin level is also raised[69]. Likewise, if fetal hyperinsulinaemia is provoked by the administration of chlorpropamide to the pregnant rat there is an increase of fetal plasma somatomedin[69]. We have shown that fetuses of mildly diabetic mother rats have increased cartilage metabolic activity and raised plasma somatomedin activity[70].

The justification for extending the link between insulin and fetal growth to peptides other than IGF-I and -II comes from Susa *et al.*[10], who had observed that fetal rhesus monkeys receiving chronic insulin infusions not only grew faster but had disproportionate development of the liver and spleen. The IDM is well known, not only for his chubbiness but also for his plethora, which is due to the persistence of extra-medullary haemopoiesis and results in a high-packed cell volume and problems due to hyperviscosity and prolonged jaundice. Measurements in the hyperinsulinaemic fetal rhesus monkey model and in IDM showed that both had increased erythropoiesis and raised levels of erythropoietin in the circulation (Figure 5)[71]. The authors speculated that this might be secondary to fetal hypoxia in the IDM, but I prefer the alternative idea that erythropoietin in the fetus is stimulated directly by insulin. In this context it is noteworthy that IGF-I has been shown to stimulate erythroid colony formation from precursor cells *in vitro* independently of erythropoietin[72]. The anabolic environment of the fetus in diabetic pregnancy may thus be doubly active in stimulating erythropoiesis.

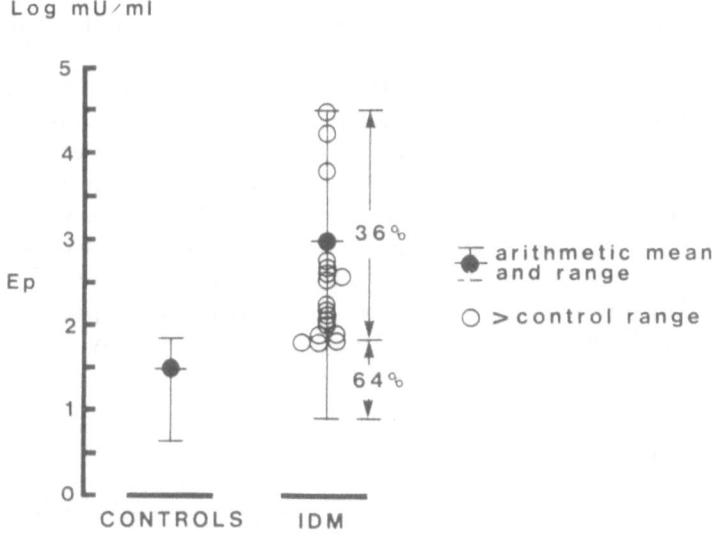

Figure 5 Human cord plasma or serum levels of erythropoietin (Ep) in control infants (n = 28) and IDM (n = 61). Arithmetic mean and range is shown, together with 22 individual IDM values that exceeded the control range. From Widness *et al.* (1981) with permission

CONCLUSIONS

By focussing on insulin and related peptide growth factors, other important endocrine controls of growth and differentiation have, of necessity, been left out. For example, the thyroid axis undoubtedly plays a vital role in prenatal development[73] and at the present state of knowledge it would be foolhardy to attempt to rank the known peptide growth factors in order of importance. Some consider that epidermal growth factor plays an important part in the overall control of fetal growth[74] and parallels have been drawn between the ontogeny of the thyroid hormones and of epidermal and nerve growth factor[75]. Alternatively, the steroid hormones have been proposed as being intimately concerned in growth and development[76]. Concerning insulin, however, the evidence shows clearly that a dual role must now be allotted to this hormone in prenatal life. In the last trimester, when the fetal B cell responds to glucose, insulin acts as a glucoregulatory hormone in an individual receiving continuous intravenous nutrition. In these circumstances the result of oversecretion is not hypoglycaemia but adiposity and this may have lifelong consequences. The other role of insulin is probably even more important and dates from the time the B cell first functions at about 10 weeks' gestation. Insulin, possibly secreted under amino acid stimulation, acts to convert a satisfactory nutrient supply into an anabolic environment within the conceptus, resulting in a wide variety of cells synthesizing and secreting growth stimulatory peptides that act in an autocrine or paracrine manner. IGF-I is probably under such control and it is possible that erythropoietin may be, in part, also. In contrast, IGF-II does not appear to be influenced by this control mechanism, but to be influenced by the placenta and a hormone or hormones secreted by it. It may be that these are two examples of a spectrum of peptide growth factor synthesis and that other hormones such as the thyroid play their part in stimulating growth factors other than IGF-I and -II. Interaction between endocrine and paracrine systems has been argued plausibly in evolutionary terms[77] and the examples reviewed here will fulfil both the remits of phylogeny and ontogeny.

ACKNOWLEDGEMENTS

The personal work quoted in the text has been carried out in collaboration with many colleagues whose names are cited in the list of references. Particular thanks are due to Dr D. J. Hill. Financial support has been received from the Medical Research Council, the British Diabetic Association, the Wellcome Trust, the Nuffield Foundation, the Trustees of the former United Sheffield Hospitals and the Hawley Trust.

References

1. Gluckman, P. D. and Liggins, G. C. (1984). The regulation of fetal growth. In Beard, R. W. and Nathanielsz, P. W. (eds.) *Fetal Physiology and Medicine: The Basis of Perinatology*. pp. 511–57. (London: W. B. Saunders)
2. Milner, R. D. G., Leach, F. N. and Jack, P. M. B. (1974). Reactivity of the fetal islet. In Sutherland, H. W. and Stowers, J. M. (eds.) *Carbohydrate Metabolism in Pregnancy and the Newborn*. pp. 83–104. (Edinburgh: Churchill Livingstone)
3. Milner, R. D. G., de Gasparo, M., Milner, G. R. and Wirdnam, P. K. (1979). Amino acids and development of the beta cell. In Sutherland, H. W. and Stowers, J. M. (eds.) *Carbohydrate Metabolism in Pregnancy and the Newborn*. pp. 133–51. (London: Springer-Verlag)
4. Milner, R. D. G. (1979). The role of insulin and glucagon in fetal growth and metabolism. In Visser, H. K. A. (ed.) *Nutrition and Metabolism of the Fetus and Infant*. pp. 3–18. (The Hague: Martinus Nijhoff)
5. Milner, R. D. G. (1981). Growth and development of the endocrine pancreas. In Davis, J. A. and Dobbing, J. (eds.) *Scientific Foundation of Paediatrics*. pp. 701–13. (London: W. Heinemann)
6. Widdowson, E. M., Crabb, D. E. and Milner, R. D. G. (1972). Cellular development of some human organs before birth. *Arch. Dis. Child.*, **47**, 652–6
7. Girard, J. R., Rieutort, M., Kervran, A. and Jost, A. (1976). Hormonal control of fetal growth with particular reference to insulin and growth hormone. In Rooth, G. and Brateby, L-E. (eds.) *Perinatal Medicine*. pp. 197–202. (Stockholm: Alquist and Wiksell)
8. Fletcher, J. M., Falconer, J. and Bassett, J. M. (1982). The relationship of body and placental weight to plasma levels of insulin and other hormones during development in fetal rabbits. *Diabetologia*, **23**, 124–30
9. Naeye, R. L. (1965). Infants of diabetic mothers: a quantitative morphologic study. *Pediatrics*, **35**, 980–8
10. Susa, J. B., McCormick, K. L., Widness, J. A., Singer, D. B., Oh, W., Adamsons, K. and Schwartz, R. (1979). Chronic hyperinsulinemia in the fetal rhesus monkey: effects on fetal growth and composition. *Diabetes*, **28**, 1058–63
11. Ktorza, A., Nurjhan, N., Girard, J-R. and Picon, L. (1983). Hyperglycaemia induced by glucose infusion in the unrestrained pregnant rat: effect on body weight and lipid synthesis in postmature fetuses. *Diabetologia*, **24**, 128–30
12. Taitz, L. S. (1983). Pathogenesis of obesity: prenatal factors. In *The Obese Child*. pp. 32–50. (Oxford: Blackwell Scientific)
13. Pettitt, D. J., Baird, H. R., Aleck, K. A., Bennett, P. H. and Knowler, W. C. (1983). Excessive obesity in offspring of Pima Indian women with diabetes during pregnancy. *N. Engl. J. Med.*, **308**, 242–5
14. Widdowson, E. M., Dauncey, M. J., Gairdner, D. M. T., Jonxis, J. H. P. and Pelikan-Filipkova, M. (1975). Body fat of British and Dutch infants. *Br. Med. J.*, **1**, 653–5
15. Blundel, T. L. and Humbel, R. E. (1980). Hormone families: pancreatic hormones and homologous growth factors. *Nature (London)*, **287**, 781–7
16. Gospodarowicz, D. (1981). Epidermal and nerve growth factor in mammalian development. *Annu. Rev. Physiol.*, **43**, 251–63
17. Raines, E. W. and Ross, R. (1982). Platelet-derived growth factor. 1. High yield purification and evidence of multiple forms. *J. Biol. Chem.*, **257**, 5154–60
18. Phillips, L. S. and Vassilopoulou-Sellin, R. (1980). Somatomedins, parts 1 and 2. *N. Engl. J. Med.*, **302**, 371–80, 438–46
19. Gospodarowicz, D., Bialecki, H. and Greenburg, G. (1978). Purification of the fibroblast growth factor activity from bovine brain. *J. Biol. Chem.*, **253**, 3736–43

20. Yanker, B. A. and Shooter, E. M. (1982). The biology and mechanism of action of nerve growth factor. *Annu. Rev. Biochem.*, **51**, 845–68
21. Goldwasser, E. (1975). The purification and properties of erythropoietin: a critical review. In Nakas, F., Fisher, J. W. and Takau, F. (eds.) *Erythropoiesis*. pp. 75–82. (Tokyo: University Press)
22. Hill, D. J., Andrews, S. J. and Milner, R. D. G. (1981). Cartilage response to plasma and plasma somatomedin activity in rats related to growth before and after birth. *J. Endocrinol.*, **90**, 133–42
23. Rechler, M. M., Schilling, E. E., King, G. S., Fraioli, F., Rosenberg, A. M., Higa, O. Z., Podskalny, J. N., Grunfeld, C., Nissley, S. P. and Kahn, C. R. (1980). Receptors for insulin and insulin-like growth factors in disease. *Adv. Biochem. Psychopharmacol.*, **20**, 489–97
24. Daughaday, W. H. (1982). Divergence of binding sites, *in vitro* action, and secretory regulation of the somatomedin in peptides IGF-I and IGF-II. *Proc. Soc. Exp. Biol. Med.*, **170**, 257–63
25. Nissley, S. P. and Rechler, M. M. (1978). Multiplication stimulating activity (MSA): a somatomedin-like polypeptide from cultured rat liver cells. *Natl. Cancer Inst. Monog.*, **48**, 167–77
26. Merimee, T. J., Zapf, J. and Froesch, E. R. (1982). Insulin-like growth factors (IGFs) in pygmies and subjects with the pygmy trait: characterization of the metabolic actions of IGF-I and IGF-II in man. *J. Clin. Endocrinol. Metab.*, **55**, 1081–8
27. Gluckman, P. D. and Butler, J. H. (1983). Parturition related changes in insulin-like growth factors -I and -II in the perinatal lamb. *J. Endocrinol.*, **99**, 223–32
28. Gluckman, P. D., Barrett-Johnson, J. J., Butler, J. H., Edgar, B. and Gunn, T. R. (1983). Studies of insulin-like growth factor I and II by specific radioligand assays in umbilical cord blood. *Clin. Endocrinol.*, **19**, 405–13
29. Bennett, A., Wilson, D. M., Lin, F., Nagashima, R., Rosenfeld, A. G. and Hintz, R. L. (1983). Levels of insulin-like growth factors I and II in human cord blood. *J. Clin. Endocrinol Metab.*, **57**, 609–12
30. Zapf, J., Waldvogel, M. and Froesch, E. R. (1975). Binding of non-suppressible insulin-like activity to human serum. *Arch. Biochem. Biophys.*, **168**, 638–45
31. D'Ercole, A. J., Wilson, D. F. and Underwood, L. E. (1980). Changes in the circulating form of serum somatomedin-C during fetal life. *J. Clin. Endocrinol. Metab.*, **51**, 674–6
32. Blethen, S. L., White, N. H., Santiago, J. V. and Daughaday, W. H. (1981). Plasma somatomedins, endogenous insulin secretion, and growth in transient neonatal diabetes mellitus. *J. Clin. Endocrinol. Metab.*, **52**, 144–7
33. Massague, J., Freidenberg, G. F., Olefsky, J. M. and Czech, M. P. (1983). Parallel decreases in the expression of receptors for insulin and insulin-like growth factor I in a mutant human fibroblast line. *Diabetes*, **32**, 541–4
34. Massague, J. and Czech, M. P. (1982). The subunit structures of two distinct receptors for insulin-like growth factors I and II and their relationship to the insulin receptor. *J. Biol. Chem.*, **257**, 5038–45
35. Hurley, T. W., D'Ercole, A. J., Handwerger, S., Underwood, L. E., Furlanetto, R. W. and Fellows, R. E. (1977). Ovine placental lactogen induces somatomedin: a possible role in fetal growth. *Endocrinology*, **101**, 1635–8
36. Daughaday, W. H., Trivedi, B. and Kapadia, M. (1979). The effect of hypophysectomy on rat chorionic somatomammotrophin as measured by prolactin and growth hormone radioreceptor assays: possible significance in maintenance of somatomedin generation. *Endocrinology*, **105**, 210–14
37. Merimee, T. J., Zapf, J. and Froesch, E. R. (1982). Insulin-like growth factor in pregnancy: studies in a growth hormone-deficient dwarf. *J. Clin. Endocrinol. Metab.*, **54**, 1101–3

38. Posner, B. I. (1974). Insulin receptors in human and animal tissue. *Diabetes*, **23**, 209–13
39. Potau, N., Rinder, E. and Ballabriga, A. (1981). Insulin receptors in human placenta in relation to fetal weight and gestational age. *Pediatr. Res.*, **15**, 798–802
40. Daughaday, W. H., Mariz, I. K. and Trivedi, B. (1981). A preferential binding site for insulin-like growth factor II in human and rat placental membranes. *J. Clin. Endocrinol. Metab.*, **53**, 282–8
41. King, G. L., Kahn, C. R., Rechler, M. M. and Nissley, S. P. (1980). Direct demonstration of separate receptors for growth and metabolic activities of insulin and multiplication-stimulating activity (an insulin-like growth factor) using antibodies to the insulin receptor. *J. Clin. Invest.*, **66**, 130–40
42. Neufeld, N. D., Scott, M. and Kaplan, S. A. (1980). Ontogeny of the mammalian insulin receptor. Studies of human and rat fetal liver plasma membranes. *Devl. Biol.*, **78**, 151–60
43. Sodoyez-Goffaux, F., Sodoyez, J. C. and De Vos, C. J. (1982). Maturation of liver handling of insulin in the rat fetus. *Diabetes*, **31**, 60–9
44. Sara, R. V., Hall, K., Misaki, M., Fryklund, L., Christensen, L. and Wetterberg, L. (1983). Ontogenesis of somatomedin and insulin receptors in the human fetus. *J. Clin. Endocrinol. Metab.*, **71**, 1084–94
45. Adams, S. O., Nissley, S. P., Kasuga, M., Foley, T. P., Jr and Rechler, M. M. (1983). Receptors for insulin-like growth factors and growth factors of multiplication-stimulating activity (rat insulin-like growth factor II) in rat embryo fibroblasts. *Endocrinology*, **112**, 971–8
46. Sandra, A. and Przybylski, R. J. (1979). Ontogeny of insulin binding during chick skeletal myogenesis *in vitro. Devl. Biol.*, **68**, 546–56
47. Thorsson, A. V. and Hintz, R. L. (1977). Insulin receptors in the newborn, increase in receptor affinity and number. *N. Engl. J. Med.*, **297**, 908–12
48. Neufeld, N. D., Kaplan, S. A. and Lippe, B. M. (1981). Monocyte insulin receptors in infants of strictly controlled diabetic mothers. *J. Clin. Endocrinol. Metab.*, **52**, 473–8
49. Ashton, I. K. and Phizackerley, S. (1981). Human fetal cartilage response to plasma somatomedin activity in relation to gestational age. *Calcified Tissue Int.*, **33**, 205–9
50. Jack, P. M. B. and Milner, R. D. G. (1975). Effect of decapitation and ACTH on somatic development of the rabbit fetus. *Biol. Neonate*, **26**, 195–204
51. Hill, D. J., Davidson, P. and Milner, R. D. G. (1979). Retention of plasma somatomedin activity in the foetal rabbit following decapitation *in utero. J. Endocrinol.*, **81**, 93–102
52. Thorburn, G. D. (1974). The role of the thyroid gland and kidneys in fetal growth. In Elliot, K. and Knight, J. (eds.) *Size at Birth*. pp. 185–200. (Amsterdam: Associated Scientific Publishers)
53. D'Ercole, A. J., Applewhite, G. T. and Underwood, L. E. (1980). Evidence that somatomedin is synthesized by multiple tissues in the fetus. *Devl. Biol.*, **75**, 315–28
54. Hill, D. J., Crace, C. R., Fowler, L., Holder, A. T. and Milner, R. D. G. (1984). Cultured fetal rat myoblasts release peptide growth factors which are immunologically and biologically similar to somatomedin. *J. Cell Physiol.* (In press)
55. Stiles, C. D., Capone, G. T., Scher, C. D., Amtoniades, H. N., Van Wyk, J. J. and Pledger, W. J. (1979). Dual control of cell growth by somatomedins and platelet derived growth factor. *Proc. Natl. Acad. Sci. USA*, **76**, 1279–83
56. Van Wyk, J. J., Underwood, L. E., D'Ercole, A. J., Clemmons, D. R., Pledger, W. J., Wharton, W. R. and Leof, E. B. (1981). The role of somatomedin in cellular proliferation. In Ritzen, N. *et al.* (eds.) *Biology of Normal Human Growth*. pp. 223–39. (New York: Raven Press)
57. Hill, D. J., Holder, A. T., Seid, J., Preece, M. A., Tomlinson, S. and Milner, R. D. G. (1983). Increased thymidine incorporation into fetal rat cartilage *in vitro* in the presence of human somatomedin, epidermal growth factor and other growth factors. *J. Endocrinol.*, **96**, 489–97

58. Kaplowitz, P. B., D'Ercole, A. J. and Underwood, L. E. (1982). Stimulation of embryonic mouse limb bud mesenchymal cell growth by peptide growth factors. *J. Cell. Physiol.*, **112**, 353–9

59. Adams, S. O., Nissley, S. P., Handwerger, S. and Rechler, M. M. (1983). Development patterns of insulin-like growth factor I and II synthesis and regulation in rat fibroblasts. *Nature (London)*, **302**, 150–3

60. Gardner, L. I. and Amacher, P. (1973). *Endocrine Aspects of Malnutrition: Marasmus, Kwashiorkor and Psychosocial Deprivation.* p. 520. (Santa Ynez, California: Kroc Foundation)

61. Milner, R. D. G. (1970)). Malnutrition and the endocrine system in man. In Benson, G. K. and Philips, J. G. (eds.) *Memoirs of the Society for Endocrinology, No. 18, Hormones and the Environment.* pp. 191–212. (Cambridge: University Press)

62. Maes, M., Underwood, L. E. and Ketelslegers, J-M. (1983). Plasma somatomedin C in fasted and refed rats: close relationship with changes in liver somatogenic but not lactogenic binding sites. *J. Endocrinol.*, **97**, 243–53

63. Fekete, M., Hill, D. J. and Milner, R. D. G. (1983). Somatomedin activity and cartilage [^{35}S] sulphate incorporation in the growth-retarded neonatal rat. *Biol. Neonate*, **44**, 114–22

64. Hill, D. J., Fekete, M., Milner, R. D. G., DePrins, F. and Van Assche, A. (1984). Reduced plasma somatomedin activity during experimental growth retardation in the fetal and neonatal rat. In Spencer, E. M. (ed.) *Insulin-like Growth Factors/ Somatomedins, Basic Chemistry, Biology and Clinical Importance.* pp. 354–62. (Berlin: Walter de Gruyter)

65. De Prins, F. A., Hill, D. J., Fekete, M., Robsen, D. J., Van Assche, F. A. and Milner, R. D. G. (1984). Reduced plasma somatomedin activity and sulphate incorporation by costal cartilage *in vitro* during experimental growth retardation in the fetal rat. *Pediatr. Res.* (In press)

66. Maes, M. and Ketelslegers, J-M. (1981). Long-term effects of diabetes on somatogenic and lactogenic receptors in rat liver. *Diabetes*, **30**, 54A

67. Foley, T. P. J., De Philip, R., Perricelli, A. and Miller, A. (1980). Low somatomedin activity in cord serum from infants with intrauterine growth retardation. *J. Paediatr.*, **96**, 605–10

68. Hill, D. J. and Milner, R. D. G. (1980). Increased somatomedin and cartilage metabolic activity in rabbit fetuses injected with insulin *in utero*. *Diabetologia*, **19**, 143–7

69. Heinze, E., Thi, C. N., Vetter, U. and Fussganger, R. D. (1982). Inter-relationship of insulin and somatomedin activity in fetal rats. *Biol. Neonate*, **41**, 240–5

70. Hill, D. J., Sheffrin, R. A. and Milner, R. D. G. (1982). Raised plasma somatomedin activity and cartilage metabolic activity (^{35}S sulphate uptake *in vitro*) in the fetus of mildly diabetic pregnant rats. *Diabetologia*, **23**, 270–4

71. Widness, J. A., Susa, J. B., Garcia, J. F., Singer, D. B., Sehgal, P., Oh, W., Schwartz, R. and Schwartz, H. C. (1981). Increased erythropoiesis and elevated erythropoietin in infants born to diabetic mothers and in hyperinsulinemic rhesus fetuses. *J. Clin. Invest.*, **67**, 637–42

72. Kurtz, A., Jelkman, W. and Bauer, C. (1982). A new candidate for the regulation of erythropoiesis: insulin-like growth factor I. *FEBS Lett.*, **149**, 105–8

73. Nathanielsz, P. W. (1976). The fetal thyroid. In Beard, R. W. and Nathanielsz, P. W. (eds.) *Fetal Physiology and Medicine: The Basis of Perinatology.* pp. 215–31. (London: W. B. Saunders)

74. Thorburn, G. D., Waters, M. J., Young, I. R., Dolling, M., Buntine, D. and Hopkins, P. S. (1981). Epidermal growth factor: a critical factor in fetal maturation. In Elliott, K. and Whelan, J. (eds.) *The Fetus and Independent Life.* pp. 172–98. (London: Pitman)

75. Walker, P., Weichsel, M. E., Jr, Eveleth, D. and Fisher, D. A. (1982). Ontogenesis of nerve growth factor and epidermal growth factor in submaxillary glands and nerve growth factor in brains of immature male mice: correlation with ontogenesis of serum levels of thyroid hormones. *Pediatr. Res.*, **16**, 520–4
76. Csaba, G. (1977). Hormonal regulation: morphogenetic and adaptive systems. *Biol. Rev.*, **52**, 295–303
77. Roth, J., LeRoith, D., Shiloach, J., Rosenzweig, J. L., Lesniak, M. A. and Havrankova, J. (1982). The evolutionary origins of hormones, neurotransmitters, and other extracellular chemical messengers. *N. Engl. J. Med.*, **306**, 523–7

SECTION 4

Normal and
Abnormal Growth

Chairman: P. H. W. RAYNER

9

NORMAL GROWTH IN INFANCY, CHILDHOOD AND ADOLESCENCE

M. A. PREECE

In describing the growth of a normal child it is important to consider both the typical pattern and the manner in which this may vary in the population. It is also important to discuss skeletal growth in the context of the events of puberty as this is a time of great importance in the completion of normal skeletal development. In this chapter the growth of the typical male and female are first described, followed by an evaluation of normal variation.

THE PATTERN OF NORMAL GROWTH

The normal height growth curve

(1) *Distance curve*

Figure 1(a) shows the height growth curve for a typical boy and girl from birth to 19 years[1]. This type of growth curve is usually referred to as the height attained or distance curve and is the most commonly used representation. It contains all the relevant information about growth in height of any individual child and represents the typical pattern of most elements of skeletal growth. Other dimensions, such as leg length, may differ in absolute size and exact timing of events, but their growth curves still have essentially the same shape.

(2) *Velocity curve*

In Figure 1(b) growth data is represented in a different way. Here, the distance data is converted into height velocity in centimetres per year. This is calculated from the distance data by dividing the difference between two height measurements, as near to 1 year apart as possible, by the exact time elapsed between them. The calculated velocity is plotted at the midpoint of the time interval over which it was measured to give the velocity curve. This representation of growth is particularly useful as it shows more detail of the growth process and, of course, is more immediate. The growth velocity in any 1 year is a more sensitive measure of events that have occurred in that year than is the height distance measurements at the same time. The latter are measurements subsumed from all previous heights before them. Thus the velocity curve may show rather dramatic changes in growth due to disease, where the simpler distance curve would obscure them.

In general there are three epochs of growth: early, rather fast growth before the age of 3 years; a relatively unchanging pattern of growth during the preschool and primary school years; and then the adolescent growth spurt.

During the first year of life the infant has an average height velocity of about 25 cm/year. However, this is a time when the velocity is changing dramatically and shorter time periods should be studied. The velocity during the first 3 months is 40.0 cm/year in boys and 36.0 cm/year in girls, dropping to 14.5 cm/year and 15.9 cm/year, respectively, by the last 3 months of that year[1]. During the next 3 years there is a further deceleration to achieve a rather constant velocity of about 5–6 cm/year. This continues with gentle slowing until puberty.

The first 3 years are also the time of increasing canalization of the growth curve. At birth the length of the baby is mostly determined by maternal size; father's height is poorly correlated with the child's. During the next 2–3 years the influence of father's genetic make-up progressively increases until there is equal influence by both parents. This phenomenon can result in some rather bizarre growth patterns where mother and father have very different heights. For example, when the child is born to a very tall mother but short father, the initially large baby will tend to grow unusually slowly until the genetically expected channel is achieved[2].

There is little difference between boys and girls before 10 years of age. Then the typical girl starts her adolescent growth spurt and for a few years is taller than the same aged boy. Some 2 years later the boy starts his spurt and by the age of 14 is the taller. The major differences in mature height between men and women (12.5 cm in the UK) is established at puberty. About 10 cm comes from the extra 2 years of prepubertal growth of boys and 2.5 cm from their more intense growth spurt.

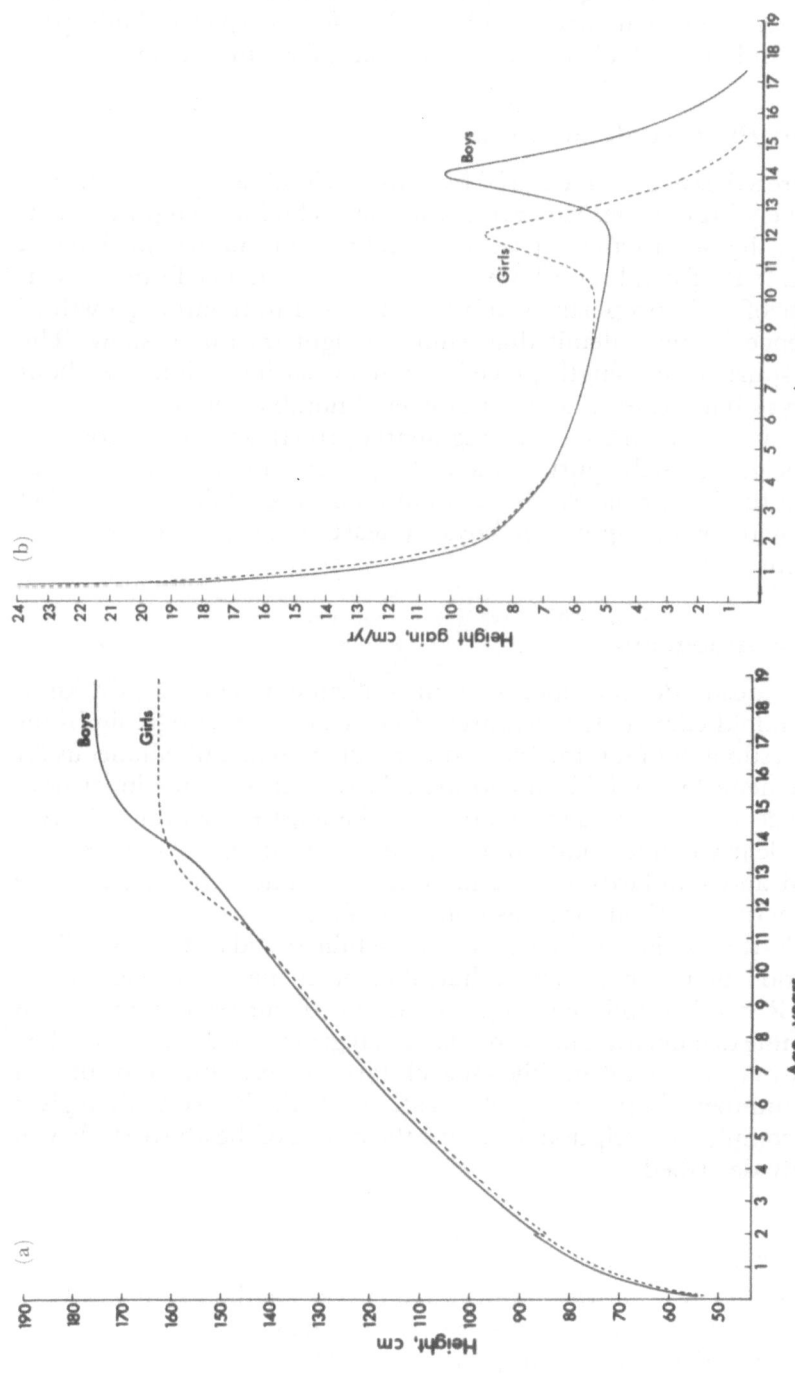

Figure 1 The height distance (a) and velocity (b) curves of a typical boy (solid line) and girl (broken line). From Tanner *et al.*[1] with permission

In many endocrinological applications the measurement of height alone gives insufficient detail and it is helpful to separate body proportions and also to look at muscle, bone and fat individually.

The growth of trunk and limb

Trunk growth is usually measured by sitting height[3], although alone it is of relatively little value. However, when subischial leg length is calculated by the subtraction of sitting height from stature we have a measurement of trunk and lower limbs which together form a useful indicator of body proportions and may be used to monitor growth at adolescence in more detail than simple height measures allow. The growth spurt in leg length precedes that for sitting height by about 1.5 years in both sexes. There is, however, a notable difference between the sexes in the intensity of the segmental growth spurts. In boys the sitting height growth spurt is about 25% more intense than in girls, although the leg spurts are about equal[4]. This is explained by the fact that growth of the spine, in boys at least, is largely testosterone-dependent.

Tissue components

Here we mostly depend upon measures of subcutaneous fat thickness using skinfold calipers for measures of body fat or X-rays of limbs for indirect estimates of fat, muscle and bone diameters. Subcutaneous fat measurements by skinfold calipers are relatively demanding in terms of experience as these measures tend to be the most error-prone. Nevertheless, clearly defined patterns of subcutaneous fat growth have been reported and standards are available for use. They are clinically the most practical method for measurements of fat.

The X-ray method is limited in its usefulness today because of the recognition that X-rays can be harmful, particularly in longitudinal studies. Recently published longitudinal growth curves[5] obtained at an earlier time demonstrate patterns of normal growth of these tissues. The method may be useful in following children whose disease justifies a limited number of serial X-ray observations. As the X-ray method gives a more complete description of events, the results of the above study will be briefly described.

(1) *Bone diameters*

In Figure 2(a) are shown the distance curves for the mean widths of humerus and tibia from the age of 3 years onwards. These data, together with those in Figure 2(b) and (c) are taken from Tanner *et al.*[5], where details of methods and further analysis may be found.

The humerus in boys is on average slightly wider than the girls' until the female adolescent spurt starts. For about 2 years the means are then equal, after which the boys' greater growth spurt commences. In tibia width there is no sex difference before the onset of puberty, but by maturity both bones show a 13% greater width in the male than in the female.

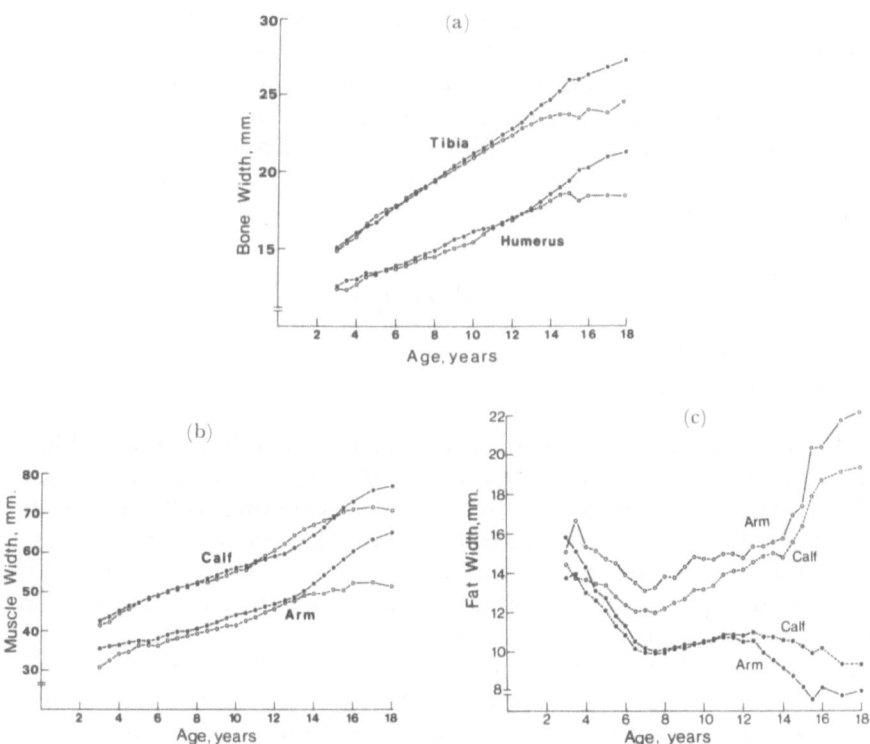

Figure 2 Distance curves of growth for limb bone (a), muscle (b) and fat (c) diameters for boys (filled circles) and girls (open circles). From Tanner *et al.*[5] with permission

(2) *Limb muscle*

In Figure 2(b) where calf and arm muscle widths are illustrated, it can be seen that before puberty the curves are very similar to those for bone, although the sex difference in the arm is somewhat greater for muscle. At puberty there is a marked growth spurt in both limb muscles in boys; in girls the arm muscle increases only slightly, while the calf muscle comes to exceed that of boys between the ages of 11 and 15. By full maturity the male preponderance is much greater in the arm (about 20%) than in the calf (10%).

(3) *Limb fat*

Figure 2(c) shows the widths of the fat layer again for arm and calf. At both sites boys have less fat than girls from age 4 onwards. The difference is increased during childhood and particularly so at puberty. In both sexes fat width falls from age 3 to about 7 and then starts to rise. In boys the rise is replaced from about 12 to 18 years by a further loss which is greater in the arm than in the calf. In girls fat accumulates fairly continuously except for a period during puberty from 10 to 12 years of age when arm fat remains fairly constant; note the marked increase in fat in postpubertal girls. Essentially the same pattern is seen when triceps skinfold is used as a measure of limb fat. The changes tend to be less dramatic but clearly reflect the same events.

NORMAL VARIATION IN GROWTH

Height standards

(1) *Population standards*

In Figure 3 are shown the British standards for height for boys[6]. These are standards with the shape of the growth curve derived from analysis of normal longitudinal data. The range of normality, reflected by the centiles, was, however, calculated from a much larger cross-sectional set of data so that the centiles conform to the shape of the individual child's growth but with an overall spread to encompass the entire population. This is important as longitudinal data is nearly always collected from a selected population of children leading to an underestimate of population variance. The usual centiles, namely the 3rd, 10th, 25th, 50th, 75th, 90th and 97th centiles, are drawn to give guidance as to the normal variation in size, but an alternative would be the use of ± 1, 2 or even 3 standard deviations.

In the figure are two small shaded areas above the 97th and below the 3rd centiles at the time of the adolescent growth spurt. These areas allow for the greater variance at this time in cross-sectional standards. Thus a child who is seen for the first time and whose height lies in one of these areas may be quite normal and just a little delayed or advanced in his growth. A second visit will clarify the situation as if his growth is normal, then his curve of growth will be closer to normal on subsequent visits.

It is conventional for children to be measured lying down until the age of 2 years and standing thereafter. For this reason there is a small discontinuity in the standards at the age of 2 years as a child measured supine is about 1 cm taller than when measured standing. At this time of change-over from the supine to standing measurement it is important that on at least two occasions both measurements are taken so that a correction can be made. Alternatively, it could be argued that children should be measured supine at all times, particularly when dealing with populations of children who are in the younger age groups. It would not be a major problem to adjust the standards accordingly and in some countries this is routine.

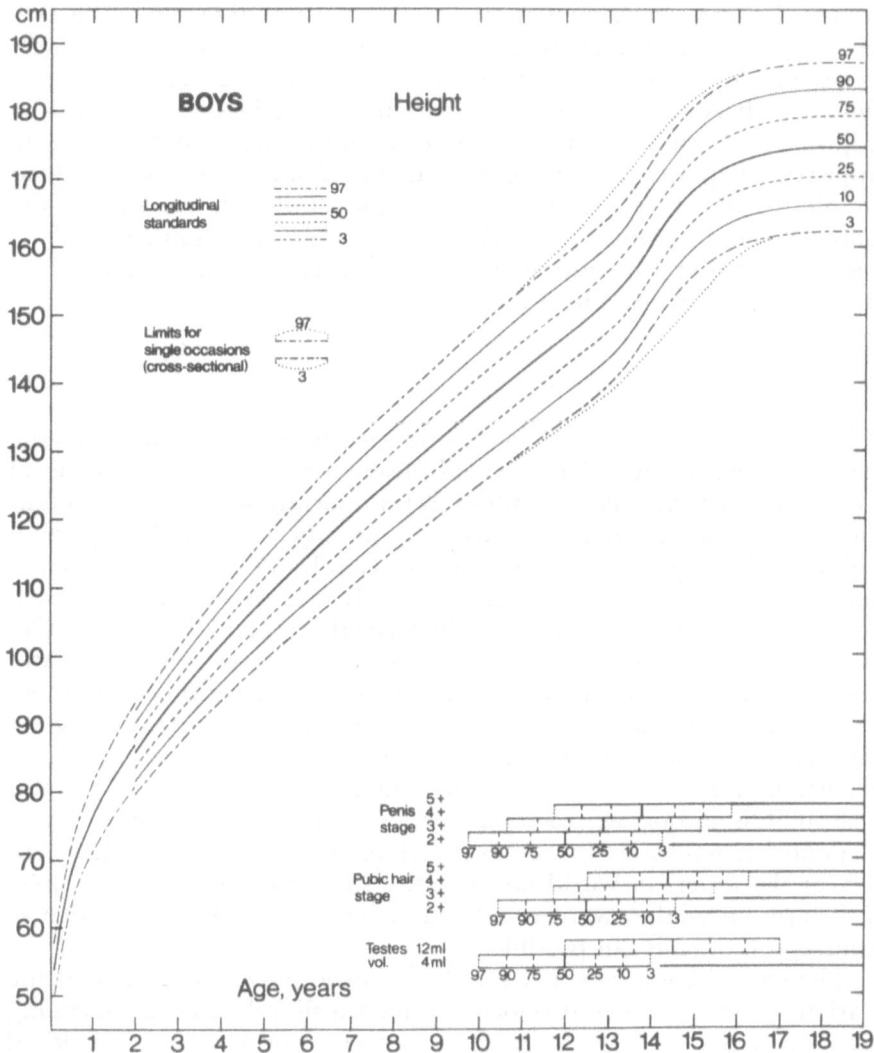

Figure 3 British standards for height for boys. From Tanner and Whitehouse[6] with permission

(2) *Correction for midparental height*

The standards on the previous page are derived from population surveys; they can be made more accurate for a given child if the heights of the parents are taken into account. The easiest way of doing this is to plot the parents' centiles at the right-hand edge of the chart; age 19 for these standards. This is quickly done by plotting the actual height of the like-sexed parent and the father's height minus 12.5 cm, or the mother's height plus 12.5 cm for the unlike-sexed parent. The 12.5 cm is the mean difference between adult men and women in the UK. This should be adjusted appropriately in other countries according to local data. The approximate position of the family 3rd and 97th centiles may be added by plotting the height of the midparental centile (the average of the parents' centiles), and this height ± 8 cm, which is obtained from the residual standard deviation for height, after allowing for parents' heights[7] (4.25 cm) multiplied by 1.88.

Height velocity standards

Figure 4 shows the standards for height velocity for boys. Once again the data is based on pure longitudinal observations and the extremes of normality are indicated by centiles. It is important to make two qualifications. In the first place it must be remembered that these normal values and the positions of the various centiles are based on velocity measurements taken over a whole year. If measurements were taken over a shorter time then the spread between the 3rd and the 97th centiles would be greater. This is because measurement errors assume greater importance as a percentage of the measured change and because there are substantial variations in growth velocity in any one year. This aspect has been explored more fully by Marshall[8], who has developed centiles for height velocity based on 3- and 6-monthly velocity data. For this reason it is important to interpret cautiously growth velocities in patients when they are based upon periods of measurements of less than 1 year. In a perfect world no velocities should be compared to these standards unless they were calculated over a full year, but in practice, of course, this often is not possible.

The second comment that should be taken into account is that the various centiles for height velocity do have a slightly different meaning than do height centiles. On average over a year or more any individual child who is growing normally should have a height velocity somewhere near the 50th centile for the population. If a child is to maintain his position on, say, the 10th centile for height, he should grow somewhere near the 40th centile for velocity. Similarly, a child who is maintaining his position on the 90th centile will have to grow at a slightly above average velocity but only at about the 60th centile. The child persistently growing at a 10th centile velocity will steadily fall further and further behind his peer group and some become distinctly short.

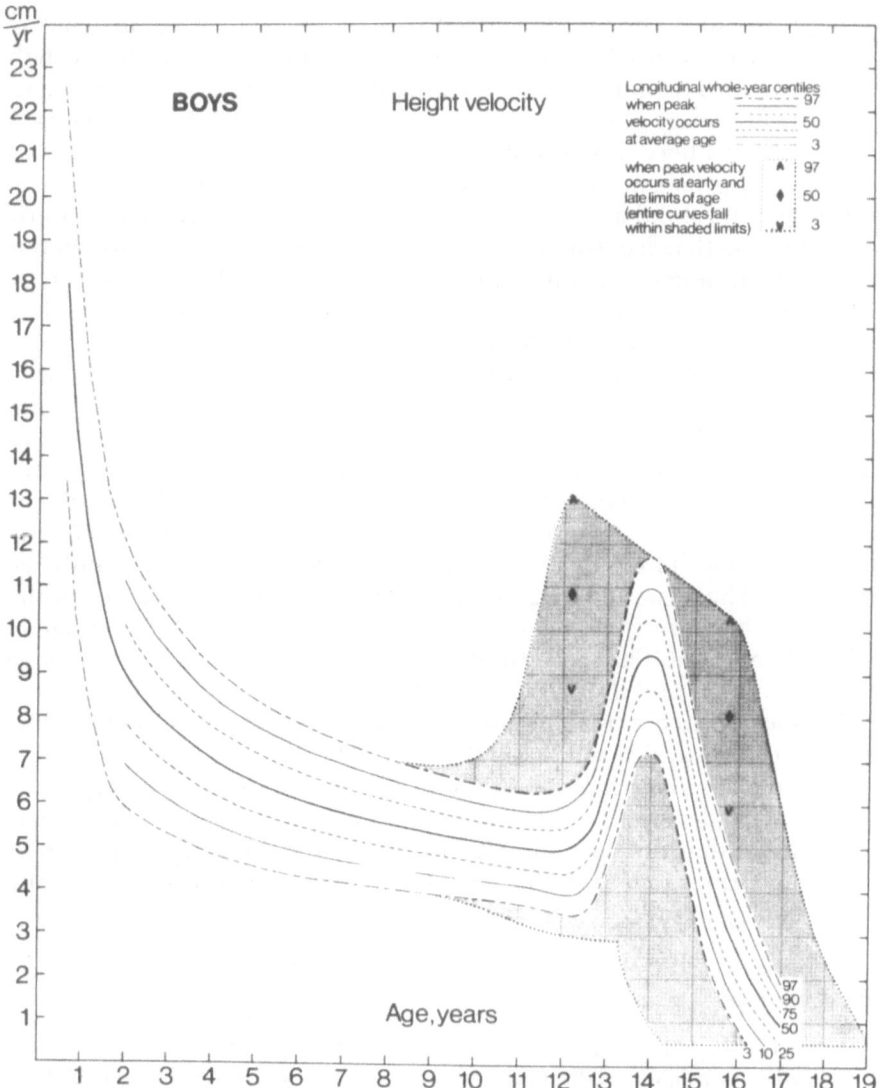

Figure 4   British standards for height velocity for boys. From Tanner and Whitehouse[6] with permission

In Figure 4 it will be seen that there are two large grey areas flanking the adolescent growth spurt. The centiles for the adolescent growth spurt are those for a child whose growth spurt occurs at an average age, i.e. 14 years in boys. However, there is a normal variation in this age of attaining the peak growth spurt. This is approximately ± 2 years about the mean and the grey shaded areas take this into account. In an individual case the growth spurt should occur within the grey area with a shape similar to the centile centred at 14 years. Note that, particularly in boys, earlier growth spurts tend to be more intense and later growth spurts less so. The same effect is seen in girls but to a less marked extent.

There are many other standards available for different measurements not illustrated here. Longitudinal standards exist for sitting height and subischial leg length[9] and cross-sectional standards for such measurements as biacromial and bi-iliac diameters and skinfold thickness. Variation in growth exists not only in the size at a given stage of growth but also in the timing of reaching different stages of growth. This latter type of variation or tempo is seen with some children growing at a slow tempo, reaching each relative part of their growth curve at later and later chronological ages compared with the average, and some children growing at a fast tempo attaining the same points but earlier than average. Standards for puberty stages have been developed and they are included on the stature standards illustrated in Figure 3. It is important to note the way in which these standards are constructed. The designation PH2, PH3, etc. represent the instant when these appearances first become visible. This is almost never observable; the doctor can only see that a child has attained PH2 but not yet PH3. We therefore describe the subject as being in PH2 + and the standards give the centiles for age of *being in* that stage. Thus a boy in PH2 + and aged 13.0 years is just above the 25th centile and thus a little older than average for that stage, albeit quite normal. In contrast, a similar boy aged 15.0 years would be below the 3rd centile and suspiciously delayed.

A convenient *aide-mémoire* is to note that for all the events of puberty the standard deviation for the age of attaining an event is close to 1 year. This means that the normal range of age for reaching an event such as menarche, expressed as the 95% confidence limits, is approximately the mean age ± 2 years.

References

1. Tanner, J. M., Whitehouse, R. H. and Takaishi, M. (1966). Standards from birth to maturity for height, weight, height velocity and weight velocity: British children, 1965. *Arch. Dis. Child.*, **41**, 454–71
2. Smith, D. W., Truog, W., McCann, J. J., Rogers, J. E., Greitzer, L. G., Skinner, A. L. and Harvey, M. A. S. (1976). Shifting linear growth during infancy and the genetics of growth in infancy. *J. Pediatr.*, **89**, 225–30
3. Cameron, N. (1978). The methods of auxological anthropometry. In Falkner, F. and Tanner, J. M. (eds.) *Human Growth.* pp. 35–90. (New York: Plenum Press)
4. Preece, M. A. (1981). The development of skeletal sex differences at adolescence. In Russo, P. and Gass, G. (eds.) *Human Adaptation.* pp. 3–13. (Sydney: Department of Biological Sciences, Cumberland College of Health Sciences)

5. Tanner, J. M., Hughes, P. C. R. and Whitehouse, R. H. (1981). Radiographically determined widths of bone, muscle and fat in the upper arm and calf from age 3 to 18 years. *Ann. Hum. Biol.*, **8**, 495–518

6. Tanner, J. M. and Whitehouse, R. H. (1976). Clinical longitudinal standards for height, weight, height velocity and weight velocity and the stages of puberty. *Arch. Dis. Child.*, **51**, 170–9

7. Tanner, J. M., Goldstein, H. and Whitehouse, R. H. (1970). Standards for children's height at ages 2–9 years, allowing for height of parents. *Arch. Dis. Child.*, **45**, 755–62

8. Marshall, W. A. (1971). Evaluation of growth rate in height over periods of less than one year. *Arch. Dis. Child.*, **46**, 414–20

9. Tanner, J. M. (1978). Human growth standards: construction and use. In Gedda, L. and Parisi, P. (eds.) *Auxology: Human Growth in Health and Disorder.* pp. 109–21. (London: Academic Press)

10

INVESTIGATION AND MANAGEMENT OF ABNORMAL GROWTH

M. A. PREECE

As a general principle, all chronic paediatric diseases may cause stunting of growth. By and large if a child's poor growth is due to a general system disease, such as chronic renal failure, the primary condition will have already produced symptoms that outweigh the growth problems. These disorders therefore tend to present not because of short stature but because of some other anxiety. This is, however, not an absolute rule. There are one or two notorious exceptions to which the clinician must be alert. Probably the most important, in terms of frequency with which it occurs, is coeliac syndrome, which quite commonly presents because of short stature with no overt gastro-intestinal symptoms[1]. Indeed the gastro-intestinal system is a particular trap as Crohn's disease may present with short stature and particularly delayed puberty.

With these important exceptions the children presenting with abnormal growth (and the vast majority will be those who are short as opposed to tall) are going to fall into three groups. On the one hand, there will be those children where there is in fact little wrong in the medical sense. These are usually children from relatively small families, often with growth delay, where reassurance and occasionally more specific measures can readily solve the problem. The second group comprises the patients with one of the dysmorphic syndromes, including the bone dysplasias and some chromosomal abnormalities. Finally, there are the endocrine disorders, where short stature may frequently be the presenting symptom and where accurate diagnosis and management are of great importance.

As many of the endocrine problems are being discussed in other sections of this book, I will confine myself to the general approach to diagnosis and then discuss the management of growth hormone deficiency, as this is the only endocrine cause of short stature which is not covered elsewhere.

CLINICAL ASSESSMENT OF SHORT STATURE

Here there are five broad questions that need to be answered when a patient presents to an outpatient clinic with a complaint of short stature:

Is the child really short?
Is the child growing slowly?
Is the poor growth of pre- or postnatal onset?
Is there growth delay?
Are there any specific stigmata?

We will now discuss each of these in turn.

Is the child really short?

This may seem a silly question to start with but it is surprising how often children are referred to a clinic with a mistaken view of their height. The most common reason for this is that the child is indeed small for the population but not for the family, and the importance of inheritance has not been explained in the past. An alternative problem, which should be totally avoidable, is where the anxieties have been raised by health officials because of completely inadequate measurement in a routine examination, usually at school.

With the use of the growth standards described in the previous chapter and adequate measuring techniques, it should be perfectly possible to answer this question fairly easily. It is, however, important to take note of the technique of measurement as the very best standards in the world are useless if the patient is being measured in an inaccurate way. Sadly this is an aspect of outpatient assessment which is often left to the most junior member of staff so that measurements may be inaccurately taken by a host of different people on different occasions. Somebody who has been properly trained to measure children, be it doctor, nurse or other individual, is essential in any clinic which is seeing children with problems of growth. The equipment should also be adequate for the job it is being asked to perform and able to provide repeatable measurements with an accuracy of the order of 2 mm. The measurement of growth velocity is an essential part of growth assessment but virtually impossible if measurement error is substantial, as these errors start to multiply when serial measurements are being considered.

It is also important to ensure that the standards being used are appropriate for the race of the child being examined. Seldom is it possible to have standards specific for each racial type but, by being aware of the problem, suitable adjustment can be made in the clinical situation. One great help in this direction, and an essential to accurate measurement, is the interpretation of parental heights providing, as it were, family specific standards. This has been discussed in the previous chapter.

Is the child growing slowly?

Assuming that on the first visit it is clear that the child is indeed smaller than would be expected for the family and that there is no obvious explanation or other clinical clue to guide one to immediate specific investigations, assessment of growth velocity is an important subsequent step. There is little point in measuring a child over shorter periods than 3 months as, with the possible exception of very early life, the growth velocity is too low to be measurable with any accuracy over shorter periods. Even the 3-month measurement is probably insufficient in all but the most extreme cases and it is often necessary to allow 6 months or more to elapse between the measurements before one can form a real impression of the child's growth rate. This is obviously very difficult for parents to understand because of the delay it introduces and often one is forced into accepting that the velocity is indeed low over a relatively short period. Here one must be particularly aware of the problems of seasonal variation[2] which can lead to seriously misleading results.

Is the poor growth of pre- or postnatal onset?

The answer to this question will, by and large, depend on the assessment of birth weight and length. Sadly, birth length is rarely measured with any accuracy in this country and we are usually dependent upon weight. More recently it has become increasingly common to have direct evidence of poor intra-uterine growth from sequential ultrasound measurements. A low birth weight for gestational age suggests that growth failure commenced *in utero* and is more typically seen in children with short stature due to dysmorphic or chromosomal syndromes. On the other hand, a normal birth weight, suggesting normal intra-uterine growth followed subsequently by poor growth velocity, is generally more typical of the endocrine disorders.

Is there growth delay?

Usually growth failure associated with general paediatric disease and endocrine disorders is associated with some degree of growth delay.

There is also, of course, the common problem of constitutional delay of growth and development. Assessment of delay in the child of peri-pubertal age range can be conveniently made clinically by the assessment of pubertal stages (see previous chapter). In the younger child some other objective assessment of maturation is clearly required. Bone age as a measure of skeletal maturity is by far the most useful technique, usually depending upon the left hand and wrist for its assessment.

Are there any specific clinical stigmata?

This should include such aspects as body proportions, body composition and the presence of specific clinical signs. The use of measurements of sitting height and subischial leg length and comparison with appropriate standards provides a useful screening test for many of the bone dysplasias, although by no means all are associated with disproportion.

Body composition is difficult to assess in a detailed manner as it sometimes requires quite invasive methods. A simple clinical assessment of skinfold thickness does, however, give some idea of total body fat and can be a helpful addition to clinical assessment. By and large, children with endocrine abnormalities have excessive subcutaneous fat, whereas in the dysmorphic syndromes normal amounts of fat are usual.

Other more specific clinical findings may be especially helpful. Here is not the place for a detailed list of such abnormalities, but examples would include the presence of small external genitalia in a male, suggesting pituitary abnormalities, and *café au lait* spots or axillary freckling, suggesting neurofibromatosis.

After answering these five questions one should be in a position to form an assessment of the direction for further investigation. In a child who is short, growing slowly, tending to be fat but otherwise of quite normal appearance and with growth delay, clearly the endocrine abnormalities would be uppermost in one's mind. Alternatively, a child who was certainly short but growing normally, with prenatal onset of growth failure and no growth delay, one might be more inclined to think of a dysmorphic syndrome. Severe disproportion with very short limbs suggests one of the bone dysplasias, perhaps hypochondroplasia.

LABORATORY AND OTHER INVESTIGATIONS

The manner in which these are carried out depends, to some extent, on the local situation. Much of the investigation of children with growth problems can be carried out on an outpatient or day-case basis, doing a limited number of investigations at a time and waiting for results before proceeding to the next step. In contrast, there are sometimes occasions where it is more desirable to perform a battery of investigations without intermediate results. My own prejudice is to avoid the latter approach where possible as many of the tests are discomforting to the child and best avoided if not necessary. Here I will discuss the various investigations under the four broad headings of the most likely diagnoses that are being pursued; of course, there would usually be overlap.

GENERAL INVESTIGATIONS

Here one is aiming to identify children with growth problems secondary to some other disorder, such as some of the more subtle renal disorders, particularly tubular. These should include:

(1) haemoglobin and blood film,
(2) plasma electrolytes and creatinine,
(3) plasma calcium and phosphate,
(4) serum iron,
(5) red blood cell folate,
(6) erythrocyte sedimentation rate.

Any abnormalities in these results would naturally lead to appropriate specific studies.

GASTRO-INTESTINAL INVESTIGATIONS

As this forms the largest group of covert general paediatric diseases presenting with short stature they are grouped alone. The results from the above investigations may further suggest a gastro-intestinal cause, although not necessarily. If there is any doubt of diagnosis, jejunal biopsy to exclude coeliac disease is essential and barium meal and follow-through to exclude Crohn's disease.

GENETIC/DYSMORPHIC SYNDROMES

Here the emphasis is much more on detailed clinical assessment, but there are two major investigations: skeletal survey and karyotype analysis. In respect of the latter there should be a particularly low threshold in performing this investigation in girls with short stature and no obvious diagnosis. Turner syndrome is notorious for being quite subtle at times, and although it is not usually considered in the treatable groups of diseases, there is no doubt that earlier diagnosis leads to more satisfactory counselling of the patient and the more sympathetic handling of the problems in the teenage years.

ENDOCRINE SYNDROMES

Here we are involved in two aspects. On the one hand, we are interested in making the diagnosis and defining any possible endocrine abnormality leading to short stature and, on the other hand, in those found to have an endocrine abnormality we wish to decide the extent of this. The latter point is particularly relevant where pituitary disease is found, as it is important to know not only about the growth hormone status but also about the other aspects of pituitary function for optimum management.

Although it is often possible, and indeed desirable, to combine pituitary investigations, it is probably easier to consider the different endocrine axes independently in the first instance. However, as the many endocrine systems have already been considered in some depth in other parts of this book, here only the assessment of growth hormone status is discussed. Some comments about combined investigations will follow later.

Investigation of growth hormone deficiency

In many ways this is still one of the least satisfactory hormone systems to investigate. As is the case in many endocrine systems, growth hormone is secreted in a pulsatile manner, most frequently during sleep. The use, therefore, of a basal growth hormone level is of no value whatsoever and some form of provocation test is still required. These tend to fall into two broad categories: those for screening purposes and those for definitive diagnosis. Even in the latter case, however, it is important to emphasize that no biochemical investigations alone can really make this diagnosis and it really must be combined with the clinical and auxological assessment for any reliable result. A general description of provocation tests will be found in Milner and Burns[3].

The use of screening tests has had varying degrees of popularity and their value rather depends upon the patient population that any one clinic is seeing. As even the best screening tests have a rather high percentage of false positive results, many people feel that they are not worth the extra tests involved. However, with this cautionary comment, the best screening test is now probably the use of controlled exercise, with blood being taken for growth hormone estimation 20 minutes after the cessation of the exercise. This is only really practical in children over the age of about 8 where good co-operation may be obtained, and the exercise is best administered by the use of a bicycle ergometer. It is important that for each child the exercise produces a significant degree of fatigue, with elevation of the pulse rate and sweating. There seems to be little value in a blood sample taken before the start of the exercise as the only thing of importance is whether the postexercise value is in excess of 15 mU/l. If it is, then a diagnosis of growth hormone deficiency is excluded, whereas if it falls below this value further definitive investigations are required.

In the area of definitive tests for growth hormone deficiency the situation is still more confusing. For many years the insulin hypoglycaemia test has been the lynchpin of such investigations. The insulin is usually given at a dose of 0.1 mg/kg body-weight intravenously and blood is taken at 15 minute intervals for 90 minutes. The blood sugar should fall to 2.2 mmol/l or lower. Given that this occurs, a rise in growth hormone to a peak of < 7 mU/l strongly suggests severe growth hormone deficiency, whereas a rise to a peak of between 7 and 15 mU/l is suggestive of a partial deficiency. Peak values in excess of 15 mU/l almost certainly exclude the diagnosis. Two further tests have assumed progressively greater prominence as alternatives to insulin hypoglycaemia: the arginine infusion and oral clonidine tests. Arginine hydrochloride is given at a dose of 500 mg/kg body-weight over a 30 minute infusion and blood samples taken at 30 minute intervals up to 150 minutes. In the clonidine test, oral clonidine at a dose of 0.15 mg/m^2 is given and samples taken at 15 minute intervals for 150 minutes. In both tests the criteria for severe or partial growth hormone deficiency are the same as for insulin hypoglycaemia.

Most people now consider that at least two definitive tests are required for a diagnosis of growth hormone deficiency and these are often combined, particularly as a composite of the insulin hypoglycaemia and arginine infusion tests. In this situation the insulin may be given first, followed by the arginine infusion or vice versa. In many situations double-testing is of value, but equally it seems to be an unnecessary adornment in a child who has the full auxological and clinical appearance of the diagnosis and an unequivocal result in the first definitive test.

There are two further tests that should be mentioned. In the first place the use of insulin hypoglycaemia or arginine may be very difficult in the very young, rather fat child. A useful accessory test is intramuscular glucagon in a dose of 100 μg/kg, but blood samples must be taken at 30 minute intervals for as long as 3 hours as the peak growth hormone response may be late. It has the advantage that the glucagon is given intramuscularly and the blood samples may be taken by capillary sampling, obviating the need for any form of intravenous line. The second test, or rather modification of an earlier test, is sex hormone priming of insulin hypoglycaemia. In patients who are in the immediate prepubertal age range with bone ages in excess of 10 'years' in boys or girls and little or no sign of puberty, there is often a blunting of the growth hormone response to conventional provocation[4]. With the onset of spontaneous puberty this transient apparent growth hormone deficiency is restored to normal and no growth hormone replacement is required. At the present time the best way of modifying the existing provocation test is the use of a single intramuscular dose of 100 mg of mixed testosterone esters in boys about 3–5 days before the growth hormone provocation, and in girls the administration of ethinyl oestradiol in a daily dose of 100–200 µg/day for 3 days prior to the test. Although not free of false positive results this modification does seem to improve the discrimination of the conventional test.

It would be inappropriate to discuss the diagnosis of growth hormone deficiency without mention of overnight blood sampling during sleep. Although this technique is in many ways still in its infancy, the use of sleep as one of the most physiological stimuli to growth hormone secretion is gaining in popularity. It requires the patient to be in hospital overnight and in its most rigorous form requires EEG monitoring to allow staging of sleep. However, it has been shown[5] that it can be a practical alternative and a particularly attractive one to those who believe in being as physiological as possible in testing for any hormone deficiency.

Commonly, one is faced with a patient where one suspects an endocrine cause, most usually growth hormone deficiency, and one needs to investigate pituitary function to assess whether there is more than one deficiency and to get a better idea of the aetiological cause. It is now possible to get a very thorough impression of pituitary function by the use of a pituitary cocktail consisting of insulin hypoglycaemia administered at the same time as intravenous boluses of LHRH and TRH. Thus the growth hormone, thyroid and gonadal axes are studied, and as plasma cortisols can be measured at the same time, the pituitary–adrenal axis is also investigated. Hypoglycaemia is a potent stimulus to ACTH release and thus helps to define the ACTH–cortisol status.

We have just alluded to the use of releasing factors (TRH and LHRH) in the investigation of the appropriate axes. More recently the possibility of using growth hormone releasing factor (GRF) has become possible[6]. While requiring much evaluation this may eventually prove to be a very useful test to discriminate between the hypothalamic and pituitary causes of growth hormone deficiency.

Having defined a pituitary defect, be it growth hormone deficiency in an isolated form or as part of a multiple pituitary hormone deficiency, it is still important to decide on the aetiological cause. In a situation where growth hormone is deficient alone the most likely diagnosis is idiopathic growth hormone deficiency, with a number of rare specific causes also being possible[7]. On the other hand, if there are multiple pituitary hormone deficiencies it becomes progressively more likely that the condition is due to a structural lesion of the pituitary or hypothalamus. One is most anxious in this situation to exclude the possibility of a tumour, such as a craniopharyngioma, and skull radiography and computerized axial tomography are important aspects of investigation.

THE MANAGEMENT OF GROWTH HORMONE DEFICIENCY

When growth hormone deficiency is part of more extensive hypo-thalamo–pituitary dysfunction, the other hormone systems require appropriate supplementation. Here we will simply consider the problem of growth hormone.

There are a number of different regimes for growth hormone therapy in different countries of the world. In the United Kingdom it is general to give growth hormone in a dose of 4 IU three times per week by intramuscular injection, under the auspices of the Health Services Human Growth Hormone Committee. In other countries dosages are tailored to body size, usually using weight, the doses typically being in the range 50–100 mIU of growth hormone per kg of body weight given three times weekly. In many countries the dose has to be given at suboptimal levels because of poor supplies of material.

Figure 1 shows a typical response of a boy treated for many years with exogenous growth hormone and his growth curve is quite typical of children who respond satisfactorily. He has isolated growth hormone deficiency and therefore there were no other problems of hormone supplementation but, in essence, these should not alter the situation when necessary. Thyroid and adrenal insufficiencies are relatively easy to identify and treat, although in the case of the latter the dose of replacement steroids should be kept to a minimum[7]. The situation as far as the gonadotrophin–gonadal axis is concerned is always more difficult and identification of a gonadotrophin-deficient child before the age appropriate for puberty is exceedingly difficult, even with the use of the LHRH test. However, the possibility must always be borne in mind and appropriate supplementation instituted if necessary.

Final outcome of children with growth hormone deficiency is still less than optimal[8, 9], but in many cases the reason for this can be related to late diagnosis and hence late commencement of treatment. In other patients, particularly if the diagnosis of growth hormone deficiency is due to a structural lesion of the pituitary or hypothalamus, the ultimate outcome is modified by the complications and it is always important to ensure an optimal orchestration of the various hormone replacements at the relevant time.

More recently there has been a debate as to whether growth hormone replacement should be continued in adult life. At the present time supplies of growth hormone really preclude this possibility, even if it was thought to be of value. In the future, with the possibilities of relatively unlimited supplies of growth hormone due to its synthesis by recombinant DNA techniques, this whole question may need to be readdressed.

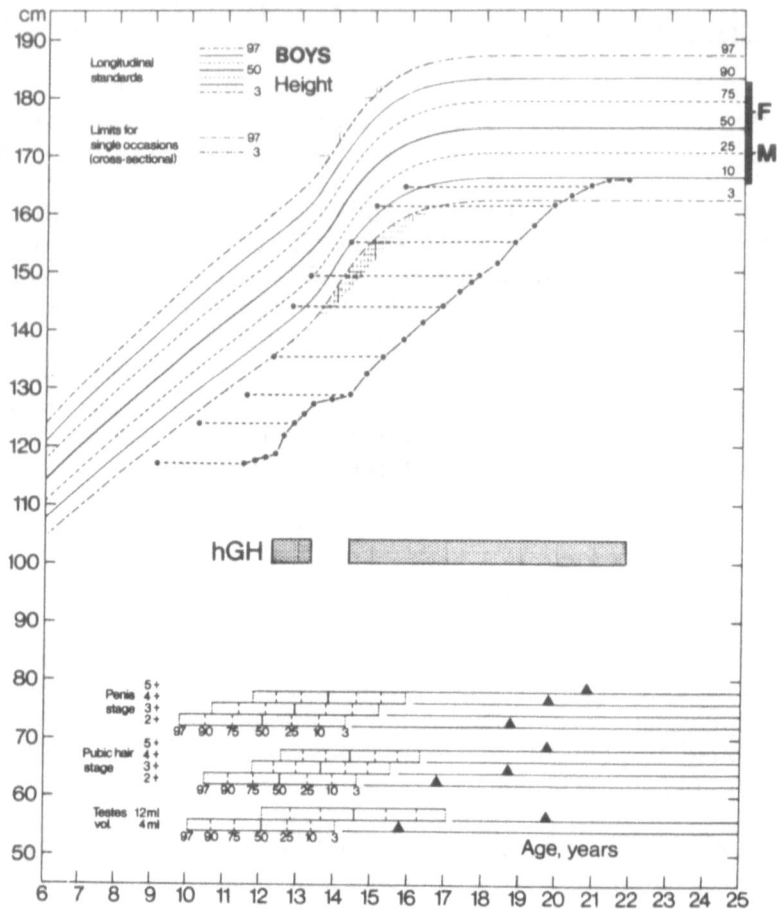

Figure 1 The height curve of a boy with IGHD, treated for 9 years. The parents' centiles are marked on the right-hand axis (M, mother; F, father) and the adjacent heavy vertical bar indicates the target limits for his mature height

References

1. Groll, A., Candy, D. C. A., Preece, M. A., Tanner, J. M. and Harries, J. T. (1980). Short stature as the primary manifestation of coeliac disease. *Lancet*, **2**, 1097–9
2. Marshall, W. A. (1975). The relationship of variations in children's growth rates to seasonal climatic variations. *Ann. Hum. Biol.*, **2**, 243–50
3. Milner, R. D. G. and Burns, E. C. (1982). Investigation of suspected growth hormone deficiency. *Arch. Dis. Child.*, **57**, 944–7
4. Eastman, C. J., Lazarus, L., Stuart, M. C. and Casey, J. H. (1971). The effect of puberty on growth hormone secretion in boys with short stature and delayed adolescence. *Aust. NZ J. Med.*, **2**, 154–9
5. King, J. M. and Price, D. A. (1983). Sleep-induced growth hormone release-evaluation of a simple test for clinical use. *Arch. Dis. Child.*, **58**, 220–2

6. Grossman, A., Savage, M. O., Wass, J. A. H., Lytras, N., Sueiras-Diaz, J., Coy, D. H. and Besser, G. M. (1983). Growth hormone-releasing factor in growth hormone deficiency: demonstration of a hypothalamic defect in growth hormone release. *Lancet*, **2**, 137–8

7. Preece, M. A. (1981). Growth hormone deficiency. In Brook, C. G. D. (ed.) *Clinical Paediatric Endocrinology*. pp. 285–304. (Oxford: Blackwell Scientific Publications)

8. Burns, E. C., Tanner, J. M., Preece, M. A. and Cameron, N. (1981). Final height and pubertal development in 55 children with idiopathic growth hormone deficiency, treated for between 2 and 15 years with human growth hormone. *Eur. J. Pediatr.*, **137**, 155–64

9. Burns, E. C., Tanner, J. M., Preece, M. A. and Cameron, N. (1981). Growth hormone treatment in children with craniopharyngioma: final growth status. *Clin. Endocrinol.*, **14**, 587–95

SECTION 5

Normal and
Abnormal Puberty

Chairman: C. C. FORSYTH

11

ENDOCRINE ASPECTS OF NORMAL PUBERTAL DEVELOPMENT

P. C. SIZONENKO

Puberty is the period within the larger developmental segment of life called adolescence, during which many changes in somatic growth, maturation of gonads and development of secondary sex characteristics occur so reproduction of the species can be maintained. Several review articles have summarized the endocrinologic and metabolic changes observed during this period[1-11].

Onset of puberty is not an isolated event but the result of several phenomena. The sequence of changes is not fully understood, but important information is now available, in particular on the neuroendocrine aspects of puberty. The hypothalamo–hypophyso–gonadal axis is very active during fetal life, in particular when sexual differentiation of the fetus takes place, and at the immediate postnatal period, at 2 months of age, when a rise of sex steroids occurs. Following the second year of age a quiescent period expands until 10 years of age, when the hypothalamo–hypophyso–gonadal axis is at rest. This phase of development has often been called the juvenile period.

After 10 years of age a reactivation of the hypothalamo–pituitary axis happens: pubertal development starts. The central nervous system plays a key role in this reactive phase. The neuroendocrine control is exerted by the arcuate nucleus located in the mediobasal hypothalamus (Figure 1). The arcuate nucleus contains neurones secreting GnRH (gonadotrophin-releasing hormone). The secretion of GnRH is modulated by extrahypothalamic neurones and cortical biogenic amines. Stress and nutrition play an important role in the onset of puberty.

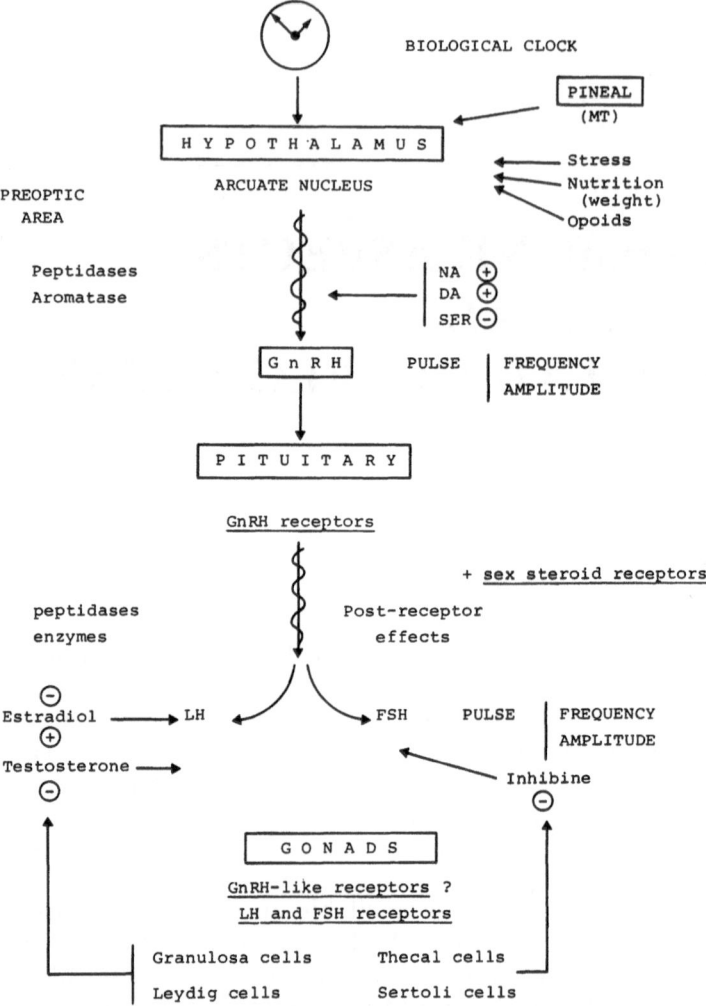

Figure 1 Neuroendocrine axis involved in pubertal development. Under the influence of a biological clock and the stimulating or inhibiting effect of cerebral factors like biogenic amines (norepinephrine [NA], dopamine [DA] and serotonin [SER]) or opiates, environmental factors like stress, nutrition and the pineal gland (secreting in particular melatonin [MT]), the hypothalamus secretes gonadotrophin-releasing hormone (GnRH) by pulses of higher amplitude and/or frequency. GnRH induces synthesis and stimulates secretion of pituitary gonadotrophins (LH and FSH). These hormones are also secreted in a pulsatile fashion. Acting on the ovary or the testis, they induce the ripening of the follicle or spermatogenesis and the secretion of oestradiol or testosterone. In turn, oestradiol and testosterone act on the hypothalamo–pituitary axis through negative (and in addition, in the girl, positive) feedback mechanism. Inhibin, secreted by the testis and the follicle, also plays a role in the feedback mechanism. GnRH, LH and FSH act on target-cells through specific receptors. Reproduced with authorization from Sizonenko et al.[17]

In girls, the mean age of first budding of the breast is 10.9 years (with a range of 8–13 years); menarche occurs at 12 years 9 months (with a range of 10–16 years).

In boys, the first growth of testis is observed at a mean age of 11.5 years (range 9–14 years). Adult genitalia is observed from 14.5 to 18 years, with a mean age of 15 years. (Emission of spermatozoa in the urine has been observed at a median age of 14.5 years[12, 13].)

Numerous factors influence the age of onset of puberty and its development. Some are endogenous or genetic, like familial delay in pubertal development. Others are exogenous, like nutrition or sport. According to Frish and Revelle[14], nutritional factors play an important role in the onset of puberty. Many studies have shown that menarche is related to a critical body composition (in particular fat content) and a

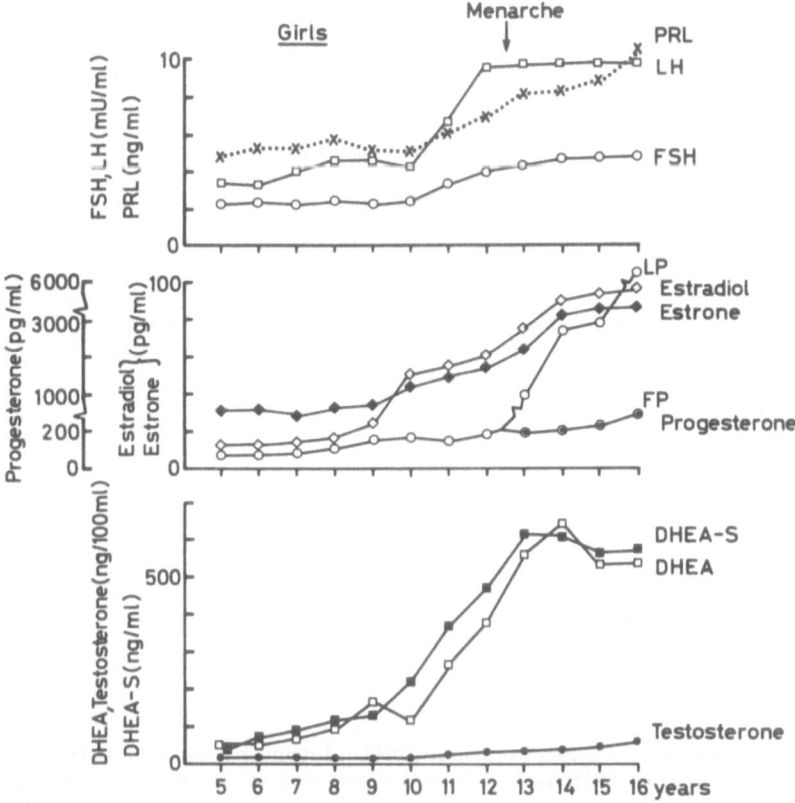

Figure 2 Changes of plasma prolactin (PRL), luteinizing hormone (LH), follicle-stimulating hormone (FSH), oestradiol, oestrone, progesterone (before puberty and after menarche), dehydroepiandrosterone (DHEA), dehydroepiandrosterone sulphate (DHEA-S) and testosterone before, during and after puberty in normal girls. LP and FP represent progesterone levels during luteal phase (open circles) and follicular phase (closed circles) after menarche. Reproduced with authorization from Sizonenko[10]

critical weight. The mean critical weight is 47.8 kg for American girls and most of the European girls. However, this 'critical weight' theory reflects most probably a temporal relationship rather than a real cause–effect relationship of the cerebral 'appetite' and 'onset of puberty' centres.

Plasma hormonal changes have been analysed by many authors since 1972. These changes are schematically drawn in Figure 2 for girls and in Figure 3 for boys.

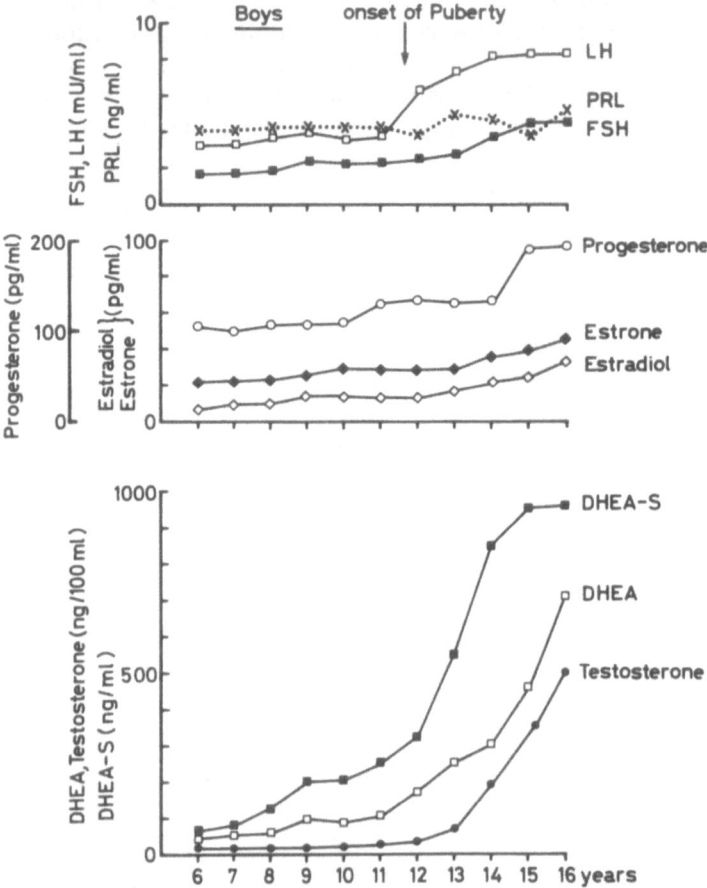

Figure 3 Changes of plasma prolactin (PRL), luteinizing hormone (LH), follicle-stimulating hormone (FSH), progesterone, oestrone, oestradiol, dehydroepiandrosterone (DHEA), dehydroepiandrosterone sulphate (DHEA-S) and testosterone before, during and at end of puberty in normal boys. Reproduced with authorization from Sizonenko[10]

In girls, from 10 years of age, plasma concentrations of FSH, LH and prolactin increase steadily (Figure 2). This increase in gonadotrophins leads to an increase in oestradiol and oestrone. It is only after menarche that progesterone increases during the second part of menstrual cycle, when ovulation occurs. The first ovulatory cycle appears 8–10 months after menarche, and ovulatory cycles follow thereafter (Figure 4). Plasma levels of adrenal androgens, dehydroepiandrosterone and its sulphate increase early, from 7 years of age. Testosterone mainly, from ovarian origin, is secreted in a low level, as Δ_4-androstenedione, the origin of which is both ovarian and adrenal.

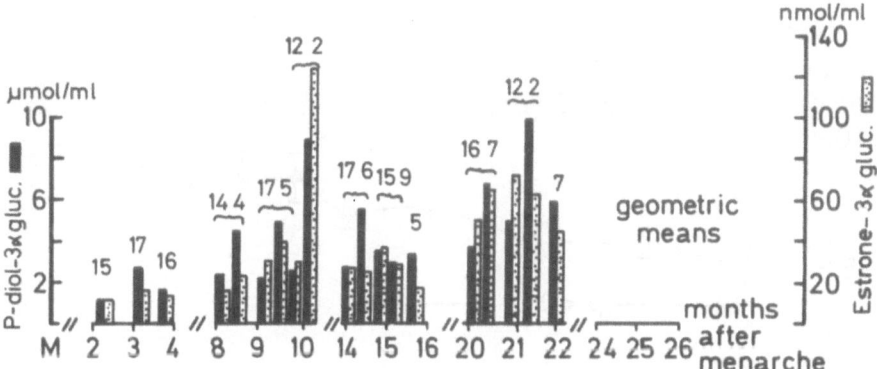

Figure 4 Mean changes in urinary concentrations of pregnanediol-3α-glucuronide (P-diol-3α-gluc) and oestrone-3α-glucuronide (oestrone-3α-gluc) in 24 girls followed during the 2 years after the onset of menarche. The number of samples analysed is indicated above the bars. The evaluation of geometric mean urinary concentrations of pregnanediol-3α-glucuronide shows that first ovulation seems to appear 10 months after menarche (P-diol-3α-gluc > 5 μmol/l). Urinary oestrone-3α-glucuronide steadily increases during the postmenarchial period to reach mean values of 50–70 nmol/ml 20 months after menarche. Reproduced with authorization from Sizonenko and Aubert[15]

In boys, a similar pattern is observed; plasma gonadotrophins rise from 11 years (Figure 3). Plasma prolactin remains similar throughout pubertal development, contrary to what is seen in girls. Plasma testosterone rises markedly from 12 years (above 25 ng/100 ml), reaching adult levels by 15 years (500 ng/100 ml). A slight increase in plasma oestradiol and oestrone is observed mainly at the late stages of puberty. Similarly to girls, plasma adrenal androgens rise 3 years before gonadarche (at 8 years).

Longitudinal studies of the endocrine changes occurring during pubertal development have given new knowledge. In particular, it has been clearly shown that plasma prolactin increases during puberty in girls, mostly during the first menstrual cycles, simultaneously with the increasing level of oestradiol (Figure 5). The occurrence of breast development was associated with the achievement of similar plasma levels of oestradiol in normal girls, in girls with premature adrenarche (premature development of public and axillary hair) and in girls with delayed puberty (onset of breast at a mean age of 12.5 years, instead of 10.5 in normal girls): 20.5 ± 2.5, 25.9 ± 3.2 and 22.5 ± 1.9 pg/ml, respectively. Similarly, the mean levels of dehydroepiandrosterone achieved at the time of appearance of pubic hair is comparable in girls with premature adrenarche or delayed puberty or in normal girls (190 ± 31, 209 ± 43, 186 ± 31 ng/100 ml, respectively, mean $\pm$ SEM).

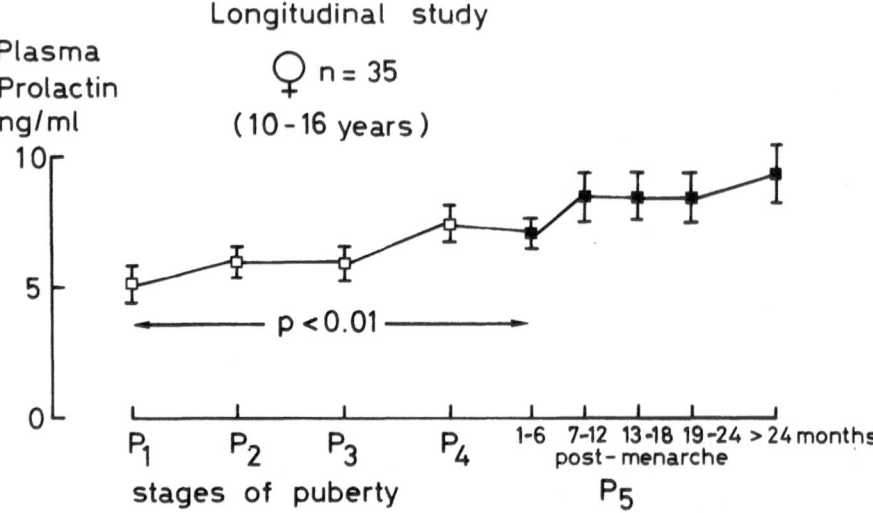

Figure 5 Pattern of change of plasma prolactin in relation to stage of pubertal development. Menstruating girls (P_5), designated by closed squares, were classified according to the time elapsed since onset of menses. Reproduced from Aubert *et al.* with authorization[16]

Plasma concentration of oestrone in plasma of girls between chronological age of 7–10 years remained unchanged, plasma oestrone level (30 pg/ml) being higher than plasma oestradiol (10 pg/ml). From 11 years, plasma oestrone rises progressively (Figure 6). Plasma oestradiol rises also from 9.5 years, reaching by 10 years the level of oestrone. Then, the two oestrogens increase steadily during the pubertal development, reaching a plateau at 12.5 years with very comparable levels for both of them. A similar pattern is observed for plasma oestrone and oestradiol when analysed in correlation with bone age. The first significant rise of oestrone is observed between 10 and 11 years. Oestrone levels are normal in Turner's syndrome and are slightly elevated in girls with premature adrenarche. Although oestrone mainly comes from the adrenal cortex before pubertal age, the pattern of oestrone is not similar to that of the adrenal androgens, as observed in normal children. Later on, the ovary may play a role in the secretion of oestrone, and/or the rate of aromatization of adrenal androgens or the rate of interconversion of oestradiol to oestrone is modified.

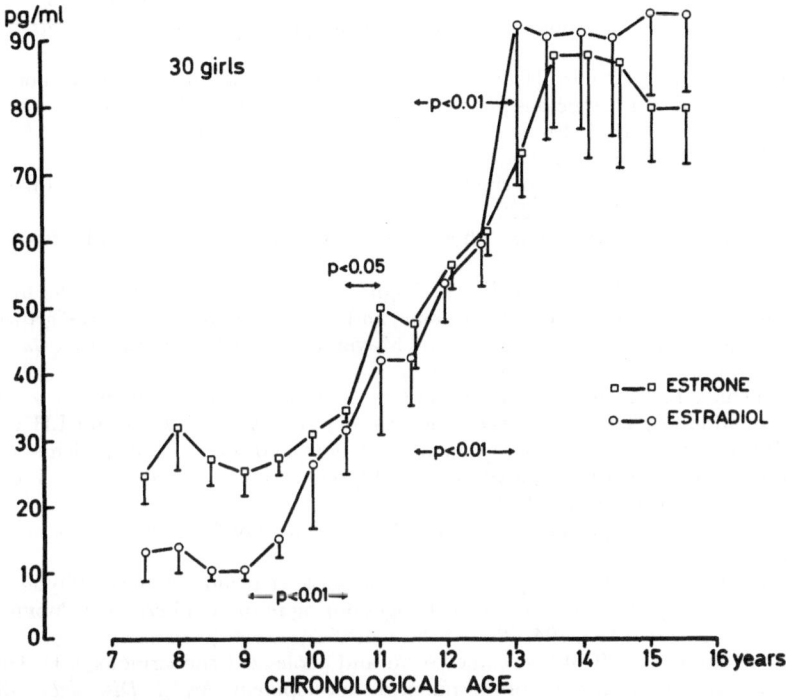

Figure 6 Mean plasma levels ($\pm$ SEM) of oestrone (E_1) and oestradiol (E_2) in 30 normal girls followed longitudinally every 6 months from 7 to 16 years during pubertal development

CONCLUSION

A general scheme of the presently known neuroendocrine events occurring with the onset of puberty has been described. Indirect experiments, both in the animal and human, suggest that the arcuate nucleus located in the mediobasal hypothalamus secretes GnRH by pulses (with increasing amplitude, and probably frequency). GnRH stimulates the secretion of gonadotrophins (LH and FSH) with maturation of the ovary and the testis, ripening of the follicle or spermatogenesis and secretion of oestradiol or of testosterone. Prolactin rises in the girl. The maturation of the adrenal cortex (adrenarche) occurs 3 years before the maturation of the gonad (gonadarche).

References

1. Sizonenko, P. C. and Burr, I. M. (1972). Problèmes physiologiques de la puberté. III. Les fonctions hypophysaires. *Arch. Fr. Pédiatr.*, **29**, 203–20

2. Sizonenko, P. C., Lewin, M. and Burr, I. M. (1972). Problèmes physiologiques de la puberté. II. Les sécrétions endocriniennes périphériques. *Arch. Fr. Pédiatr.*, **29**, 185–201
3. Reiter, E. O. and Kulin, H. E. (1972). Sexual maturation in the female: normal development and precocious puberty. *Pediatr. Clin. N. Am.*, **19**, 581–603
4. Root, A. W. (1973a). Endocrinology of puberty. I. Normal sexual maturation. *J. Pediatr.*, **83**, 1–19
5. Root, A. W. (1973b). Endocrinology of puberty. II. Aberrations of sexual maturation. *J. Pediatr.*, **83**, 187–200
6. Visser, H. K. A. (1973). Some physiological and clinical aspects of puberty. *Arch. Dis. Child.*, **48**, 169–82
7. Blizzard, R. M., Thompson, R. G., Baghdassarian, A. *et al.* (1974). The interrelationship of steroids, growth hormone, and other hormones on pubertal growth. In Grumbach, M. M., Grave, G. D. and Mayer, F. E. (eds.) *The Control of the Onset of Puberty.* pp. 342–59. (New York: Wiley)
8. Sizonenko, P. C. and Paunier, L. (1975). Hormonal changes in puberty. III. Correlation of plasma dehydroepiandrosterone, testosterone, FSH and LH with stages of puberty and bone age in normal boys and girls and in patients with Addison's disease or hypogonadism or with premature or late adrenarche. *J. Clin. Endocrinol. Metab.*, **41**, 894–904
9. Forest, M. G. (1975). Differentiation and development of the male. *Clin. Endocrinol. Metab.*, **4**, 569–96
10. Sizonenko, P. C. (1978a). Pre-adolescent and adolescent endocrinology. Physiology and physiopathology. I. Hormonal changes during normal pubertal development. *Am. J. Dis. Child.*, **132**, 704–12
11. Sizonenko, P. C. (1978b). Pre-adolescent and adolescent endocrinology. II. Hormonal changes during abnormal pubertal development. *Am. J. Dis. Child.*, **132**, 797–805
12. Richardson, D. W. and Short, R. V. (1978). Time of onset of sperm production in boys. *J. Biosoc. Sci.*, Suppl. **5**, 15–25
13. Hirsch, M., Shemesh, J., Modan, M. and Lunenfeld, B. (1979). Emission of spermatozoa: age of onset. *Int. J. Androl.*, **2**, 289–98
14. Frish, R. E. (1974). Critical weight at menarche: initiation of the adolescent growth spurt in girls and control of puberty. In Grumbach, M. M., Grave, G. D. and Mayer, F. E. (eds.) *The Control of the Onset of Puberty.* pp. 403–23. (New York: Wiley)
15. Sizonenko, P. C. and Aubert, M. L. (1984). Pituitary gonadotrophins, prolactin and sex steroids secretions in prepuberty and puberty. In Grumbach, M. M., Aubert, M. L. and Sizonenko, P. C. (eds.) *The Control of the Onset of Puberty. II.* (London: Academic Press) (In press)
16. Aubert, M. L., Sizonenko, P. C., Kaplan, S. L. and Grumbach, M. M. (1977). The ontogenesis of human prolactin from fetal life to puberty. In Crosignani, P. G. and Robyn, C. (eds.) *Prolactin and Human Reproduction.* pp. 9–15. (London: Academic Press)
17. Sizonenko, P. C., Lang, U. and Aubert, M. L. (1982). Neuroendocrinologie de la puberté. *Ann. Endocrinol.*, **43**, 453–64

12

THE EFFECTS OF CANCER TREATMENT ON GROWTH AND SEXUAL DEVELOPMENT

S. M. SHALET

There are a number of factors which may adversely affect growth in children treated for cancer. These include direct radiation damage to the long bones[1] and spine[2], malnutrition and steroid therapy. Additional factors which may well be important are cytotoxic drugs[3] and the presence of residual tumour. In recent years there has been an increasing interest in abnormalities of growth which result from the endocrine complications of cancer treatment. There are two main reasons for the increased attention. Firstly, the types of cancer in which these endocrine complications may occur are common and, secondly, the endocrine causes of impaired growth are eminently treatable, i.e. hypothyroidism and growth hormone deficiency.

A number of children who received neck irradiation for Hodgkin's disease and other lymphoma have abnormal thyroid function tests. In predominantly adult series the frequency of thyroid dysfunction varies markedly. Fuks et al.[4] found elevated serum thyroid-stimulating hormone (TSH) and normal serum thyroxine (T_4) levels in 44% of their patients and raised TSH plus low T_4 levels in an additional 20%. Schimpff et al.[5] found almost identical results, with 41% having an isolated elevation of the serum TSH and a further 25% TSH elevation and a low T_4 level. The dose of irradiation to the neck received by the patients studied by these two groups ranged between 4000 and 5000 cGy over 4–5 weeks. Not unexpectedly, the incidence and severity of radiation-induced thyroid dysfunction appears to be lower in patients receiving less than 4000 cGy to the neck[6]. The inclusion of a TRH stimulation test to amplify minor abnormalities in basal TSH secretion has revealed a further group of patients who show an exaggerated TSH response to TRH but normal basal serum T_3 and T_4 concentrations[6,7].

The early Stanford studies[8] suggested that there was a higher incidence of thyroid dysfunction following neck irradiation in young patients. Glatstein et al.[8] found a 48% incidence of TSH elevation among patients under 20 years of age but a 33% rate for older patients. Other groups[5,9] have found the age at irradiation to be irrelevant.

The bulk of accumulated data regarding radiation-induced hypothyroidism is derived from studies performed in patients treated for lymphoma or head and neck cancer. These individuals have generally received doses of irradiation in the range of 3000–5000 cGy given in multiple fractions over several weeks. Sklar et al.[10] have recently shown that the incidence of thyroid dysfunction is similar following a single dose of 750 cGy. They studied thyroid function in 27 long-term survivors of bone marrow transplantation in childhood. Twenty-three patients received single-dose whole-body or total lymphoid irradiation (750 cGy) and 10 developed thyroid dysfunction within a median time of 13 months, two of whom had low T_4 as well as raised TSH levels.

The treatment of hypothyroidism (raised TSH, low T_4), whether it be due to radiation-induced thyroid damage or any other cause, is thyroxine. It is not clear whether all patients with compensated thyroid dysfunction (raised TSH, normal T_4) should also receive lifelong thyroxine replacement therapy. Support for this view is derived from the observation that an elevated TSH level in the presence of irradiation-damaged thyroid tissue is known to be carcinogenic. Therefore, it is argued that TSH suppression may lessen the recognized potential for development of post-irradiation thyroid carcinoma. However, this is based on animal data and there is no conclusive evidence in man that a raised TSH level has a carcinogenic role in the presence of radiation-induced thyroid damage. Furthermore, virtually all of these patients have had relatively high-dose irradiation to the neck for lymphoma and there is no convincing evidence that such patients have an increased risk of developing thyroid cancer. However, there are a large number of children who have received a significant but lower dose of irradiation to the thyroid gland as a result of the spinal field component of whole CNS irradiation for medulloblastoma and acute lymphoblastic leukaemia. These children, not infrequently, show evidence of compensated thyroid dysfunction and have a greater theoretical risk of developing thyroid cancer in later years.

Considerable debate has been generated over whether compensated thyroid dysfunction actually represents a mild but significant form of hypothyroidism[11] or merely a biochemical abnormality. More recently, Ridgway et al.[12] have shown that patients with compensated thyroid dysfunction have alterations in the cardiac systolic time interval which can be changed significantly by thyroxine replacement in doses which reduce the previously raised TSH level into the normal range. These data support the concept that such patients have a subclinical or very mild form of primary hypothyroidism which can be corrected by thyroxine. If, however, thyroid hormone replacement therapy is not instituted in patients with compensated thyroid dysfunction following radiation damage, then clinical examination and biochemical assessment of thyroid function should be performed at least annually.

GROWTH IMPAIRMENT IN CHILDREN TREATED FOR BRAIN TUMOURS

Short stature is an extremely common complication following the treatment of brain tumours in childhood[13,14]. The brain tumours include gliomas, ependymomas and medulloblastomas, all lesions which do not directly involve the hypothalamic–pituitary axis. The treatment of these tumours may include neurosurgery, cranial or craniospinal irradiation and chemotherapy. Poor growth in children receiving whole CNS irradiation was not too surprising as it has been recognized for a number of years that spinal irradiation may impair spinal growth[2]. However, some children who were small had received only cranial irradiation, suggesting that other adverse factors which affected growth were important. Several years after treatment, many of these children were found to be biochemically growth hormone (GH)-deficient, although hypothalamic–pituitary function was normal immediately after surgery and before radiotherapy[15]. Subsequently, it was shown that a strong correlation[16] existed between the dose of irradiation received by the hypothalamic–pituitary axis and the GH response to a standard pharmacological stimulus (insulin tolerance test). Furthermore, Czernichow et al.[17] described a high incidence of GH deficiency in children who received a significant radiation dose to the hypothalamic–pituitary axis during radiotherapy for extracranial tumours.

It has not yet been possible to define a radiation dose to the hypothalamic–pituitary region above which GH deficiency ensues and below which no pituitary dysfunction follows. However, it appeared that a radiation dose in the 2500–3000 cGy range (16 fractions over 3 weeks) was required to impair the GH response to insulin hypoglycaemia in childhood[16]. A prospective study[18] in children treated for brain tumours, each of whom received a radiation dose of 2700 cGy or greater (16 fractions over 3 weeks) to the hypothalamic–pituitary region, indicated that the majority of such patients will show impaired GH responses to an insulin tolerance test within 2 years, but an occasional patient may not become GH-deficient for several years after radiotherapy (Figure 1).

An earlier retrospective study[19] had shown that patients who received less than 3500–4000 cGy (16 fractions over 3 weeks) irradiation to the hypothalamic–pituitary axis during childhood retained normal anterior pituitary function, except for GH secretion, between 8 and 32 years later. However, if the radiation dose is significantly greater then multiple pituitary hormonal deficiencies may ensue[20,21].

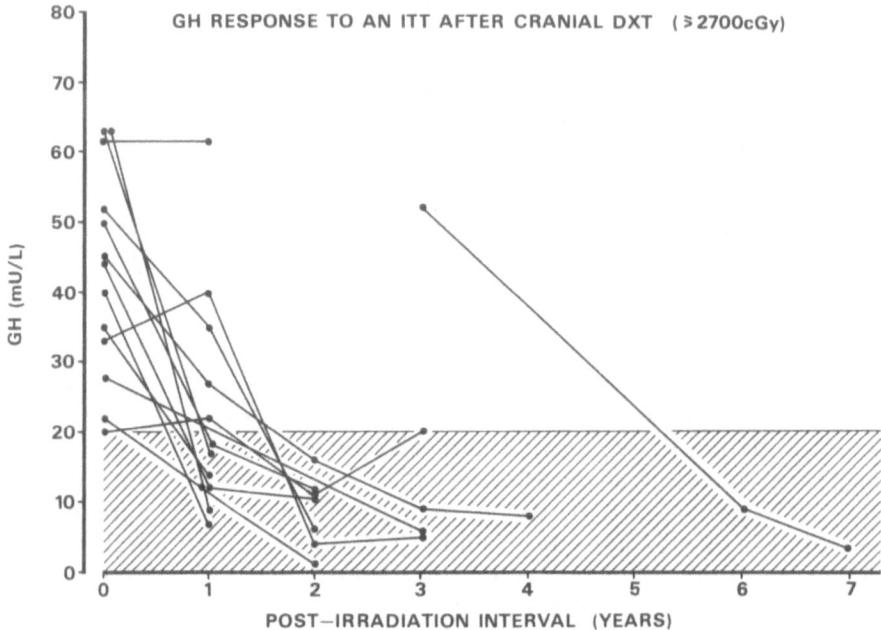

Figure 1   Peak growth hormone responses to insulin hypoglycaemia in 14 children with brain tumours, each of whom received a radiation dose of 2700 cGy (3 weeks) or greater to the hypothalamic–pituitary region

Apart from spinal irradiation and GH deficiency, there are other factors which may impair growth in children treated for brain tumours. During the first year after surgery and radiotherapy for a brain tumour, most children grow poorly[18]. The poor growth is independent of the development of GH deficiency[18]. Possible adverse factors include recurrent tumour, chemotherapy and malnutrition.

GROWTH IMPAIRMENT IN CHILDREN TREATED FOR ACUTE LYMPHOBLASTIC LEUKAEMIA (ALL)

Following the observation that radiation-induced GH deficiency may complicate the treatment of brain tumours in childhood, various groups studied GH secretion in children who had received prophylactic cranial irradiation several years earlier as part of their therapy for ALL. Initially there was disagreement about whether or not GH secretion was blunted in such children, but it soon became apparent that an important variable in these studies was the effective biological dose of radiation reaching the hypothalamic–pituitary axis[22,23]. Shalet et al.[23] showed that 14 out of 17 children (Group 1) who received cranial irradiation in a dose of 2500 cGy in 10 fractions over 16 days had a subnormal GH response to an ITT, whereas only one out of nine children (Group 2) who received a dose of 2400 cGy in 20 fractions over 4 weeks showed an impaired GH response to the same stimulus (Figure 2).

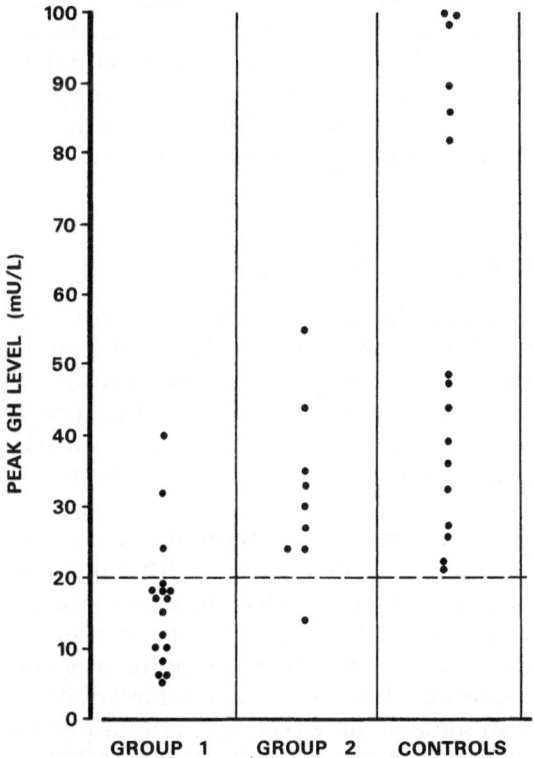

Figure 2 Peak growth hormone responses to insulin hypoglycaemia in controls and in children who had received cranial irradiation, either in a dose of 2500 cGy in 10 fractions over 16 days (Group 1) or 2400 cGy in 20 fractions over 4 weeks (Group 2)

The children in both groups were studied several years after their chemotherapy had been completed and at a time when they were in clinical and haematological remission. Those in Group 1 showed a normal growth velocity and serum somatomedin activity with no evidence of bone age retardation, which suggested that the normal physiological requirements of GH secretion had been met despite the blunted GH responses to certain pharmacological stimuli.

These results illustrate why so few ALL children who previously received the cranial radiation dose used in Group 1 actually require GH therapy. More recently, it has been shown that the dose of cranial irradiation required to prevent CNS leukaemic infiltration can safely be lowered from 2400 cGy to 1800 cGy[24], a dose which is unlikely to impair GH secretion either physiologically or in response to pharmacological stimuli.

At diagnosis it has been claimed that ALL children are significantly taller than the normal population[25]. However, Berry *et al.*[26] have suggested that a significant number of ALL children under 4 years of age are short at presentation. Whatever the height at diagnosis it is clear that these children show a definite but small loss of potential height following therapy. The author[27] attributes this to the effects of cytotoxic drugs and steroids. However, other workers[28] believe that the small loss in height is due to radiation-induced transient GH deficiency.

GROWTH HORMONE THERAPY

Shalet *et al.*[29] treated six children with radiation-induced GH deficiency with GH. These children were treated between 3 and 10 years after cranial irradiation for a brain tumour. The mean growth during the pretreatment year was 3.7 cm and during the first year of GH therapy was 7.9 cm. Similar increases in growth velocity with GH therapy have been described in other children with radiation-induced GH deficiency[20, 30].

Unfortunately, there are no long-term studies of the effects of GH therapy in a large number of children with radiation-induced GH deficiency. In the Manchester growth clinic over the last 6 years we have treated 20 such children with GH therapy for varying lengths of time. Our data suggest that there has been a significant growth response to GH therapy in children who received cranial irradiation alone, but the growth response in some of those receiving craniospinal irradiation has been less satisfactory. The majority of the former children had received a radiation dose of 3500 cGy or greater (16 fractions over 3 weeks) to the hypothalamic–pituitary axis. Nearly all the children who received craniospinal irradiation had been treated for medulloblastoma. The radiation dose was usually lower in these children and, in most cases, it was in the region of 3000 cGy (16 fractions over 3 weeks) or less. The explanation for the varied growth responses to GH therapy in this group may be that not all these children were clinically GH-deficient, despite subnormal GH responses to pharmacological stimuli.

The data in the children treated for brain tumours and ALL had led the author to speculate that not only is GH the first anterior pituitary hormone to be affected by radiation damage to the hypothalamic–pituitary axis but that the biochemical manifestation of impaired GH secretion is dependent on the severity of radiation damage. At the lower radiation doses the GH response to insulin hypoglycaemia is blunted, with increasing radiation dosage the GH response to arginine stimulation is impaired[23, 31], followed by diminution of pulsatile GH secretion.

The first studies on daily GH production following radiation to the hypothalamic–pituitary axis have now been published. Chrousos et al.[32] assessed anterior pituitary function in two groups of monkeys who received either 2400 cGy or 4000 cGy cranial irradiation in 10 fractions over 2 weeks. They substantiated the observation in humans that impairment of the GH response to insulin hypoglycaemia was a particularly early feature of radiation-induced damage to the hypothalamus. However, their other observations in the animals treated with 4000 cGy contradicted the hypothesis put forward above. One year after radiation they found a marked decrease in both frequency and amplitude of GH secretory spikes through 24 hours despite a normal GH response to stimulation by L-dopa or arginine. This suggests that an irradiated patient may have an alteration in the GH secretory pattern resulting in suboptimal growth, although GH responses to certain standard pharmacological stimuli remain normal.

Further points worthy of consideration are the effects of GH therapy on the primary tumour and the possibility of treating children with radiation-induced GH deficiency with growth hormone-releasing factor.

Out of the 20 children in the Manchester growth clinic who received GH therapy for radiation-induced GH deficiency following treatment of a brain tumour, only two have developed a recurrence of their original brain tumour (one ependymoma and one medulloblastoma). A further two had a recurrence in the year of assessment before they ever received GH.

There are 10 children in the UK who received GH therapy for radiation-induced GH deficiency following the treatment of ALL. Only two have had a relapse of ALL whilst on GH therapy, and in one of these the probable precipitating factor was an attack of measles (personal communication, Health Services Human Growth Hormone Committee).

The recent identification and isolation of a growth hormone-releasing factor produced by a pancreatic tumour has stimulated enormous interest. Subsequent immunocytochemical and biochemical analysis has demonstrated the presence of the same material in the hypothalamus. In patients with radiation-induced hypothalamic–pituitary dysfunction evidence has accumulated that the hypothalamus is more radiosensitive than the pituitary[21,23,31]. This means that it may be possible to treat children with radiation-induced GH deficiency with growth hormone-releasing factor when more material becomes available[33].

GONADAL FUNCTION

The major cause of gonadal dysfunction in children treated for malignant disease is direct damage to the gonad by either radiation or chemotherapy. However, it should be remembered that irradiation to the hypothalamic–pituitary area may lead to gonadotrophin deficiency or hyperprolactinaemia, both of which may prevent normal pubertal development and impair subsequent reproductive function[34].

CHEMOTHERAPY

There are a number of reports[35–37] of testicular damage following single-agent cytotoxic drug therapy in childhood. The alkylating agents, in particular, may cause gonadal damage and the two drugs which have been incriminated most often are cyclophosphamide and chlorambucil. More recently, the effects of combination chemotherapy on the gonadal function of children treated for ALL or Hodgkin's disease have been studied.

Lendon et al.[38] examined testicular histology in 44 boys treated with combination chemotherapy for ALL. Nearly all of their patients had received their chemotherapy when prepubertal and the mean tubular fertility index (percentage of seminiferous tubules containing identifiable spermatogonia) was 50% of that in age-matched controls. The two drugs predominantly responsible for the testicular damage were cyclophosphamide and cytosine arabinoside ($> 1\,g/m^2$). However, Lendon et al.[38] did find a significant improvement in testicular tubular morphology with increasing time after completion of chemotherapy. Investigation of testicular morphology in these 44 boys showed no evidence of Leydig cell dysfunction[39], thereby implying that these boys would undergo normal pubertal development.

Severe testicular damage is much more common following the use of combination chemotherapy for Hodgkin's disease rather than ALL. Presumably this is a reflection of the capacity of the individual drugs used in these combinations to inflict tubular damage. Sherins et al.[40] found germinal aplasia and very high serum follicle-stimulating hormone (FSH) levels in boys who had received MOPP (mustine, vincristine, procarbazine and prednisolone) therapy for Hodgkin's disease when pubertal. They also studied six boys who received the same treatment but who were prepubertal when they received their chemotherapy and at the time of the study and found that serum FSH, luteinizing hormone (LH) and testosterone concentrations were appropriate for their age. Whitehead et al.[41] also found evidence of severe damage to the germinal epithelium in patients who received MOPP therapy during childhood. Six patients provided semen for analysis between 2.4 and 8 (mean 5.3) years after completion of chemotherapy and were found to be azoospermic. The four boys studied whilst still prepubertal showed normal basal gonadotrophin levels and gonadotrophin responses to luteinizing hormone-releasing hormone (LHRH). However, one subject treated when prepubertal showed normal serum gonadotrophin levels in prepubertal life but an evolving pattern of abnormally-elevated gonadotrophin levels in early puberty, despite the increasing length of time since the completion of chemotherapy. These results emphasized an earlier observation[39] that severe testicular damage in prepubertal life may co-exist with completely normal gonadotrophin levels.

In the study of Sherins et al.[40], nine out of 13 pubertal Ugandan boys developed gynaecomastia after MOPP therapy for Hodgkin's disease. They suggested that the gynaecomastia was an accentuation of the transient breast development observed normally in early puberty but enhanced by a relative decrease in serum testosterone. Alternatively, the marked prevalence of gynaecomastia in the Ugandan boys may have reflected their improved nutritional status once they came under medical care. Whitehead et al.[41] were unable to substantiate these observations as they noted gynaecomastia in only one out of 12 British pubertal boys who were similarly treated with MOPP for Hodgkin's disease. Furthermore, although three prepubertal boys showed subnormal testosterone responses after stimulation with human chorionic gonadotrophin (HCG), all nine late-pubertal or adult males, who had received MOPP earlier in childhood, had normal testosterone levels and had progressed through puberty without disturbance.

There have been relatively few studies on the effects of cytotoxic drugs on ovarian function in the prepubertal and pubertal female. Most studies[35, 42, 43] found no evidence of menstrual dysfunction in women who had received cyclophosphamide for renal disease during childhood. Less encouraging was the morphological study of Miller et al.[44] in which the autopsy of a 13-year-old girl, who had received cyclophosphamide for 29 months, revealed ovaries totally lacking in follicles.

Siris et al.[45] examined the effects of childhood leukaemia and combination chemotherapy on pubertal development and reproductive function in 35 girls and women. Twenty-eight patients underwent normal pubertal maturation in a median time of 74 months after diagnosis of leukaemia and 49 months of chemotherapy. Only three patients showed evidence of primary ovarian dysfunction. None of these three had received cyclophosphamide and, interestingly, only nine out of the 35 females had received this drug. The main drugs used were vincristine, methotrexate, 6-mercaptopurine and steroids, although one of the three girls with primary ovarian dysfunction had also received busulphan. The author has observed definite biochemical evidence of ovarian failure (raised serum FSH level) in four out of 12 prepubertal girls who had received combination chemotherapy for ALL. All four had received cyclophosphamide. Three of the four have undergone normal pubertal development with the previously elevated serum FSH level dropping into the normal range, while the fourth girl remains prepubertal. This clearly indicates that ovarian damage has occurred in some of these patients but that recovery of ovarian function is not uncommon. The ability of cytotoxic chemotherapy to cause profound but transient effects on gonadal function in both sexes was emphasized in a recent study[46] in which children received daunorubicin, vincristine and L-asparaginase as their induction chemotherapy for ALL. The changes were more striking in the boys: serum testosterone fell, gonadotrophin concentrations doubled and there was a decrease in testicular volume within 3 weeks of induction chemotherapy. Subsequently all hormone values returned to normal and the testes increased in size within a further 3 weeks.

Apart from the possibility of reversible gonadal damage, a further difficulty in establishing the incidence of ovarian damage was indicated by the studies of Conte et al.[47]. They found normal basal gonadotrophin levels and gonadotrophin responses to LHRH in 50% of girls with gonadal dysgenesis between 6 and 9 years of age. Therefore, in both sexes reliance on abnormal gonadotrophin levels for the detection of primary gonadal damage during prepubertal life will seriously underestimate the true incidence of such damage. The morphological evidence that such gonadal damage occurs is, however, just as convincing in the female[48] as in the male. The impairment in follicular maturation in such patients may prove reversible with time, but if a serious depletion of primordial follicles has occurred following exposure to cytotoxic drugs in childhood then a premature menopause may be a long-term sequel.

RADIATION

It is known that the normal adult testis is extremely sensitive to the effects of external radiation[49]. The threshold dose of irradiation required to damage the germinal epithelium in childhood is unknown, although a little more information has become available in the last few years. Shalet et al.[50] studied testicular function in 10 men aged between 17 and 36 years, who had received irradiation for a nephroblastoma during childhood. The dose of scattered irradiation to the testes ranged from 268 to

983 cGy (20 fractions over 4 weeks). Eight subjects had either oligo- or azoospermia (sperm count 0–5.6 million/ml) and seven of these had an elevated FSH level. One patient showed evidence of Leydig cell dysfunction with a raised serum LH level and a low plasma testosterone concentration; however, in retrospect, it was apparent that he was the only one studied who showed evidence of renal impairment. Therefore the abnormal LH and testosterone concentrations may have been due to chronic renal failure rather than radiation damage to the Leydig cells.

Subsequently, we have studied testicular function in six boys who required testicular irradiation (2400 cGy over 21 days) for leukaemic infiltration of the testes (ALL relapse). Before irradiation the testosterone response to HCG stimulation was normal in those studied. After irradiation there was no testosterone response to HCG stimulation. In addition to the testicular irradiation these boys also received a further year's combination chemotherapy. Our earlier results[39] had shown that such chemotherapy when used alone did not affect Leydig cell function; however, we cannot exclude the possibility that chemotherapy contributed to the Leydig cell damage by acting synergistically with testicular irradiation. Similar results have recently been reported by Brauner et al.[51].

These results suggest that a fractionated dose of irradiation to the testes of between 268 and 983 cGy (20 fractions over 4 weeks) does not impair Leydig cell function, whilst a much higher dose of 2400 cGy (21 days) causes Leydig cell failure.

Radiation-induced testicular damage in man, during treatment of cancer, has usually resulted from multiple fractionated radiation. The successful application of bone marrow transplantation to the treatment of several potentially fatal disorders in childhood has stimulated interest in the effects of single-dose radiation on gonadal function. These boys receive between 750 and 1000 cGy total lymphoid or whole-body irradiation in a single fraction and short-term high-dose chemotherapy. Preliminary reports[52] suggest that the radiation is responsible for severe Leydig cell dysfunction as well as damage to the germinal epithelium.

Unfortunately, no treatment is available for radiation-induced damage to the germinal epithelium, however, failure of pubertal development due to Leydig cell damage can be corrected by androgen replacement therapy (Figure 3).

When girls and adult women are irradiated, the response of the ovary involves a fixed population of cells which, once destroyed, cannot be replaced. Effects on fertility are most readily explained on the basis of reduction in this fixed pool of oocytes. Not unexpectedly, the dose of irradiation required to destroy all the oocytes in the ovary is larger in younger rather than older women. While a permanent menopause can be caused by a total radiation exposure of about 600 cGy in women 40 years or more in age[53], radiotherapists' estimates of the 50% probability level for permanent sterility is approximately 2000 cGy over a 6-week period in young women[54]. The threshold dose of irradiation required to induce such damage in the prepubertal female may be larger in view of the greater number of oocytes in this age group.

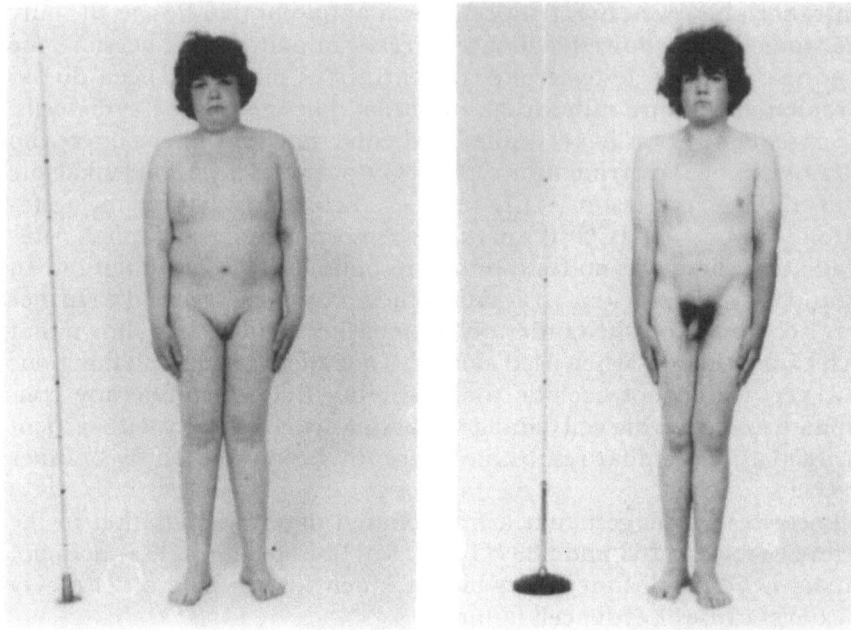

Figure 3 (a) A boy of 13 years and 6 months who, at age 5 years, had a testicular tumour removed followed by scrotal irradiation (3000 cGy over 35 days). He showed no sign of pubertal maturation and a completely absent testosterone response to HCG. (b) Same boy after receiving androgen replacement therapy for 15 months. Note the change in body habitus and the pubertal maturation

Shalet *et al.*[55] studied ovarian function in 18 females treated for abdominal tumours in childhood. Treatment consisted of abdominal irradiation in each case (2000–3000 cGy over 25–44 days) and chemotherapy in seven cases. Only one girl received a cytotoxic drug (cyclophosphamide) known to damage the ovary. All 18 showed very high FSH levels and low oestradiol levels typical of primary ovarian failure. The clinical manifestations of ovarian failure in these young women included amenorrhoea or oligomenorrhoea and poor or absent breast development. Sex steroid replacement therapy will induce breast development (Figure 4) and prevent the subsequent development of osteoporosis. Stillman *et al.*[56] studied a much larger number of long-term survivors of childhood cancer. They found evidence of ovarian failure in 17 out of 25 patients who received an ovarian radiation dose of between 1200 and 5000 cGy and in five out of 35 who received between 90 and

1000 cGy. The abdominal radiotherapy consisted of multiple fractions, but the number of fractions and duration of therapy were not stated. Himelstein-Braw et al.[57] have studied the morphological changes in the irradiated ovaries from girls who died of malignant disease. The dose of irradiation received by these patients was similar to that received by the patients studied by Shalet et al.[55]. Follicle growth was inhibited in all cases and the number of oocytes was markedly reduced in most.

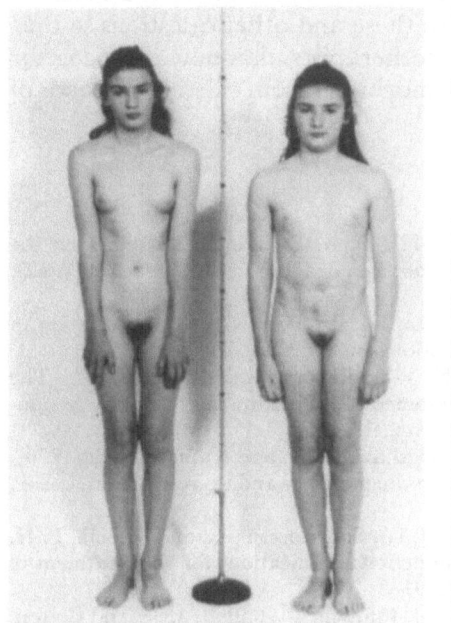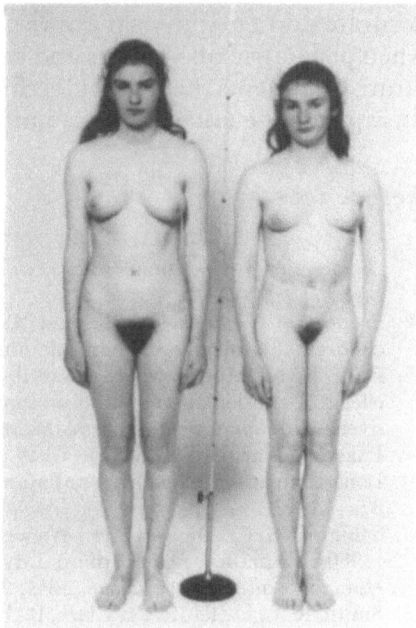

Figure 4 (a) Identical twin girls of 12 years and 6 months; the patient (on the right) had a hysterectomy and oophorectomy when aged 2 years and 6 months for a uterine tumour. Note the complete lack of breast development in the patient. (b) Same girls 3 years later. The patient has received 2 years' oestrogen replacement therapy. Note the excellent breast development

The number of reports concerned with the effects of chemotherapy and irradiation in childhood on subsequent gonadal function remains small. It is still not known if the vulnerability of the gonad to radiation- or chemotherapy-induced damage varies with pubertal status or is age-dependent. Newer cytotoxic drugs or combinations of such drugs may damage the gonad and only continued surveillance of gonadal function in these patients will allow such damage to be detected. More recently, Rappaport et al.[34] described three girls with primary ovarian failure following treatment for medulloblastoma in childhood. They attributed the ovarian failure to radiation-induced damage associated with spinal irradiation. However, they mentioned that all three girls received adjuvant chemotherapy without providing any details of which cytotoxic drugs were received. Subsequently, Brown et al.[58] and Ahmed et al.[59] have shown that gonadal failure in children treated for medulloblastoma may be caused by either radiation damage or adjuvant chemotherapy with nitrosoureas (BCNU and CCNU). Whether or not there is a synergistic interaction between radiation- and chemotherapy-induced damage is unknown; neither is it clear if gonadal dysfunction in children treated for medulloblastoma is reversible. There is a need for accurate and unequivocal answers to these and other questions so that when paediatric oncologists and radiotherapists plan new protocols for future treatments the true endocrine morbidity from existing methods of therapy can be taken into account.

References

1. Gonzalez, D. G. and Van Dijk, J. D. P. (1983). Experimental studies on the responses of growing bones to X-ray and neutron irradiation. *Int. J. Radiat. Oncolol. Biol. Phys.*, **9**, 671–7
2. Probert, J. C., Parker, B. R. and Kaplan, H. S. (1973). Growth retardation in children after megavoltage irradiation of the spine. *Cancer*, **32**, 634–9
3. Price, D. A., Morris, M. J., Rowsell, K. V. and Morris Jones, P. H. (1981). The effects of anti-leukaemic drugs on somatomedin production and cartilage responsiveness to somatomedin *in vitro*. *Pediatr. Res.*, **15**, 1553
4. Fuks, Z., Glatstein, E., Marsa, G. W., Bagshaw, M. A. and Kaplan, H. S. (1976). Long-term effects of external radiation on the pituitary and thyroid glands. *Cancer*, **37**, 1153–61
5. Schimpff, S. C., Diggs, C. H., Wiswell, J. G., Salvatore, P. C. and Wienik, P. H. (1980). Radiation-related thyroid dysfunction: implications for the treatment of Hodgkin's disease. *Ann. Intern. Med.*, **92**, 91–8
6. Smith, R. E., Adler, R. A., Clark, P., Brink-Johnsen, T., Tulloh, M. E. and Cotton, T. (1981). Thyroid function after mantle irradiation in Hodgkin's disease. *J. Am. Med. Assoc.*, **245**, 46–9
7. Shalet, S. M., Rosenstock, J. D., Beardwell, C. G., Pearson, D. and Morris Jones, P. H. (1977). Thyroid dysfunction following external irradiation to the neck for Hodgkin's disease in childhood. *Radiology*, **28**, 511–15
8. Glatstein, E., McHardy-Young, S., Brast, N., Eltringham, J. R. and Kriss, J. P. (1971). Alterations in serum thyrotropin (TSH) and thyroid function following radiotherapy in patients with malignant lymphoma. *J. Clin. Endocrinol. Metab.*, **32**, 833–41
9. Nelson, D. F., Reddy, K. V., O'Mara, R. E. and Rubin, P. H. (1978). Thyroid abnormalities following neck irradiation for Hodgkin's disease. *Cancer*, **42**, 2553–62
10. Sklar, C. A., Kim, T. H. and Ramsay, N. K. C. (1982). Thyroid dysfunction among long-term survivors of bone marrow transplantation. *Am. J. Med.*, **73**, 688–94
11. Fowler, P. B. S. (1977). Premyxoedema—a cause of preventable coronary heart disease. *Proc. R. Soc. Med.*, **70**, 297–9
12. Ridgway, E. C., Cooper, D. S., Walker, H., Rodbard, D. and Maloof, F. (1981). Peripheral responses to thyroid hormone before and after L-thyroxine therapy in patients with subclinical hypothyroidism. *J. Clin. Endocrinol. Metab.*, **53**, 1238–42
13. Bamford, F. N., Morris Jones, P. H., Pearson, D., Ribeiro, G. G., Shalet, S. M. and Beardwell, C. G. (1976). Residual disabilities in children treated for intracranial space-occupying lesions. *Cancer*, **37**, 1149–51

14. Onoyama, Y., Abe, M., Takahashi, M., Yabumoto, E. and Sakamoto, T. (1975). Radiation therapy of brain tumours in children. *Radiology*, **115**, 687–93

15. Shalet, S. M., Beardwell, C. G., Morris Jones, P. H. and Pearson, D. (1975). Pituitary function after treatment of intracranial tumours in children. *Lancet*, **2**, 104–7

16. Shalet, S. M., Beardwell, C. G., Pearson, D. and Morris Jones, P. H. (1976). The effect of varying doses of cerebral irradiation on growth hormone production in childhood. *Clin. Endocrinol.*, **5**, 287–90

17. Czernichow, P., Casohin, O., Rappaport, R., Flamant, F., Sarrazin, D. and Schweisguth, O. (1977). Sequelles endocriniennes des irradiations de la tête et du cou pour tumeurs extracraniennes. *Arch. Fr. Pediatr.*, **34**, 154–64

18. Shalet, S. M., Beardwell, C. G., Aarons, B. M., Pearson, D. and Morris Jones, P. H. (1978). Growth impairment of children treated for brain tumours. *Arch. Dis. Child.*, **53**, 491–4

19. Shalet, S. M., Beardwell, C. G., MacFarlane, I. A., Morris Jones, P. H. and Pearson, D. (1977). Endocrine morbidity in adults treated with cerebral irradiation for brain tumours during childhood. *Acta Endocrinol.*, **84**, 673–80

20. Perry-Keene, D. A., Connelly, J. F., Young, R. A., Wettenhall, H. N. B. and Martin, F. I. R. (1976). Hypothalamic hypopituitarism following external radiotherapy for tumours distant from the adenohypophysis. *Clin. Endocrinol.*, **5**, 373–80

21. Samaan, N. A., Vieto, R., Schultz, P. N., Maor, M., Meoz, R. T., Sampiere, V. A., Cangir, A., Ried, H. L. and Jesse, R. H. (1982). Hypothalamic, pituitary and thyroid dysfunction after radiotherapy to the head and neck. *Int. J. Radiat. Oncol. Biol. Phys.*, **8**, 1857–67

22. Swift, P. G. F., Kearney, P. J., Dalton, R. G., Bullimore, J. A., Mott, M. G. and Savage, D. C. L. (1978). Growth and hormonal status of children treated for acute lymphoblastic leukaemia. *Arch. Dis. Child.*, **53**, 890–4

23. Shalet, S. M., Price, D. A., Beardwell, C. G., Morris Jones, P. H. and Pearson, D. (1979). Normal growth despite abnormalities of growth hormone secretion in children treated for acute leukaemia. *J. Pediatr.*, **94**, 719–22

24. Nesbitt, M. E., Sather, H. N., Robison, L. L., Ortega, J., Littman, P. S., D'Angio, G. J. and Hammond, G. D. (1981). Presymptomatic central nervous system therapy in previously untreated childhood acute lymphoblastic leukaemia: comparison of 1800 rad and 2400 rad. *Lancet*, **1**, 461–6

25. Broomhall, J., May, R., Lilleyman, J. S. and Milner, R. D. G. (1983). Height and lymphoblastic leukaemia. *Arch. Dis. Child.*, **58**, 300–1

26. Berry, D. H., Elders, M. J., Crist, Wm., Land, V., Lui, V., Sexauer, A. C. and Dickinson, L. (1983). Growth in children with acute lymphocytic leukaemia: a pediatric oncology group study. *Med. Pediatr. Oncol.*, **11**, 39–45

27. Shalet, S. M. and Price, D. A. (1981). Effect of treatment of malignant disease on growth in children. *Arch. Dis. Child.*, **56**, 235

28. Griffin, N. K. and Wadsworth, J. (1980). Effect of treatment of malignant disease on growth in children. *Arch. Dis. Child.*, **55**, 600–3

29. Shalet, S. M., Whitehead, E., Chapman, A. J. and Beardwell, C. G. (1981). The effects of growth hormone therapy in children with radiation-induced growth hormone deficiency. *Acta Paediatr. Scand.*, **70**, 81–6

30. Richards, G. E., Wara, W. M., Grumbach, M. M., Kaplan, S. L., Sheline, G. E. and Conte, F. A. (1976). Delayed onset of hypopituitarism: sequelae of therapeutic irradiation of central nervous system, eye and middle ear tumours. *J. Pediatr.*, **89**, 533–9

31. Dickinson, W. P., Berry, D. H., Dickinson, L., Irvin, M., Schedewie, H., Fiser, R. H. and Elders, M. J. (1978). Differential effects of cranial radiation on growth hormone response to arginine and insulin infusion. *J. Pediatr.*, **92**, 754–7

32. Chrousos, G. O., Poplack, D., Brown, T., O'Neill, D., Schwade, J. and Bercu, B. B. (1982). Effects of cranial radiation on hypothalamic–adenohypophyseal function: abnormal growth hormone secretory dynamics. *J. Clin. Endocrinol. Metab.*, **54**, 1135–9
33. Editorial (1983). Growth-hormone-releasing factor. *Lancet*, **2**, 143
34. Rappaport, R., Brauner, R., Czernichow, P., Thibaud, E., Renier, D., Zucker, J. M. and Lemerle, J. (1982). Effect of hypothalamic and pituitary irradiation on pubertal development in children with cranial tumours. *J. Clin. Endocrinol. Metab.*, **54**, 1164–8
35. Lentz, R. D., Berstein, J., Steffes, M. W., Brown, D. R., Prem, K., Michael, A. F. and Vernier, R. L. (1977). Postpubertal evaluation of gonadal function following cyclophosphamide therapy before and during puberty. *J. Pediatr.*, **91**, 385–94
36. Penso, J., Lippe, B., Ehrlich, R. and Smith, F. G. (1974). Testicular function in prepubertal and pubertal male patients treated with cyclophosphamide for nephrotic syndrome. *J. Pediatr.*, **84**, 831–6
37. Guesry, P., Lenoir, G. and Broyer, M. (1978). Gonadal effects of chlorambucil given to prepubertal and pubertal boys for nephrotic syndrome. *J. Pediatr.*, **92**, 299–303
38. Lendon, M., Hann, I. M., Palmer, M. K., Shalet, S. M. and Morris Jones, P. H. (1978). Testicular histology after combination chemotherapy in childhood for acute lymphoblastic leukaemia. *Lancet*, **2**, 439–41
39. Shalet, S. M., Hann, I. M., Lendon, M., Morris Jones, P. H. and Beardwell, C. G. (1981). Testicular function after combination chemotherapy in childhood for acute lymphoblastic leukaemia. *Arch. Dis. Child.*, **56**, 275–8
40. Sherins, R. J., Olweny, C. L. M. and Ziegler, J. L. (1978). Gynaecomastia and gonadal dysfunction in adolescent boys treated with combination chemotherapy for Hodgkin's disease. *N. Engl. J. Med.*, **299**, 12–16
41. Whitehead, E., Shalet, S. M., Morris Jones, P. H., Beardwell, C. G. and Deakin, D. P. (1982). Gonadal function after combination chemotherapy for Hodgkin's disease in childhood. *Arch. Dis. Child.*, **57**, 287–91
42. Pennisi, A. J., Grushkin, C. M. and Lieberman, E. (1975). Gonadal function in children with nephrosis treated with cyclophosphamide. *Am. J. Dis. Child.*, **129**, 315–18
43. Etteldorf, J. N., West, C. D., Pitcock, J. A. and Williams, D. L. (1976). Gonadal function, testicular histology and meiosis following cyclophosphamide therapy in patients with nephrotic syndrome. *J. Pediatr.*, **88**, 206–12
44. Miller, J. J., Williams, G. F. and Leissring, J. C. (1971). Multiple late complications of therapy with cyclophosphamide, including ovarian destruction. *Am. J. Med.*, **50**, 530–5
45. Siris, E. S., Leventhal, B. G. and Vaitukaitis, J. L. (1976). Effects of childhood leukaemia and chemotherapy on puberty and reproductive function in girls. *N. Engl. J. Med.*, **294**, 1143–6
46. Beck, W., Schwarz, S., Heidemann, P. H., Jentsch, E., Stubbe, P. and Konig, A. (1982). Hypergonadotrophic hypogonadism, SHBG deficiency and hyperprolactinaemia: a transient phenomenon during induction chemotherapy in leukaemic children. *Eur. J. Pediatr.*, **138**, 216–20
47. Conte, F. A., Grumbach, M. M., Kaplan, S. L. and Reiter, E. O. (1980). Correlation of luteinizing hormone-releasing factor-induced luteinizing hormone and follicle-stimulating hormone release from infancy to 19 years with the changing pattern of gonadotropin secretion in agonadal patients: relation to the restraint of puberty. *J. Clin. Endocrinol. Metab.*, **50**, 163–8
48. Himelstein-Braw, H., Peters, H. and Faber, M. (1978). Morphological study of the ovaries of leukaemic children. *Br. J. Cancer*, **38**, 82–7

49. Rowley, M. J., Leach, D. R., Warner, G. A. and Heller, C. G. (1974). Effect of graded doses of ionising radiation on the human testis. *Radiat. Res.*, **59**, 665–78

50. Shalet, S. M., Beardwell, C. G., Jacobs, H. G. and Pearson, D. (1978). Testicular function following irradiation of the human prepubertal testis. *Clin. Endocrinol.*, **9**, 483–90

51. Brauner, R., Czernichow, P., Cramer, P., Schaison, G. and Rappaport, R. (1983). Leydig-cell function in children after direct testicular irradiation for acute lympho-blastic leukemia. *N. Engl. J. Med.*, **309**, 25–8

52. Thomas, E. D. (1982). The experience with 'late effects' after marrow transplan-tation. Presented at the *Eulep Symposium*, pp. 11–16, August 27–28, Commission of European Communities, Luxembourg

53. Lushbaugh, C. G. and Casarett, G. W. (1976). The effects of gonadal irradiation in clinical radiation therapy: a review. *Cancer*, **37**, 1111–20

54. Lushbaugh, C. G. and Ricks, R. C. (1972). Some cytokinetic and histopathologic considerations of irradiated male and female gonadal tissues. In *Frontiers of Radiation Therapy and Oncology*. Vol. 6, pp. 224–48. (Baltimore: Karger, Basel and University Park Press)

55. Shalet, S. M., Beardwell, C. G., Morris Jones, P. H., Pearson, D. and Orrell, D. H. (1976). Ovarian failure following abdominal irradiation in childhood. *Br. J. Cancer*, **33**, 655–8

56. Stillman, R. J., Schinfield, J. S., Schiff, I., Gelber, R. D., Greenberger, J., Larson, M., Jaffe, N. and Li, F. P. (1981). Ovarian failure in long-term survivors of childhood malignancy. *Am. J. Obstet. Gynecol.*, **139**, 62–6

57. Himelstein-Braw, R., Peters, H. and Faber, M. (1977). Influence of irradiation and chemotherapy on the ovaries of children with abdominal tumours. *Br. J. Cancer*, **36**, 269–75

58. Brown, I. H., Lee, T. J., Eden, O. B., Bullimore, J. A. and Savage, D. C. L. (1984). Growth and endocrine function in children treated for medulloblastoma. *Arch. Dis. Child.*, **58**, 722–7

59. Ahmed, S. R., Shalet, S. M., Campbell, R. H. A. and Deakin, D. (1984). Primary gonadal damage following treatment of brain tumours in childhood. *J. Pediatr.*, **103**, 562–5

199

SECTION 6

Miscellaneous Disorders

Chairman: J. FARQUHAR

13

SOME ASPECTS OF THE GENETICS OF PAEDIATRIC ENDOCRINOLOGY

R. HARRIS

INTRODUCTION

The traditional classification of disease into 'multifactorial' (a large assembly of common and important disorders) or 'genetic' (a collection of fascinating but rare footnotes) is outdated and misleading. Diabetes and congenital adrenal hyperplasia provide excellent examples of diseases which no longer fit comfortably into this anachronistic paradigm. They also demonstrate the diagnostic resolving power of medical genetics. Diabetes mellitus, once called 'the geneticist's nightmare', is a common 'multifactorial' found at all ages but presenting clinically in many different ways. Congenital adrenal hyperplasia (CAH) is a rare but genetically seemingly rather simple disorder of infants. Diabetes, like many other multifactorial disorders, becomes a collection of aetiologically different entities when 'split' by genetic, clinical and epidemiological scrutiny, while the apparent genetic simplicity of CAH hides considerable heterogeneity and overlap with endocrinologic disorders of adult life. These diseases illustrate well the need for precision in diagnosis without which it is difficult or impossible to design effective, preventive and therapeutic strategies in medicine.

I cannot attempt here a comprehensive review of genetics in relation to paediatric endocrinology. Some aspects have already been discussed by others in this volume and up-to-date references to the genetics of disorders of the pituitary gland, thyroid, parathyroid, gonads and internal reproductive ducts, as well as diabetes and CAH, can be found at the end of this section.

IDENTIFICATION OF GENETIC FACTORS IN DISEASE—GENETIC MARKERS

A common environment may partially explain disease clustering in families and, conversely, healthy individuals may have disease suscept-ibility genes which have not yet expressed themselves. 'Heritability' is sometimes used to describe the probability of familial recurrence when it is not possible to disentangle genetic and environmental factors common to family members. However, the aim of medical genetics is to identify, when possible, individual genes as distinct from multifactorial determi-nation and heritability. The operation of individual 'major' genes can be identified in the human by observing one or more of the following:

(1) A characteristic distribution of disease amongst family members which is consistent with 'Mendelian' inheritance; autosomal dominant, recessive or X-linked.
(2) A numerical or structural 'chromosomal' abnormality, although this is not necessarily heritable.
(3) Evidence of gene 'activity' in the form of a specific metabolic process.
(4) Identification of a specific 'gene product', usually a protein variant.
(5) The presence of a unique DNA or mRNA sequence.
(6) A closely 'linked' genetic marker.

'Genetic markers' indicate directly or indirectly the presence of dis-ease susceptibility genes. The ultimate genetic marker is the nucleotide sequence of a structural gene, but this does not indicate when or how the gene will express itself. Identification of the gene product (e.g. globin, enzyme or hormone) is a more certain guide to the activity of structural genes but may give little information about their genetic and environ-mental controls. In clinical genetics the crucial step is the one which transforms latent genetic predisposition into disease itself. The term 'penetrance' is used for the proportion of individuals possessing a disease susceptibility gene who are clinically recognizable.

With these concepts in mind we can now consider the genetics of CAH and diabetes mellitus.

CONGENITAL ADRENAL HYPERPLASIA (CAH)

Autosomal recessive inheritance of CAH was demonstrated by Barton Childs et al.[1]. They used segregation analysis which corrected the bias which is inevitable when families can only be identified after at least one case has occurred. Many families in which both parents carry a gene for CAH have by chance only normal children while families with two or more affected children tend to be over-represented. The genetic 'marker' was the 25% recurrence rate in siblings which is characteristic of the 3 : 1 ratio of healthy to affected expected under recessive inheritance. In Maryland, USA, where this study was carried out, the frequency of infantile CAH was reported to be only 1 : 67 000 live births, giving an estimated gene frequency of 0.0039 and a carrier frequency of 1 : 129. Later studies in other parts of the world suggest that this is an under-estimate (Table 1) partly attributable to incomplete ascertainment of males in whom virilization may be overlooked or from infantile death from unrecognized salt-wasting, a continuing possibility if there is no family history to alert the paediatrician to the diagnosis.

Table 1   Estimated incidence of CAH (21-OH deficiency)

	Patient/live births
Maryland, USA	1 : 67 000
Zurich, Switzerland	1 : 5041
Birmingham, England	1 : 7255
Wisconsin, USA	1 : 15 000
Alaska, USA	1 : 700*
Yupik Eskimo, USA	1 : 245
Toronto, Canada	1 : 13 000*
Munich, Germany	1 : 9831
Tyrol, Austria	1 : 8991
All of Switzerland	1 : 15 472

* Corrected for both variants: salt-wasting and salt-sparing.
Adapted from New et al.[1]

When the specific deficiency of the enzyme 21-hydroxylase was ident-ified as a cause of CAH it was realized that congenital virilization could also result from other, rarer inherited enzyme deficiencies, from maternal virilizing tumours or from the ingestion of synthetic progestins (Table 2). Later studies demonstrated that 21-hydroxylase deficiency (21-OH) was associated also with quite different endocrinological disorders or even with clinical normality.

VARIABILITY OF EXPRESSION OF 21-OH DEFICIENCY

There is wide variation in the way that 21-OH deficiency is expressed even when other causes of CAH are excluded. Precise classification of the syndromes attributable to 21-OH deficiency is still imperfect but has benefited from several biochemical and genetic advances. These include the use of the 'synacthen' test and the exploitation of the discovery of the close genetic linkage between 21-OH and HLA. In the synacthen test ACTH is given by injection following adrenal suppression with oral dexamethasone. In 21-OH deficient homozygotes very high levels of circulating 17-hydroxyprogesterone result and there is excellent discrimination in affected families from heterozygotes and normals. However, complementary HLA studies are required reliably to distinguish heterozygote carriers and homozygote normals.

Table 2   Causes of congenital virilization

	Clinical features		
	Salt-wasting	Hypertension	Virilization
(1) *Fetal deficiencies of steroidogenesis*			
21-OH { simple virilizing	−	−	+
{ salt-wasting	+	−	+
11β-hydroxylase	−	+	+
3β-hydroxysteroid dehydrogenase	+	−	−
cholestrol desmolase	+	−	−
17α-hydroxylase	−	+	−
18-hydroxylase	+	−	−
18-dehydrogenase of 18-hydroxy- corticosterone	+	−	−
17-hydroxysteroid dehydrogenase	−	−	+
(2) *Maternal ingestion of virilizing hormones*	−	−	+
(3) *Maternal virilizing tumour*	−	−	+

Adapted from New *et al.*[2]

HLA AND 21-OH DEFICIENCY

Genes coding for HLA-B and for 21-OH deficiency are located close together on the short arm of chromosome No. 6. The HLA region contains at least four antigen loci (HLA-A, -B, -C and -D(DR)) and the structural loci for the complement components Properdin B(Bf), C2 and C4. In addition to 21-OH deficiency, susceptibility to many other diseases is inherited with HLA[3]. Each HLA locus is highly polymorphic coding for many alternative antigens. Individuals may be homozygous and have only one antigenic product of each locus, or heterozygous, when they will have two. Because of close linkage the HLA region is usually inherited intact as a haplotype. Providing that genetic recombination does not occur, the genetic information for 21-OH deficiency is transmitted with the same HLA-B antigen to all close relatives. In our experience all affected sibling pairs have been HLA-B identical (Table 3). Consequently, knowledge of the HLA-B antigens of an affected child allows accurate prediction of the 21-OH genotype of relatives (including fetuses prenatally); those that share both HLA-B antigens with the patient will be 21-OH deficiency homozygotes, heterozygotes share one

B antigen and homozygote normals share neither. Genetic marker linkage studies of this kind are of value in families when one is unable to identify with certainty the presence of the disease gene but where readily identifiable gene products from a closely linked locus on the same chromosome are present. This strategy will be applied generally when markers can be found conveniently close to major disease loci and these are likely to be plentiful in the form of DNA restriction fragment length polymorphisms[5] (see below).

Table 3 21-OH deficiency (CAH) and HLA in sibling pairs

	Haplotypes shared		
	Two (HLA identical)	One (haplo-identical)	None (HLA different)
Both siblings clinically affected with CAH	10	0	0
One sibling clinically normal, one affected	1*	27	13
Expected	25%	50%	25%

* Biochemically 21-OH-deficient.
Modified from Gordon[4].

LINKAGE AND ASSOCIATION

Linkage cannot be used reliably to study unrelated individuals because the disease gene may be linked to different markers in different families. Any one marker is an unreliable guide outside those families in which the linkage relationships have been established. The 'hitch-hiker' gene (e.g. HLA antigen) is readily identified but not the 'driver' (e.g. 21-OH deficiency). During any one genetic journey the hitch-hiker and driver may well ride together, but the next time one identifies the hitch-hiker he may be in a different car altogether. In a family, genetic marker and disease gene may travel through the generations together, but there is no certainty that the marker will be coupled to the disease gene in individuals selected at random in the population. This is because of recombination which occurs even between closely linked genetic loci. The frequency of recombination is related to the distance between the two loci. When there is a tendency for disease to occur preferentially in individuals with a particular marker (referred to as population 'association') it is assumed that either there is a selective advantage involved or that insufficient generations have passed to have achieved equilibrium. There are associations between 'classical' 21-OH deficiency and HLA-B47, and between 'late onset' and 'cryptic' varieties with HLA-B14 and A28 (see below and Table 4). Population associations are characteristic of HLA related diseases and this will be discussed further in relation to diabetes mellitus.

Table 4   HLA antigen frequencies amongst unrelated individuals with 21-OH deficiency

	CAH (40)	Hyper-responders** (13)	Controls (176)
HLA-A28	3 (7.5)	5 (38.5)*	6.8
HLA-B8	3 (7.5)*	5 (38.5)	20.5
HLA-B14	3 (7.5)	5 (38.5)*	5.1
HLA-Bw47	5 (12.5)†	0	0.6

** 'Cryptic' or 'late onset'—see text.
*$p < 0.05$, †$p < 0.001$.
Modified from Gordon[3].

RECENT ADVANCES IN 21-OH DEFICIENCY

Improved biochemical analysis and HLA typing, used to complement each other, have made the following contributions to our understanding of CAH:

(1) 21-OH deficiency is genetically linked to HLA, but other forms of CAH that have been studied in this way are not. This confirms their genetic separateness and also illustrates the value of using linked genetic markers.

(2) Reliable identification is now possible of 21-OH deficiency carriers *in families*, employing a combination of biochemical and HLA tests.

(3) HLA identity with a clinically affected sibling has allowed the diagnosis of males with previously unsuspected 21-OH deficiency. Some homozygote males with the salt-sparing variety may not otherwise be recognized, and although they may sometimes be fertile, their adrenal cortical hyperplasia is potentially premalignant without corticosteroid treatment.

(4) Both the salt-sparing and the salt-wasting varieties of 21-OH deficiency are linked to HLA-B. Although these varieties tend not to occur in the same families, we have found HLA and biochemically proven 21-OH-deficient but clinically normal homozygote males who have escaped diagnosis in childhood although their sisters had severe infantile salt-wasting.

(5) New evidence suggests that genetic control involves two 21-OH deficiency loci, one producing deficiency limited to the adrenal cortical zona fasciculata and is salt-sparing, the other results in

deficiency also in the zona glomerulosa and leads to salt-wasting by blocking aldosterone production. Progress is now being made with *in vitro* characterization of microsomal 21-OH.

(6) Two additional genetic variants of 21-OH deficiency have been defined by the relative blood levels of 17-hydroxyprogesterone following the synacthen test. The late onset ('acquired') 21-OH deficiency allele is characterized by levels as high as those found in 'classical' 21-OH homozygotes. The clinical features are variable and have so far been noted in young women when they include inconstant hirsutes, acne, menstrual irregularity and relative infertility. There is also a 'cryptic' allele with similar biochemical findings but without clinical manifestations. Because the clinical features of the 'late onset' variety are so variable it is not clear how much overlap there is with the 'cryptic' variety, especially since both are found more commonly in individuals with the HLA-B14 antigen. These variants are quite common in the population but have also been reported in relatives of children with CAH. It is believed that there are several different genotypes which result in an exaggerated 17-hydroxyprogesterone response in the synacthen test. Homozygotes (or mixed heterozygotes) with two different 21-OH deficiency alleles are associated with HLA-B14 and have been called 'late onset' and 'cryptic'. The 'classical' allele is associated with HLA-Bw47 and produces CAH in the homozygote state, although there is much variability, especially in males. It can be seen that HLA studies have been particularly informative in confirming these genetic variants (Table 4).

DIABETES MELLITUS

James Neel described diabetes as the 'geneticist's nightmare' because family clustering and twin data strongly suggested a genetic basis for diabetes, but there was no general agreement about the most likely mode of inheritance. There were several reasons and these provide a paradigm for the future resolution of similar confusion in other common human diseases:

(1) Continuing ignorance of the basic defect.
(2) Lack of a generally agreed definition of diabetes mellitus.
(3) Inconstant clinical presentation in terms of symptoms, age of onset and natural history. Some features used for classification, e.g. obesity, may disappear.
(4) Environmental change, e.g. diet, may not be recognized.
(5) Only a small proportion of those with the diabetic genotype may be identifiable at any one time and prospective studies are necessary to account for all affected relatives.

(6) When a disease is common it is difficult to know what part chance, a common environment and a similar genotype have played.

The term 'diabetes mellitus' includes a variety of different diseases having only glucose intolerance in common (Table 5). The separation of the various types of diabetes (as with other multifactorials) depends on a combination of different methods, including family, twin, metabolic, immunological, genetic marker and epidemiological studies. Without this 'splitting' it is impossible to identify risk factors and offer genetic counselling.

Table 5   Classification of diabetes mellitus

(1) *Insulin dependent (type I)*
    Formerly called 'juvenile onset type', 'ketosis prone' and 'brittle'. Family history uncommon. HLA associated with immunological phenomena and insulinopenia. 'Insulin . . . to preserve life'

(2) *Non-insulin-dependent (type II)*
    Formerly called 'maturity onset type', 'ketosis resistant', 'stable'. Family history common. Late onset (> 40), but includes maturity onset diabetes of young type ('MODY'). Obese and non-obese subtypes

(3) *Other types*
    Syndromes
    Rotter and Rimoin[6] list 45 syndromes associated with impaired glucose metabolism and these include many pathogenic mechanisms and different genetic mutations
    Drug or surgically induced
    Gestational

Adapted from Keen[7].

There were several reasons for suspecting that diabetes was not a single disease. There are many different human genetic syndromes which include abnormalities of glucose metabolism. In animals, experimental diabetes provides several genetically distinct models which resemble different types of human diabetes and there is evidence of human ethnic differences in the frequency and type of diabetes. The evidence for the genetic separation of IDDM and NIDDM is particularly compelling.

GENETIC SEPARATION OF IDDM AND NIDDM

The striking clinical difference has long been recognized between the ketosis prone, insulin requiring, thin, young onset diabetic and the maturity onset, non-ketotic and frequently obese diabetic. The evidence that these are in fact genetically distinct is broadly as follows:

(1) Providing allowance is made for the late onset of the disease, monozygotic twins are nearly 100% concordant for diabetes with onset over age 40 compared with dizygotics in whom concordance is about 50%. In contrast, concordance for diabetes with onset below 40 years does not exceed 50% amongst monozygotic twins and is 5–10% in dizygotics. These observations suggest that environmental factors are also important in juvenile onset diabetes.

(2) There is little increase in the frequency of NIDDM amongst the older relatives of Caucasian patients with IDDM.

(3) Juvenile onset diabetes is associated with islet cell destruction and insulinopenia and with the absolute requirement for therapeutic insulin. In maturity onset diabetes hyperinsulinaemia is generally found.

(4) There are clinical and familial associations between IDDM and Addison's disease, some thyroid disorders and pernicious anaemia, with an increased frequency of antibodies to thyroid, gastric mucosa, intrinsic factor and adrenal. These are not characteristic of NIDDM. There is direct evidence for autoimmunity in IDDM in the form of specific cell mediated and antibody immunity to pancreatic islet cells.

(5) Although NIDDM usually occurs in the over 40s, a distinct entity, maturity onset diabetes of the young ('MODY'), has been recognized.

(6) The use of genetic markers including HLA has confirmed the separateness of IDDM (see below).

INHERITANCE OF NIDDM

Although the situation is not entirely clear, a high concordance in monozygotic twins implies a mainly genetic causation and the approximately 50% recurrence in siblings is consistent with autosomal dominant inheritance. Onset is generally delayed until middle age so that early death and unrecognized disease will obscure the pattern of inheritance in families. It is likely that NIDDM is not a single disease and further research, including molecular genetics, is needed for the resolution of this additional heterogeneity. There is no association with HLA and other genetic markers, including chlorpropamide-induced alcohol flushing, have not produced consistent results in different studies.

INHERITANCE OF IDDM

IDDM occurs in about 5–10% of siblings. Children are as likely to develop IDDM as are siblings, and this is unlike autosomal recessive inheritance where risk is largely limited to the siblings (excluding consanguinous families). Small recurrence risks evenly distributed amongst first-degree relatives are the hallmark of 'multifactorial' determination in which the operation of 'major' genes cannot be discerned. However, the association of HLA with IDDM '. . . was found to offer the most important new information on the genetics of diabetes in this century'[7] because it showed the activity of 'major' genes by the use of genetic markers.

HLA AND IDDM

The relationship between HLA and diabetes was first observed in the increased frequency of HLA B8, B15 and B18 amongst diabetics. Later, stronger associations were found with HLA, DR3 and DR4 (Table 6).

Table 6   HLA-IDDM associations in Caucasian populations

Number of studies		Patients		Controls		Relative risk	p
		Total	% Range	Total	% Range		
B8	18	1785	19–60	13349	2–29	2.56	1^{-10}
B15	17	1769	4–50	13175	2–26	2.05	1^{-10}
B18	13	1244	5–59	6577	5–50	1.69	4×10^{-8}
DR3	11	436	27–76	874	15–35	3.32	1×10^{-10}
DR4	11	436	51–83	874	5–32	6.55	1×10^{-10}

$$\text{Relative risk} = \frac{\text{Patients positive}}{\text{Controls negative}} \times \frac{\text{Controls positive}}{\text{Patients negative}}.$$

Tables 6, 7 and 8 adapted from Svejgaard[8].

Andrew Cudworth, with John Woodrow from Liverpool, studied HLA antigen sharing in siblings, both of whom have IDDM, and provided strong evidence for diabetes susceptibility genes linked to HLA (Table 7). Since each child inherits one paternal and one maternal No. 6 chromosome (haplotype), pairs of siblings taken at random should share 0, 1 or 2 parental chromosomes in the ratio of 1:2:1. However, over 90% of pairs of diabetic siblings have at least one of the parental haplotypes in common (Table 7). Although this strongly supports the hypothesis that genes for IDDM are linked to HLA on chromosome No. 6, the frequency of two haplotypes sharing falls short of the 100% expected under autosomal recessive inheritance, as we saw earlier in 21-OH (see also Table 9).

212

Table 7 HLA haplotype shared by sibling pairs affected with IDDM

Number of shared haplotypes	Number of sibling pairs			
	Eighth workshop	Other data	Total	Per cent
2	78	76	154	58.6
1	49	48	97	36.9
0	7	5	12	4.6
Total	134	129	263	

GENETIC PROBLEMS IN IDDM

In spite of the important new information which has come from studying HLA there is still uncertainty about the mode of inheritance of IDDM. This results from the factors which were summarized at the beginning of this section and from reduced penetrance, confusion between linkage and association and heterogeneity within the disorder.

REDUCED PENETRANCE

Penetrance was earlier defined as the proportion of individuals possessing a disease susceptibility genotype who also have the disease phenotype. In IDDM, penetrance is unknown, but the evidence from monozygotic twin studies suggests 15–50% concordance. Since concordant monozygotic twin pairs are more likely to be reported, 15% is the better estimate of penetrance of the IDDM genotype 'in families'. Penetrance may be different in individuals selected at random in the general population because their exposure to precipitating environmental factors may be less than within a 'diabetic family'.

LINKAGE AND ASSOCIATION

There is evidence for both linkage and association between HLA antigen genes and IDDM as detailed above and it is likely that HLA antigens themselves play a part in the immunological phenomena leading to autoimmune disease because of their function in regulating immunological cell interactions. It is not known at present whether the relationship between HLA and IDDM depends on linkage with as yet undiscovered disease genes, analogous to 21-OH, or upon the functions of HLA antigens.

HETEROGENEITY WITHIN IDDM

Heterogeneity implies the existence of aetiologic subtypes and will confound attempt to determine the genetics of IDDM. The evidence for heterogeneity is:

(1) The existence of rare syndromes, for example optic atrophy and diabetes mellitus and epiphyseal dysplasia and juvenile diabetes.

(2) Autoimmune phenomena are not found in all individuals with IDDM and this tends to run true in families.

(3) Because DR3 homozygotes and DR4 homozygotes have a lower relative risk than the DR3/DR4 heterozygote (Table 8), it is believed that there are at least two separate HLA-related diabetes genes. Further evidence for this is provided by persistent islet cell antibodies and antipancreatic cell mediated immunity, but lack of antibody response to exogenous insulin which is characteristic of the B8/DR3 form of IDDM. In the B15/DR4 form, antibodies to exogenous insulin are common, but other autoimmune disease and islet cell antibodies are unusual. DR3/DR4 heterozygotes have features of both forms of IDDM.

Table 8   Increased risk in DR3/DR4 heterozygotes

HLA-DR type	IDDM (n = 108) (%)	Controls (n = 260) (%)	Relative risk
3,—	9.3	12.3	3.7
3,X	6.5	11.5	2.7
4,—	22.2	11.2	9.7
4,X	7.4	15.4	2.4
3,4	36.1	3.8	45.8

3,— only DR3, presumed DR3/DR3 homozygote. X presence of second DR antigen not DR4.
4,— similarly.

IMPORTANCE OF THE ENVIRONMENT IN AETIOLOGY OF IDDM

The twin studies referred to earlier suggested a large environmental component in the aetiology of IDDM because concordance in identical twins was only 15–50%. The epidemiology of IDDM includes marked seasonal variation in incidence, while antibodies directed against various viruses, notably Coxsackie and mumps, are found more commonly in children who have recently developed IDDM than in normal controls. One published report demonstrated Coxsackie B4 virus in the pancreas of a child who had died of IDDM. Prospective studies of siblings of children with IDDM demonstrated how frequently complement fixing beta cell antibodies anticipated the clinical appearance of IDDM.

POSSIBLE MODES OF INHERITANCE OF IDDM

Genetic susceptibility probably depends on several genes interacting with environmental agents to trigger off an autoimmune process leading to diabetes.

(1) Autosomal dominant. This is not consistent with the excess of affected siblings who share two parental haplotypes (Table 7).

(2) Autosomal recessive inheritance. This is consistent with haplotype sharing among affected sibs, only if the population gene frequency (q) is about 0.3. The frequency of homozygotes (q^2) would then be 0.09, which contrasts with the observed frequency of IDDM in the population of about 0.003. This would require that only 3% of homozygotes should become diabetic (penetrance $= 0.03$). In families, diabetes recurs in about 5% of siblings whereas it would be expected in 25% (penetrance $= 0.2$). Simple autosomal recessive inheritance is unlikely because of the very high gene frequency, low penetrance and difference between the penetrance in the population and siblings.

(3) Gene dosage model. This proposes that penetrance is greater in homozygotes compared with heterozygotes but cannot explain the high relative risk for DR3/DR4 heterozygotes.

(4) The most attractive model at present is that of Hodge et al.[9], which proposes that there are three alleles at an HLA-linked diabetic locus. These alleles are S1 (in linkage disequilibrium with DR3), S2 (in linkage disequilibrium with DR4) and s, the normal allele which does not confer susceptibility to diabetes. This model fits

Table 9   Haplotype sharing: CAH and IDDM contrasted

	Two (%)	One (%)	None (%)
Observed			
CAH (21-OH)	100	0	0
Late onset or 'cryptic' 21-OH	100	0	0
IDDM 58.6%	36.9	4.6	
Expected for			
Autosomal recessive	100	0	0
Rare autosomal dominant	50	50	0

most of the data and does not make any unreasonable assumptions of reduced penetrance. It does not, however, take into account the additional evidence for diabetic genes which are not linked to HLA.

EVIDENCE FOR TWO (OR MORE) UNLINKED LOCI PREDISPOSING TO IDDM

HLA-DR3 and HLA-DR4 are associated with many autoimmune diseases and it is not clear what confers organ and disease specificity on such HLA related susceptibility. It is possible that an additional locus or loci confers specificity. This additional genetic information could be closely linked to HLA or elsewhere in the genome, as has been proposed by Hodge et al.[8], in their report on a possible linkage between IDDM and the Kidd blood group system.

GENETIC COUNSELLING IN DIABETES

As in all genetic counselling an accurate diagnosis is essential. IDDM, NIDDM, MODY and the various syndromes each have their own specific risks of recurrence which will be of the same type of diabetes. In spite of much new information, risk estimation is still largely empirical and recurrence risks can only be used in the population from which they are derived. In general, the risk to IDDM siblings is between 5 and 10%, but this prediction can, to some extent, be made more precise by HLA studies. HLA identical siblings have an approximately 15% risk (higher if they also have complement fixing antibodies against their islet cells). Siblings who share none of the patient's HLA antigens have a risk which is below 1%. Although in NIDDM the average risk for clinical disease is probably not greater than 5–10% for first-degree relatives (25% for an abnormal glucose tolerance test), risks rise progressively with age. In MODY the risk is 50% to first-degree relatives, but the much better prognosis should be emphasized.

THE FUTURE

Rigorous genetic analysis of IDDM is bedevilled by the reduced penetrance of the putative diabetic genome such that the majority of genetically predisposed individuals remain healthy. Some means are clearly required to identify directly the genotype in the absence of full-blown disease. It is likely that recombinant DNA technology will here, as elsewhere, make major contributions in the future[5]. Knowledge of the molecular biology of the HLA region is quickly accumulating[10], while preliminary evidence from a restriction fragment length polymorphism (RFLP) suggests that DR4 may have different linkage relationships in diabetics compared with normal[11]. One may surely also anticipate important therapeutic applications of DNA technology in endocrinology, e.g. the production of insulin and other protein hormones by 'genetic engineering'. In the meantime, using such genetic markers as are available to define a high risk cohort, it is profitable to study other phenomena, including subtle changes in glucose metabolism and complement fixing islet cell antibodies, to identify those most likely to become diabetic. Any promising means for prevention would then be tested in controlled trials in these highest risk children. It has already been suggested that the HLA identical healthy siblings of children with IDDM might be given immunosuppression to prevent autoimmune destruction of their islet cells. This apparently works well in experimental rats[12], but many would feel the need for extreme caution before embarking on a prolonged course of immunosuppression in young, growing individuals, even using Cyclosporin A. Perhaps investigations now in progress (Bottazzo, this volume) will eventually permit the specific ablation of the clone of T cells responsible for islet cell destruction.

References

1. Childs, B., Grumbach, M. M. and van Wyk, J. J. (1956). Virilizating adrenal hyperplasia: genetic and hormonal studies. *J. Clin. Invest.*, **35**, 213–22
2. New, M. I., Dupont, B., Pang, S., Pollack, M. and Levine, L. S. (1981). An update of congenital adrenal hyperplasia. In *Recent Progress in Hormone Research*. Vol. 37. (New York: Academic Press)
3. Harris, R. (1983). *HLA Antigens*. Medicine, the Monthly Add-on Series. pp. 308–34. (London: Medical Education (International) Ltd)
4. Gordon, M. (1983). A study of 21-hydroxylase deficiency syndromes. *PhD Thesis*, Manchester University
5. Botstein, D., White, R. L., Skolnick, M. and Davis, R. W. (1980). Construction of genetic linkage map in man using restriction fragment length polymorphisms. *Am. J. Hum. Genet.*, **32**, 314–31
6. Fisher, D. A., Harris, R., Jackson, C. E., New, M. I., Grumbach, K., Levine, L. S., Rimoin, D. L., Rotter, J. I. and Simpson, J. L. (1983). In Emery, A. E. H. and Rimoin, D. L. (eds.) *Principles and Practice of Medical Genetics*. pp. 1127–1240. (Edinburgh: Churchill Livingstone)
7. Keen, H., Nerup, J., Christy, M., Green, A., Hauge, M., Platz, P., Ryder, L. P., Svejgaard, A. and Thomsen, M. (1982). In Kobberling, J. and Tattersall, R. (eds.) *The Genetics of Diabetes Mellitus. Proceedings of the Serono Symposia*. Vol. 47. (London: Academic Press)
8. Svejgaard, A. (1980). *Eighth Workshop Report on Diabetes. Histocompatibility Testing. UCLA.* (Los Angeles: UCLA)
9. Hodge, S. E., Rotter, J. I. and Lange, K. L. (1980). A three-allele model for heterogeneity of juvenile onset insulin dependent diabetes. *Ann. Hum. Genet.*, **43**, 399–412

10. Lee, J. and Trowsdale, J. (1983). Molecular biology of the major histocompatibility complex. *Nature (London)*, **304**, 214–15
11. Owerbach, D., Lernmark, A., Platz, P., Ryder, L. P., Rask, L., Peterson, P. A. and Ludvigsson, J. (1983). HLA-D region beta-chain DNA endonuclease fragments differ between HLA-DR identical healthy and insulin-dependent individuals. *Nature (London)*, **303**, 815–17
12. Laupacis, A., Stiller, C. R., Gardell, C., Keown, P., Dupre, J., Wallace, A. C. and Thibert, P. (1983). Cyclosporin prevents diabetes in BB Wistar rats. *Lancet*, **1**, 10–12

14

HLA-DR EXPRESSION ON ENDOCRINE CELLS: A NEW WAY TO LOOK AT AUTOIMMUNITY

G. F. BOTTAZZO and D. DONIACH

Organ-specific autoimmunity has been demonstrated in all the defined endocrine glands except the pineal and is now being studied in the paracrine systems of the gastrointestinal tract[1] and the hypothalamus[2]. The 'autoimmune' endocrine disorders are characterized by the presence of antibodies in the patients' serum which may be detected years before the onset of clinical symptoms and are useful monitors of the lesions well before hormonal deficiencies can be measured by metabolic tests[3]. In the case of 'stimulating' antibodies that produce growth and hormone excess, and hormone receptor antibodies generally, the situation is far more complex[4].

Human autoimmune thyroiditis has been studied more extensively than any other organ-specific system and has served as a model for other similar endocrine diseases. Thyroid-specific surface antibodies were first described by Fagraeus and Jonsson[5] on viable suspensions of human cells. Khoury et al.[6] extended the immunofluorescence (IFL) work using human thyroid monolayer cell cultures. This culture system enabled them to investigate the effect of the antibodies on thyroid cells more extensively. The existence of thyroid surface antibodies was confirmed by the fine granular membrane staining seen on the surface of thyroid cells after applying the sera from patients with Hashimoto's disease to viable monolayers followed by fluoresceinated antihuman Ig. The first interesting point in the analysis of these antibodies was the high correlation between the results of the surface immunofluorescence·and the haemagglutination test for thyroid microsomal autoantibodies (McHA), implying that the same antigens are expressed both in the cytoplasm (microsomal antigens) and the surface ('microvillar' antigens) of thyroid cells. All the haemagglutinating ability was absorbed out of positive sera by living monolayers which exposed only their surface antigens. In some instances, however, a surface fluorescence was seen after complete removal of the McHA, suggesting that separate surface antibodies also exist.

In adult primary myxoedema a proportion of cases are negative for microsomal antibodies by the haemagglutination test. Preliminary results indicate that surface reactive 'microvillar' antibodies can be detected in about 25% of these negative cases. An autoimmune aetiology was suspected in some cases of congenital myxoedema[7], but the microsomal haemagglutination results in the mothers showed no correlation with the absence of thyroid function in the babies. Work in progress in our laboratory suggests the presence of 'microvillar' antibodies in some mothers in the absence of corresponding cytoplasmic specificity.

The cytotoxic effects of thyroiditis sera correlated perfectly with the microvillar expression, suggesting that surface autoantibodies play a pathogenetic role in thyroid autoimmunity. Another interesting finding was the re-expression of ABH blood group antigens on cultured thyroid monolayers[8]. These antigens are detectable in the fetal gland but are not seen on adult thyroid epithelium in cryostat sections. The significance of this modulation is at present unknown.

Surface expression of microsomal antigens is also observed in the gastric parietal cell system[9] and in addition there is a separate cell surface antigen. Cytotoxicity for parietal cells was demonstrated with unusual pernicious anaemia sera which gave negative results on stomach sections yet reacted by IFL on viable cells[10]. In the adrenal[11] and the pancreatic islet cell system the same principles apply. The important beta-cell cytotoxic antibody which damages the islets in diabetic insulitis is surface reactive[12]. Recently, cell surface antibodies to cultured melanocytes have been identified in most cases of patchy vitiligo[13], whereas cytoplasmic antibodies are very rare in this disease and were only found in severe polyendocrine conditions[14].

In the thyroiditis system these correlations were observed irrespective of whether the sera were obtained from overt autoimmune thyroid disease patients or from patients with subclinical focal thyroiditis and no detectable functional impairment. *In vivo*, therefore, there are some apparently contradictory observations with respect to the possible pathogenic role of thyroid microsomal antibodies. First, the monkeys injected with sera containing high titre of microsomal antibodies did not develop thyroiditis[15]. Second, the thyroid function of most babies born to Hashimoto mothers with high titre of microsomal antibodies remains intact despite the presence of the antibodies in their serum[16]. Third, these antibodies can be found in up to 20% of healthy middle-aged women without any detectable thyroid dysfunction[17]. Such findings cannot be explained by *in vitro* studies. The discrepancy with the situation during life can probably be attributed to the difference in the follicular conformation of the intact gland. *In vivo* thyroid epithelial cells are well organized as follicular structures surrounded by basement membranes. In these polarized acini the 'microvillar' antigen is confined to the apical border of follicular cells and is sequestered from antibodies in the blood, while *in vitro* these antigens are fully exposed and vulnerable to added antibodies and complement because the microvilli remain polarized and face the culture medium.

Considering this anatomical difference, Khoury *et al.*[18] examined the possibility of *in vivo* binding of antibodies to 'microvillar' antigens. In semi-intact follicles obtained by incomplete digestion from operated Graves' thyroid glands it was found by simply applying a fluorescein-tagged anti-Ig that antibodies were already bound to the inner border of the follicles, indicating *in vivo* attachment to the 'microvillar' antigen. These pre-existing complexes were only seen in occasional acini and the pattern was similar to that obtained with Hashimoto sera on viable disrupted half follicles and on monolayers by indirect IFL. The results suggest the presence of certain factor(s) which break the protective conformation of thyroid follicles and allow the antibodies to have access to their own autoantigens localized only inside of the thyroid acini. The investigation of these factors will certainly help to understand the pathogenesis of autoimmune thyroid disease more deeply. The major question is 'What impairs the protective mechanism?'

A first possibility is the deposition of circulating antigen–antibody complexes on the basement membrane of thyroid follicles, resulting in tissue injury[19]. Although this could explain one of the mechanisms involved in the breakdown of the follicular structure, it cannot be applied to all the cases, as many thyroid patients lack circulating or already deposited immune complexes and many cases have no circulating thyroglobulin antibodies.

The second and more attractive possibility is the appearance of autoantigens on the outer surface of thyroid follicles. If the cells expressed autoantigens on their outer surface, they could be damaged by the complement-mediated cytotoxic effect of 'microvillar' antibodies, which would lead to the entering of autoantibodies into the follicles. They could also be destroyed by cytotoxic T-lymphocytes[20], which kill the cells by recognizing antigens, together with class I major histocompatibility complexes (HLA-A, -B, -C in man), on the surface of thyroid cells. Although this phenomenon has not been proven *in vivo*, preliminary experiments suggest that this hypothesis is promising. It has been shown that the reconstituted human thyroid follicles prepared from mildly

221

digested normal tissue have the potential to become reversed and able to express 'microvillar' antigens outside reconstituted follicles[21]. This suspension culture system will allow us to explore possible factors that induce the appearance of autoantigens *in vivo* on the vascular surface of thyroid follicles.

The following crucial question still remains, however: 'How can these autoantigens be presented to helper T-lymphocytes if thyroid cells normally do not possess class II major histocompatibility molecules (HLA-DR in man) which are necessary in the presentation of antigens[22]?' Trying to answer this question, we made a hypothesis that thyroid cells themselves might act as antigen-presenting cells by expressing HLA-DR molecules together with their organ-specific autoantigens on their surface. To study this possibility we stimulated normal thyroid monolayer cells with several mitogens (phytohaemoagglutinin, pokeweed mitogen and concanavalin A) and the reaction was revealed by indirect immunofluorescence using various monoclonal antibodies to the non-polymorphic region of the HLA-DR molecule. Interestingly, normal thyroid cells negative for HLA-DR before the stimulation became DR positive both on the membrane and in the cytoplasm 24 hours after culture with mitogens[23]. This suggested the active synthesis and expression of these molecules by thyroid cells. Both the number of positive cells and the intensity of the staining increased gradually up to 7 days. This phenomenon appears to be a direct effect of mitogens on thyroid cells, as the removal of contaminating lymphocytes or macrophages from the culture did not affect the extent of the positivity.

Following these experiments we investigated the spontaneous *in vivo* expression of HLA-DR in the thyrocytes in 46 cases of autoimmune thyroid disease, using the same monoclonal DR antibodies. Thyroidectomy specimens were examined by IFL in cultures and sections[24]. On thyroid monolayers this appeared as isolated cells showing granular surface DR staining. By double fluorochrome IFL these granules were quite separate from the 'microvillar' surface staining of Hashimoto antibodies. On tissue sections of Graves' glands DR staining could be seen in a patchy distribution not strictly related to lymphoid foci. Some follicles showed only one to three stained cells whereas others appeared fully involved. The IFL was diffuse in the cytoplasm of the affected cells and was sometimes more pronounced on their outer surface. In sections from Hashimoto's glands the staining was stronger and more diffuse. This observation was confirmed on partially digested 'half melon' thyrotoxic acini where DR staining was preferentially seen on the outer side surface of the half follicles.

It appears that aberrant DR expression could be one of the earliest markers of focal thyroiditis and we are now trying to correlate this in thyrotoxic glands with the established histological features, including the number of lymphocytic foci per field, the presence of Askenazy-cell metaplasia, germinal centres, epithelial damage, fibrosis, activated T lymphocytes, dendritic reticulum cells and paracortical interdigitating antigen-presenting cells. There is a suggestion that DR expression will correlate better with the postoperative course of the disease than the traditional parameters used by previous pathologists.

These findings support our view that thyroid cells themselves have the potentiality to present their autoantigens to helper T cells, together with newly expressed HLA-DR molecules induced by as yet unidentified factors, initiating or maintaining an autoimmune response. Previous attempts made to identify 'altered' antigens were unsuccessful in thyroiditis, but the new information presented may revive the importance of the unknown environmental factors that make the cells synthesize DR antigens.

We now believe that aberrant HLA-DR expression will also be seen in other endocrine tissues affected by autoimmune inflammatory lesions. We examined one diabetic pancreas in detail[25]. There were few remaining insulin secreting cells even at the very onset of the disease. By looking at many different blocks and examining a great number of islets in various stages of disintegration, it was possible to establish the presence of DR molecules in some surviving beta-cells. They were not seen in glucagon or in somatostatin cells which remain intact in diabetic insulitis. Interestingly, class I molecules (HLA-A, -B and -C) were also increased in the diabetic islets.

Immune responses are initiated by HLA-DR positive cells, which present antigens to T cells. Based on observations that HLA-DR may be experimentally induced on thyroid epithelium, and that it is found on thyrocytes in Graves' disease, we proposed a mechanism of autoimmunity with special relevance to organ-specific diseases[26]. This involves the local aberrant expression of HLA-DR antigens by epithelial cells and their subsequent capacity to present autoantigens occurring on their surfaces to T lymphocytes. For autoantigens which T cells recognize infrequently owing to their restricted tissue location and low concentration in the circulation, T-cell tolerance is unlikely and so induction of autoreactive T cells would occur.

Because interferon (IFN-γ) is the best known inducer of DR antigen expression and viral infections may predate endocrine autoimmunity, we envisage the following sequence: local viral infection which would cause IFN production, or any other local environmental factor which would induce DR antigen expression, presentation of autoantigens, and subsequent autoimmune T-cell induction. These T cells would activate effector B and T cells. Whether the initial induction of autoimmune T cells leads to autoimmune disease would depend on a variety of other factors such as abnormalities of the suppressor T-cell pathway, reported to coexist with autoimmunity and necessary to induce autoimmune diseases in mice. This mechanism of autoimmune disease induction explains vague associations with viral infections, long latency periods before disease becomes manifest and gives a straightforward explanation for the well-documented HLA-DR association of autoimmune diseases in man.

ACKNOWLEDGEMENTS

Work in the laboratory is supported by The Wellcome Trust Foundation, The Juvenile Diabetes Foundation (USA), The British Diabetic Association and The Medical Research Council. We thank Mrs Mirtha Clark for preparing the manuscript.

References

1. Mirakian, R., Richardson, C. A., Bottazzo, G. F. and Doniach, D. (1981). Humoral autoimmunity to gut-related endocrine cells. *Clin. Immunol. Newsl.*, **2**, 161–7
2. Scherbaum, W. A. and Bottazzo, G. F. (1983). Autoantibodies to vasopressin-cells in diopathic diabetes insipidus: evidence for an autoimmune variant. *Lancet*, **1**, 801–97
3. Doniach, D. and Bottazzo, G. F. (1983). Early detection of autoimmune endocrine disorders. *Hospital Up-date*, **9**, 1145–59
4. Doniach, D., Chiovato, L., Hanafusa, T. and Bottazzo, G. F. (1982). The implications of thyroid-growth-immunoglobulins (TGI) for the understanding of sporadic non-toxic nodular goitre. *Springer Semin. Immunopathol.*, **5**, 433–46
5. Fagraeus, A. and Jonsson, J. (1970). Distribution of organ antigens over the surface of thyroid cells as examined by the immunofluorescence test. *Immunology*, **18**, 413–16
6. Khoury, E. L., Hammond, L., Bottazzo, G. F. and Doniach, D. (1981). Presence of the organ-specific 'microsomal' antigen on the surface of human thyroid cells in culture: its involvement in complement-mediated cytotoxicity. *Clin. Exp. Immunol.*, **45**, 316–28
7. Dussault, J. H. and Walker, P. (eds.) (1983). *Congenital Hypothyroidism*. (New York: M. Dekker Inc.)
8. Khoury, E. L. (1982). Re-expression of blood group ABH antigens on the surface of human thyroid cells in culture. *J. Cell Biol.*, **94**, 193–8
9. Masala, C., Smurra, G., Di Prima, M. A., Amendolea, M. A., Celestino, D. and Salsano, F. (1980). Gastric parietal cell antibodies: demonstration by immunofluorescence of their reactivity with the surface of the gastric parietal cells. *Clin. Exp. Immunol.*, **41**, 271–80
10. de Aizpurua, H. J., Cosgrove, L. J., Ungar, B. and Toh, B. H. (1983). Autoantibodies cytotoxic to gastric parietal cells in serum of patients with pernicious anaemia. *N. Engl. J. Med.*, **309**, 625–9
11. Khoury, E. L., Hammond, L., Bottazzo, G. F. and Doniach, D. (1981). Surface reactive antibodies to adrenal cells in Addison's disease. *Clin. Exp. Immunol.*, **45**, 48–58
12. Papadopoulos, G. K. and Lernmark, A. (1983). The spectrum of islet cell antibodies. In Davies, T. F. (ed.) *Autoimmune Endocrine Disease*. pp. 167–80. (New York: John Wiley)
13. Naughton, G. K., Eisinger, M. and Bystryn, J. C. (1983). Antibodies to normal human melanocytes in vitiligo. *J. Exp. Med.*, **158**, 246–51

14. Betterle, L., Mirakian, R., Doniach, D., Bottazzo, G.F., Riley, W. and MacLaren, N. K. (1984). Antibodies to melanocyte in vitiligo. *Lancet*, **1**, 159
15. Roitt, I. M. and Doniach, D. (1958). Human autoimmune thyroiditis: serological studies. *Lancet*, **2**, 1027–32
16. Parker, R. H. and Beierwaltes, W. H. (1961). Thyroid antibodies during pregnancy and in the newborn. *J. Clin. Endocrinol.*, **21**, 792–800
17. Roitt, I. M. (1981). *Essential Immunology*. 4th Edn. (Oxford: Blackwell Scientific Publications)
18. Khoury, E. L., Bottazzo, G. F. and Roitt, I. M. (1984). The thyroid 'microsomal' antibody revisited: its paradoxical binding *in vivo* to the apical surface of the follicular epithelium. *J. Exp. Med.*, **159**, 577–91
19. Kalderon, A. E.(1980). Emerging role of immune complexes in autoimmune thyroiditis. *Pathol. Ann.* (Part 1), **15**, 23–35
20. Zinkernagel, R. M. and Doherty, P. C. (1979). MHC-restricted cytotoxic T cells: studies on the biological role of polymorphic major transplantation antigens determining T-cell restriction specificity, function and responsiveness. *Adv. Immunol.*, **27**, 51–91
21. Hanafusa, T., Pujol-Borrell, R., Chiovato, L., Doniach, D. and Bottazzo, G. F. (1984). *In vitro* and *in vivo* reversal of thyroid epithelial polarity: its relevance for autoimmune thyroid disease. *Clin. Exp. Immunol.* (Submitted)
22. Dorf, M. E. (1981). *The Role of the Major Histocompatibility Complex in Immunology*. (Chichester: John Wiley)
23. Pujol-Borrel, R., Hanafusa, T., Chiovato, L. and Bottazzo, G. F. (1983). Lectin-induced expression of DR antigen on human cultured follicular thyroid cells. *Nature (London)*, **304**, 71–3
24. Hanafusa, T., Pujol-Borrell, R., Chiovato, L., Russell, R. C. G., Doniach, D. and Bottazzo, G. F. (1983). Aberrant expression of HLA-DR antigen on thyrocytes in Graves' disease: relevance for autoimmunity. *Lancet*, **2**, 1111–15
25. Bottazzo, G. F. (1984). Beta cell damage in diabetic insulitis: are we approaching a solution? *Diabetologia.*, **26**, 241–50
26. Bottazzo, G. F., Pujol-Borrell, R., Hanafusa, T. and Feldmann, M. (1983). Hypothesis: role of aberrant HLA-DR expression and antigen presentation in the induction of endocrine autoimmunity. *Lancet*, **2**, 1115–19

15

CONTROVERSIES IN DIABETES

J. D. BAUM

In 1921, Banting and Best isolated insulin and in due course their efforts were rewarded by the Nobel Prize for the discovery of the 'cure' for diabetes[1]. Over the ensuing decades insulin manufacturers developed various forms of insulin with delayed absorption characteristics which allowed a reduction in the number of daily injections[2, 3]. In 1955, Sanger completed his work on the amino acid sequence of porcine insulin, work which was again distinguished by the award of the Nobel Prize[4]. In 1968, Steiner performed the chromatographic separation of insulin crystals[5], with the identification of a range of impurities in insulin preparations which led to the development of monocomponent insulins and most recently purified preparations of human insulin[6].

Meanwhile, in 1936, Kimmelstiel and Wilson identified a lethal form of nephropathy specific to the diabetic patient[7]. This represented a single example of the wide range of microvascular complications that were being recognized among patients with long-standing insulin-requiring diabetes mellitus. Thus, while insulin prevented the rapid and fatal decline of patients presenting with diabetes, it introduced the considerable range of delayed morbidity and associated reduction in life expectancy among the survivors[8]. Sixty years after the discovery of the 'cure' for diabetes there has been little advance in the prevention of these complications.

There is still considerable controversy regarding the cause of diabetic microvascular damage. The consensus view at present is that chronic hyperglycaemia is the major factor and clinically an attempt should be made to achieve as near normal blood glucose control as is possible[9]. How this is to be accomplished remains uncertain. Which is the best insulin regimen? What is the preferred diet? Indeed, what are the objectives of management in terms of diabetic control?

While I shall touch upon these issues I shall also endeavour to indicate why I think that the very focus of these controversies has been blurred in that they have, on the whole, not been addressed to the needs of the 'free-range' diabetic child living in his normal environment under everyday conditions. I shall indicate how I think these controversies may be realistically resolved in the future and, finally, consider recent developments in the treatment and prevention of diabetes and the dilemmas that these pose in terms of the management of children with diabetes today.

TOWARDS 'GOOD DIABETIC CONTROL'

It is generally held to be axiomatic that there is a relationship between diabetic control and the risk of the complications of long-standing diabetes[9]. In this context 'diabetic control' is generally taken to mean the maintenance of blood glucose within the normal physiological range

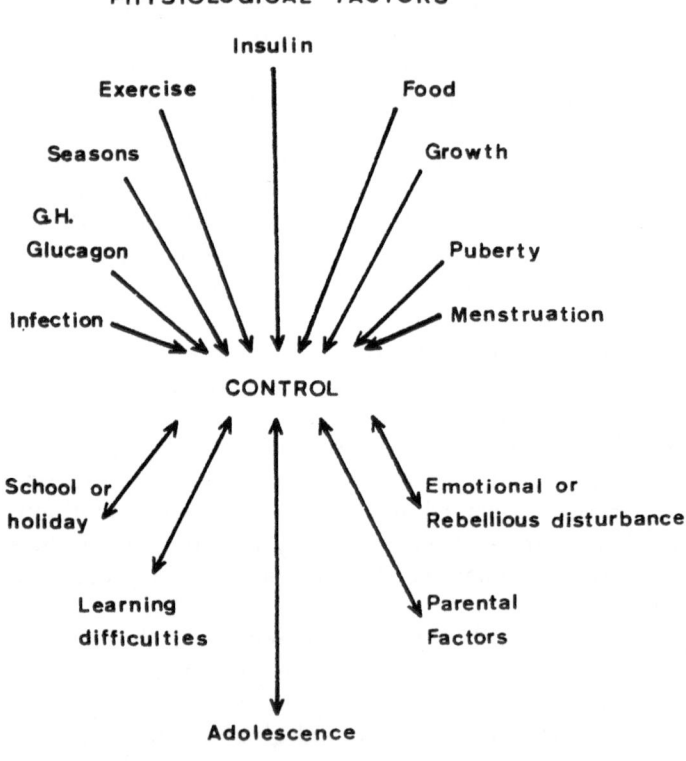

Figure 1　Factors which influence diabetic control

throughout the day and night. Among insulin-requiring diabetic children there are a multitude of factors which influence diabetic control; these can arbitrarily be divided into physiological and psychological (Figure 1). In many ways those factors labelled as psychological are the most powerful in their influence upon the day-to-day control of blood glucose. However, it is only insulin, diet and, to some extent, exercise which can be readily manipulated by the physician and patient in their joint endeavour to achieve good control.

INSULIN

While a range of insulins is available and many different regimens of therapy are used, the majority of children, particularly those who are prepubertal, prefer a simple once-daily insulin regimen such as a combined injection of Monotard* and Actrapid* insulin given some 20–30 minutes before breakfast. This regimen, which was used in Werther's studies[10], led to blood glucose profiles (Figure 2a) which are certainly no worse than those published by other authors employing alternative multiple-dose insulin regimes[11,12].

In recent years, taking advantage of Steiner's identification of C-peptide and the availability of monocomponent insulins, it has become clear that subjects with residual endogenous insulin production have more stable and more physiological blood glucose levels than those with no such reserve, whichever insulin regimen is employed. This can be seen from Werther's data[10] separating the four subjects who were C-peptide positive from the 11 subjects who were C-peptide negative, showing clearly that the children with endogenous insulin could maintain their blood glucose levels near the normal physiological range (Figure 2b).

It should be noted, however, that studies concerning the effect of insulin regimens on blood glucose concentration have usually been performed under highly artificial conditions. Thus Werther's profile represents blood glucose levels from a selected group of 15 children who had been carefully managed for 6 weeks prior to their admission to hospital for a 36-hour period, during which time a venous cannula was inserted and blood glucose samples taken for measurements. How far these or the other similar published results reflect everyday control among ordinary diabetic children remains highly questionable.

DIET

Manipulation of the daily diet represents the second most important variable which the physician and child can alter in order to influence

---

* Novo Industries.

blood glucose concentrations throughout the 24 hours. Studies from different clinics have shown that increasing the carbohydrate and fibre content of a diet leads, in general, to an improvement in blood glucose control[13,14]. The studies of Kinmonth *et al.*[15] have shown that, in

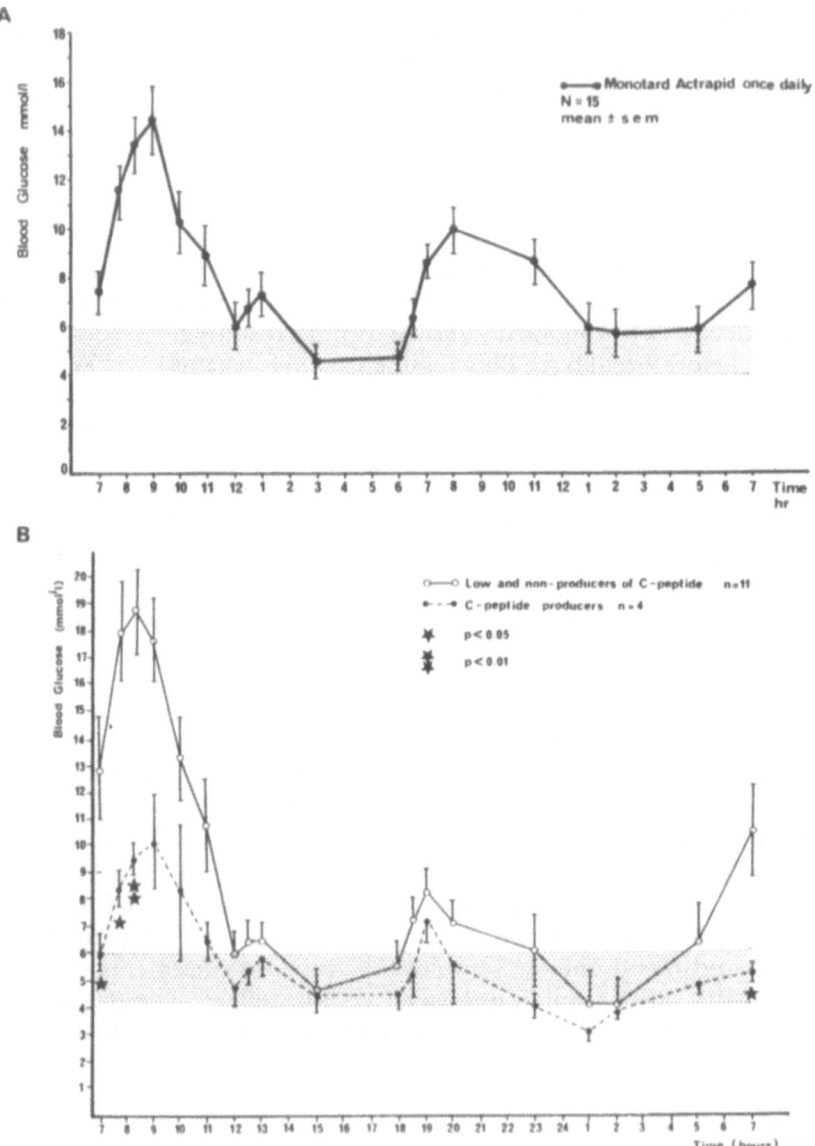

Figure 2 (A) Blood glucose profile from 15 diabetic children on Monotard and Actrapid insulin once daily[10]. Shaded area represents physiological range of blood glucose. (B) Blood glucose profiles separating out the four children with endogenous insulin reserves whose control is near the normal physiological range[10]

children, a diet including whole foods high in dietary fibre in which 55% of the energy comes from carbohydrate sources led to a great improvement in blood glucose levels throughout the 24 hours (Figure 3).

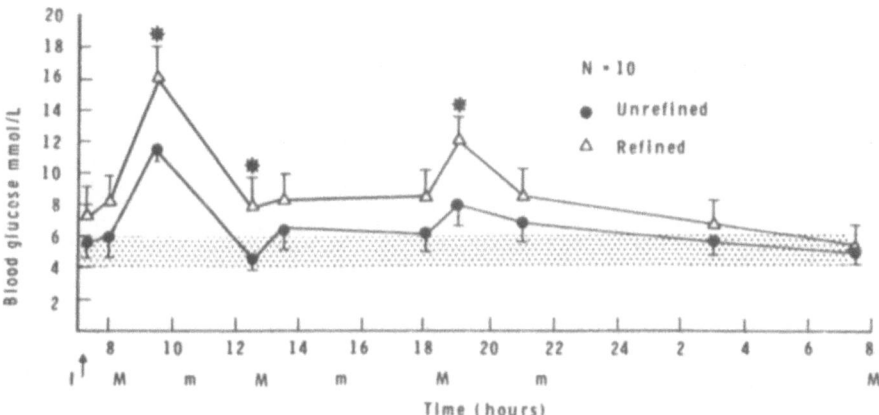

Figure 3 Blood glucose profiles from 10 diabetic children indicating that during the period on a diet high in dietary fibre the control is nearer to the normal physiological range (shown as the shaded area)[15]

These studies were performed on 10 subjects who volunteered to participate in this highly demanding clinical experiment. The children were meticulously managed on a day-to-day basis during the 3 months of the study by Dr Kinmonth and were encouraged and supported to keep to their diet throughout by a research dietitian. One may reasonably question what the effect of prescribing a high fibre, high carbohydrate diet might be on ordinary diabetic children under everyday conditions. However, it should be noted that in this study at least much of the evaluation was based on capillary blood glucose measurements performed by the children at home throughout the course of the trial.

INSULIN PUMPS

In 1978, Pickup, Keen and others published experiments in adults on the delivery of insulin by continuous insulin infusion pump as an improved means of controlling blood glucose throughout the 24 hours[16]. Since then a number of studies in adults have confirmed that a continuous subcutaneous insulin infusion can achieve blood glucose levels within the normal physiological range over prolonged periods of time[17,18]. Greene et al. have recently shown[19] that pump therapy can be applied to children and in their study of seven children the blood glucose profile on pump therapy was relatively physiological when compared with a

231

control period on optimized conventional insulin therapy (Figure 4). In particular, the blood glucose surge after breakfast, so prevalent on conventional insulin regimens, was not seen in the children on continuous subcutaneous insulin infusion.

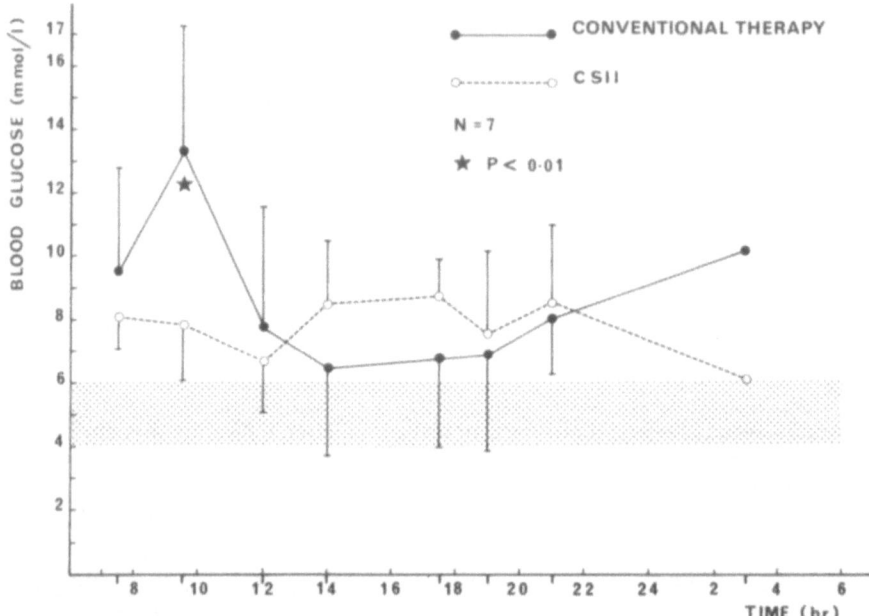

Figure 4 Blood glucose profiles from seven diabetic children indicating that on continuous subcutaneous insulin infusion (CSII), or pump therapy, the control is nearer to the normal physiological range (shown as the shaded area)[19]

Once again, before generalizing the results of this study, it is important to realize that these seven children can hardly be held to be representative of the clinic as a whole in that they volunteered to participate in the study. Moreover, they were under close supervision throughout the course of the study (a factor itself known to improve diabetic control)[20] and the study was sequential in its design. Nevertheless, the blood glucose measurements were performed at home throughout the course of the study and to this extent can be taken to reflect the blood glucose concentrations prevailing among this group of children under more or less normal living conditions.

However, Greene's study did reveal certain aspects of pump therapy which need to be considered in relation to the place of this therapy in the management of children with diabetes in the future. For example, the children were able to relax on some details of their daily diet, both in its content and frequency of snacks and meals dictated by the clock. They found that the pump led to restrictions in speed and style of dressing and, from the girls' point of view, led to certain limitations of fashion. Vigorous forms of exercise required the pump to be removed and led to the practical problems of the safe storage of the pump during sporting activities. Some of the older boys also indicated that the pump presented difficulties in relation to the spontaneity of their sexual behaviour.

A single experience with the pump in a boy with particularly unstable diabetes clearly demonstrated to us how inappropriate this form of therapy is for such subjects. In his case it became clear that his diabetes was unstable as a direct result of deliberate manipulation and that the pump offered nothing more than an addition to his repertoire.

For the time being continuous subcutaneous insulin therapy is probably best restricted to a relatively small proportion of teenagers with diabetes who are intelligent and sufficiently well organized to cope with the technical management of the pump and the frequent daily blood glucose monitoring necessary for its safe employment. In the future, as pumps become smaller and hopefully coupled to glucose sensors, the applicability of insulin pump therapy will greatly extend. For the present, however, the majority of diabetic children must be managed using conventional insulin therapy with all its imperfections.

MONITORING

The blood glucose profiles referred to above (Figures 2–4) represent those achievable under idealized conditions. We need now to ask: what are the achievable targets of control and how can these be measured among ordinary diabetic children under ordinary living conditions?

Blood glucose measurement in the home represents a direct measurement of the variable at the centre of the diabetic control controversy. There are many recommendations for the routine collection of blood glucose measurements by diabetic subjects, but these recommendations themselves have to be considered in relation to the child's age, ability and motivation to take and record such measurements. Where blood glucose measurements have been collected under normal conditions by representative diabetic children they have shown that the average child runs blood glucose concentrations which are mostly in the order of twice that of the normal physiological range (Figure 5)[21].

Glycosylated haemoglobin levels also give some idea of the magnitude and range of the imperfections of blood glucose control prevalent among diabetic children. It is a very small minority who achieve normal glycosylated haemoglobin concentrations, the majority having levels 50% or more above the normal (Figure 6). Although it has been shown that the glycosylated haemoglobin concentration correlates well with physicians' ratings and with measurements of blood glucose concentrations, how well it indicates the threshold, if one exists, above which the risks of microvascular disease begin to escalate, remains uncertain.

The measurement of daily blood glucose and glycosylated haemo-globin provides evidence not previously available which directly relates to diabetic control. We can now address the problem of the long-term storage and analysis of such data and how it interacts with the development of diabetic microvascular disease. Recent advances in micro-electronics and computer technology offer the possibility of resolving the problem of long-term data storage, retrieval and analysis.

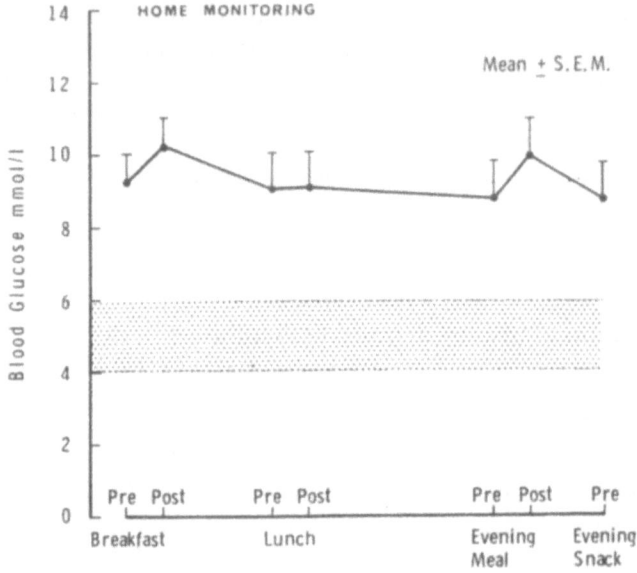

Figure 5 Blood glucose measurements collected under normal conditions by average diabetic children indicating how far the blood glucose concentrations are removed from the normal physiological range (shown as the shaded area)[21]

One recent development in blood glucose monitoring seems relevant here. A glucose reflectance meter designed for home use (Glucometer*) has recently been modified to our specifications to incorporate a real-time memory. The data collected by the diabetic subject on a day-to-day basis can be transferred automatically to a microcomputer, thereby short-circuiting the need for the patient to keep a written record of blood glucose measurements. At the same time, the system leads to an improvement in the precision of data recording in relation to time of day, preceding events, day of the week, season of the year, etc. However, whatever the refinements in data collection and storage, the prospect of evaluating such information against the development of overt diabetic microvascular disease *decades later* remains a major obstacle in the advancement of the subject.

---

*Miles Laboratories Limited.

LATENT MICROVASCULAR DISEASE

It seems possible that shorter-term outcome measures may be used in assessing the influence of blood glucose control by looking at physiological tests of the integrity of the microvascular circulation rather than awaiting the signs and symptoms of established microvascular disease.

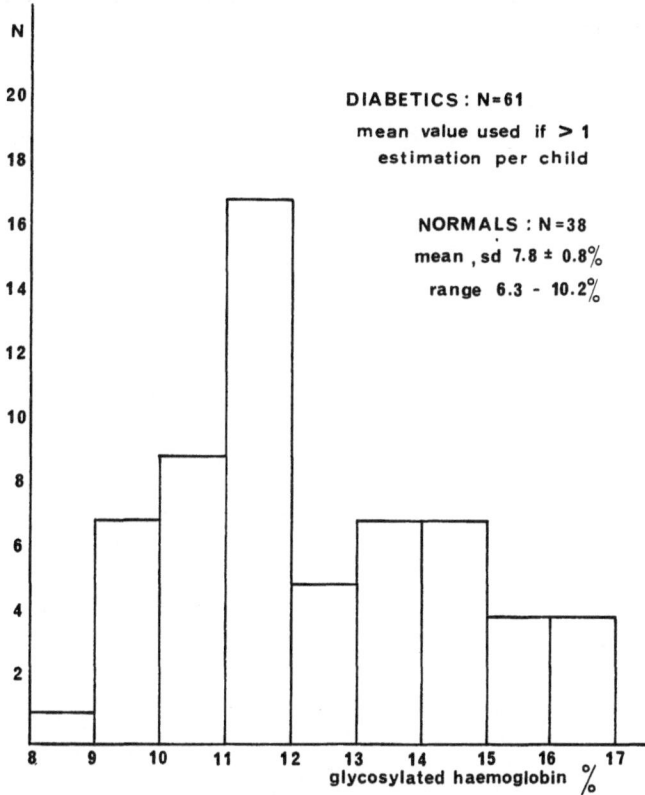

Figure 6 Glycosylated haemoglobin concentrations from 61 diabetic children indicating that the majority have levels 50% or more above the normal

There are now a number of promising approaches to the measurement of what might be called latent microvascular disease. These include: investigation of the microcirculation of the retina utilizing fluorescein angiography[22]; estimating the functional integrity of the cutaneous microcirculation of the forearm by changes in transcutaneous oxygen tension in response to vascular occlusion and subsequent flush[23]; looking at the functional behaviour of the connective tissue of the hands reflected by fixed flection deformities, as described by Rosenbloom *et al.*[24]; and the evaluation of renal microvascular health by radioimmunoassay of urinary albumin[25]. While such a range of tests are likely to be suitable as outcome measures for any study on the influence of various regimes of management, it is perhaps the measurements of urinary albumin excretion by radioimmunoassay, possibly enhanced by an exercise test, which offer the most readily available quantitation of diabetic microvascular damage (Greene, unpublished information). An example of the separation of the postexercise urinary albumin excretion among a group of diabetic children compared with a group of normal children is shown in Figure 7.

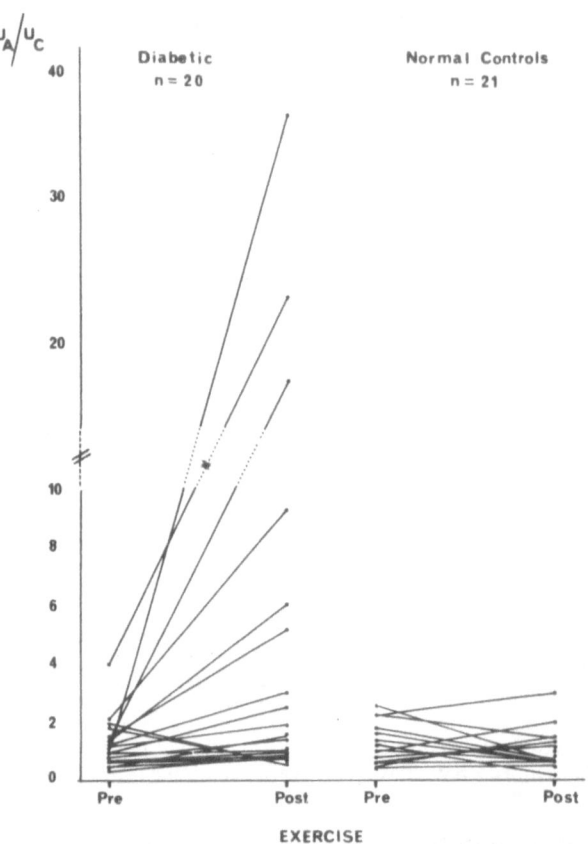

Figure 7 Urinary albumin excretion is expressed as the ratio of urinary albumin to creatinine concentration. This ratio becomes elevated in six diabetic children after exercise, while there is no change in a comparable group of normal children (Greene, unpublished information)

The availability of a battery of tests for the detection of latent microvascular disease offers the possibility of evaluating controlled trials of different therapeutic regimes (for example, pump therapy vs. conventional therapy) and also offers the possibility of evaluating early therapeutic manoeuvres, such as, for example, the use of hypotensive agents in the management of early nephropathy associated with mild hypertension.

INCIDENCE, AETIOLOGY AND PREVENTION

While the struggle for improvement in the management and evaluation of diabetes continues, a number of physicians working with diabetic children have formed the impression that the actual incidence of the disease is increasing. Two recent studies[26, 27] have supported this impression, suggesting that the disease has doubled in its incidence over the last 10 years in the United Kingdom. Figures from the Oxford Children's Diabetes Clinic possibly support this impression, even when allowance is made for any referrals to the clinic from outside its natural catchment area. This impression is not, however, shared by the notification register at the British Diabetic Association (Gamble, personal communication) which shows no changes in the incidence over the decades. However, it could be argued that the unknown variability in the rate of reporting cases of diabetes to the British Diabetic Association Register must represent a serious confounding factor. If, however, the impressions of an increasing incidence are confirmed then the question of the aetiology and the possibility of preventing type 1 diabetes mellitus must be considered as a matter of the utmost urgency.

Family studies have shown that diabetes in children is associated with particular tissue type markers which, by association with loci on chromosome 6, suggest that a disorder of the immunological regulation is closely associated with the diabetogenic process[28]. For example, the striking association between B8, B15 and DR4 with diabetes can be seen in Table 1. Furthermore, studies on islet cell antibodies lend support to an autoimmune element in the development of the disease[29]. In two studies

Tables 1a and 1b   Comparison of the frequencies (%) of HLA antigens in index: patients and controls[34]

Antigen	Patients $n = 76$	Controls $n = 180$	Antigen	Patients $n = 43$	Controls $n = 150$
A10	4.0	15.3*	DR2	2.3	30.0‡
Aw19	9.2	30.7†	DR3	46.5	19.3‡
B8	48.7	19.3‡	DR4	93.0	24.7‡
B15	39.5	8.0‡	DRw6	7.0	23.3*
B17	1.3	11.9*	DR7	0.0.	36.4*
Bw6	38.2	61.4†			

$*p < 0.05$ ⎫
$†p < 0.01$ ⎬ denote significance level for the difference between patients and controls.
$‡p < 0.001$ ⎭ Only data for antigens differing substantially in frequency are shown.

the majority of children with diabetes have been shown to be islet cell antibody positive at the time of diagnosis[30, 31]. Furthermore, islet cell antibodies have been demonstrated among family members of children with diabetes; and from among these family members a number have become frankly diabetic after the passage of months and, in some instances, years[32].

These observations raise the possibility that an early identification of the diabetogenic process may be'possible and that some medical intervention might lead to the arrest or reversal of the process. Experiments in diabetic strains of rats have shown that cyclosporin can prevent the onset of diabetes[33]. It remains to be seen whether clinically acceptable agents can be identified which will safely suppress or reverse such an autoimmune process in human subjects.

CONCLUSIONS

For the present, despite two Nobel Prizes in the field of diabetes, we are left as children's physicians with the frustration of offering our patients hope, mixed with an honest appraisal of the long-term prospects for health and disease. The details of today's management remain controversial. However, we now have the tools to resolve our uncertainties in the future, particularly with the advent of microcomputer technology.

We should not lead our patients to hope that a dramatic cure for diabetes will present itself in the immediate future. We can perhaps hope for progress towards successful islet cell transplantation or miniaturized implantable insulin delivery devices, but it is likely that these developments are still a long way off. For the present the prospect of such developments may serve to sustain the morale and fortitude of the' physician and the patient alike.

References

1. Banting, F. G., Best, G. H., Coup, J. B., Campbell, W. R. and Fletcher, A. A. (1922). Pancreatic extracts in the treatment of diabetes mellitus. *Can. Med. Assoc. J.*, **12**, 141–6
2. Hagedon, H. C., Jensen, P. N., Krarup, N. B. and Wodstrup, I. (1936). Protamine insulinate. *J. Am. Med. Assoc.*, **106**, 177
3. Hallas-Moller, K. (1945). Chemical and biological insulin studies I and II. Dissertation, Copenhagen
4. Sanger, F. (1959). Chemistry of insulin: determination of the structure of insulin opens the way to greater understanding of life process. *Science*, **129**, 1340–4
5. Steiner, D. F., Hallund, O., Rubenstein, A., Cho, S. and Bayliss, C. (1968). Isolation and properties of proinsulin, intermediate forms and other minor components from crystalline bovine insulin. *Diabetes*, **17**, 725–36
6. Moritata, K., Oken, T. and Tzuzuki, H. (1979). Semi synthesis of human insulin by tryplin-catalysed replacement of Ala-B30 by Thr in porcine insulin. *Nature (London)*, **280**, 412–13

7. Kimmelstiel, P. and Wilson, C. (1936). Intercapillary lesions in glomerulous of kidney. *Am. J. Pathol.*, **12**, 83–98

8. Deckert, T., Poulsen, J. E. and Larsen, M. (1978). Prognosis of diabetics with diabetes onset before the age of thirty-one. I. Survival, causes of death and complications. *Diabetologia*, **14**, 363–70

9. Tchbroutsky, G. (1978). Relation of diabetic control to development of microvascular complications. *Diabetologia*, **15**, 143–52

10. Werther, G. A., Jenkins, P. A., Turner, R. C. and Baum, J. D. (1980). Twenty-four-hour metabolic profiles in diabetic children receiving insulin injections once or twice daily. *Br. Med. J.*, **281**, 414–18

11. Francis, A. J., Howe, P. D., Hanning, I., Alberti, K. G. M. M. and Tunbridge, W. M. G. (1983). Intermediate acting insulin given at bedtime: effect on blood glucose concentrations before and after breakfast. *Br. Med. J.*, **286**, 1173–6

12. Ward, G. M., Simpson, R. W., Ward, E. A. and Turner, R. C. (1981). Comparison of two twice daily insulin regimens: ultralente/soluble and soluble/isophane. *Diabetologia*, **21**, 383–6

13. Simpson, H. C. R., Lonsley, S., Geekie, M. *et al.* (1981). A carbohydrate leguminous fibre diet improves all aspects of diabetic control. *Lancet*, **1**, 1–5

14. Goulder, T. T. and Alberti, K. G. M. M. (1978). Dietary fibre and diabetes. *Diabetologia*, **15**, 285–7

15. Kinmonth, A. L., Angus, R. M., Jenkins, P. A., Smith, M. A. and Baum, J. D. (1982). Whole foods and increased dietary fibre improve blood glucose control in diabetic children. *Arch. Dis. Child.*, **57**, 187–94

16. Pickup, J. C., Keen, H., Partons, J. A. and Alberti, K. G. M. M. (1978). Continuous subcutaneous insulin infusion: an approach to achieving normoglycaemia. *Br. Med. J.*, **1**, 204

17. Tamborlane, W. V., Sherwin, R. S., Gench, M. and Felig, P. (1980). Outpatient treatment of juvenile onset diabetes with a preprogrammed portable subcutaneous insulin infusion system. *Am. J. Med.*, **68**, 190–6

18. Mecklenburg, R. S. *et al.* (1982). Clinical use of the insulin infusion pump in 100 patients with Type 1 diabetes. *N. Engl. J. Med.*, **307**, 513–18

19. Greene, S. A., Smith, M. A. and Baum, J. D. (1983). Clinical application of insulin pumps in the management of insulin dependent diabetes. *Arch. Dis. Child.*, **58**, 578–81

20. Skyler, J. S., Seigler, D. E. and Reeves, M. C. (1982). A comparison of insulin regimens in insulin dependent diabetes mellitus. *Diabetes Care*, **5** (Suppl. 1), 11–18

21. Greene, S. A., Smith, M. A., Cartwright, B. and Baum, J. D. (1984). A comparison of human versus porcine insulin in the treatment of diabetes in children. *Br. Med. J.* (In press)

22. Malone, J. I., Van Cader, T. C. and Edwards, W. C. (1977). Diabetic vascular changes in children. *Diabetes*, **26**, 673–9

23. Ewald, U., Rooth, G. and Tuvemo, T. (1981). Early reduction of vascular reactivity in diabetic children detected by transcutaneous oxygen electrode. *Lancet*, **72**, 373–8

24. Rosenbloom, A. L. *et al.* (1981). Limited joint mobility in childhood diabetes mellitus indicates increased risk for microvascular disease. *N. Engl. J. Med.*, **305**, 191–4

25. Viberti, G. C. *et al.* (1982). Microalbuminuria as a predictor of clinical nephropathy in insulin dependent diabetes mellitus. *Lancet*, **1**, 1430–2

26. Stewart-Brown, S., Hasman, M. and Butler, N. (1983). Evidence for increasing prevalence of diabetes mellitus in childhood. *Br. Med. J.*, **286**, 1855–7

27. Patterson, C. C., Thorogood, M., Smith, P. G., Hensman, M. A., Clarke, J. A. and Mann, J. I. (1983). Epidemiology of type 1 (insulin dependent) diabetes in Scotland 1968–76: evidence of an increasing incidence. *Diabetologia*, **24**, 238–43

28. Cudworth, A. G. (1980). Current concepts in the aetiology of type 1 (insulin dependent diabetes mellitus). In Berlingham, A. J. (ed.) *Advanced Medicine*. Vol. 16, pp. 123–35. (London: Pitman)
29. Botazzo, G. F., Dean, B. M., Gornson, A. N., Cudworth, A. G. and Doniach, D. (1980). Complement fixing islet cell antibodies in type 1 diabetes: possible monitors of active beta-cell damage. *Lancet*, **1**, 668–72
30. Bottazzo, G. F., Mann, J. I., Thorogood, M., Baum, J. D. and Doniach, D. (1978). Autoimmunity in juvenile diabetics and their families. *Br. Med. J.*, **2**, 165–8
31. Lendrum, R. *et al.* (1976). Islet cell antibodies in diabetes mellitus. *Lancet*, **2**, 1273–6
32. Gornsoh, A. N. *et al.* (1981). Evidence for a long prediabetic period in type 1 (insulin dependent) diabetes mellitus. *Lancet*, **2**, 1363–6
33. Lampacis, A. *et al.* (1983). Cyclosporin prevents diabetes in BB Wistar rats. *Lancet*, **1**, 10–12
34. Winnearls *et al.* (1984). A family study of the association between insulin-dependent diabetes mellitus, autoantibodies and the HLA system. (Submitted for publication)

16

PRACTICAL MANAGEMENT OF DISORDERS OF CALCIUM HOMEOSTASIS

J. ALLGROVE

INTRODUCTION

Disorders of mineral homeostasis are relatively uncommon during childhood, but their recognition and diagnosis is of considerable importance, since failure to appreciate their presence may result in long periods of suffering during which time effective treatment is often available. During this discourse I shall briefly discuss the principal methods which are currently available for the investigation of these conditions and then illustrate how these investigations can be used to diagnose the cause of each of the most important disorders of calcium homeostasis in childhood, thus enabling a logical form of treatment to be instituted.

INVESTIGATIONS

The measurement of serum calcium is of paramount importance in this respect and must be undertaken if there is any possibility of hypo- or hypercalcaemia. This prevents patients being labelled as epileptic and treated for several years, often unsatisfactorily, with anticonvulsants when measurement of serum calcium would reveal that hypocalcaemia was the cause of their convulsions. At the same time, serum albumin concentrations should always be measured in conjunction with total serum calcium and a suitable adjustment made to the latter if necessary. Outside the neonatal period serum calcium remains remarkably constant throughout life, being maintained between 2.2 and 2.6 mmol/l, although it is slightly higher in early childhood than later on[1].

In contrast, serum inorganic phosphorus is considerably higher in early childhood than subsequently, and only falls to adult levels after adolescence, being highest during periods of rapid growth[2]. Likewise, alkaline phosphatase is also closely related to growth rates[2] and may normally be as much as five or six times adult levels during periods of very rapid growth. These normal variations should be taken into account when assessing parameters of mineral metabolism in childhood.

The measurement of serum magnesium should also be undertaken, particularly during the neonatal period or if malabsorption is considered to be a cause of hypocalcaemia, since hypomagnesaemia may be the cause of low serum calcium which is resistant to treatment unless the magnesium deficiency is corrected[3].

The assessment of urinary losses of minerals is important if a disorder of renal tubular function is suspected. Urinary cation excretion varies with dietary intake[4,5], but total daily losses of calcium do not usually exceed 0.1 mmol/kg bodyweight/day[6]. It is more satisfactory to express this in terms of some measure of renal function and the normal molar ratio of urinary calcium/creatinine is between 0.1 and 0.7 mmol Ca/mmol creatinine in the mid-morning sample[6]. More exact measurements of urinary calcium and magnesium excretion, which eliminate the effects of body size, renal function and serum concentrations, such as the tubular maximum rate of reabsorption expressed as a function of GFR (TmCa/GFR)[7], can be calculated if a more precise measurement of tubular function is needed.

The measurement of urinary excretion of phosphorus is most easily undertaken by assessing the fractional excretion or tubular reabsorption of phosphorus (TRP). This can be calculated from measurements of phosphorus and creatinine on *simultaneous* samples of serum and fresh urine (*not* 24-hour urine collections) according to the formula:

$$TRP = 1 - [Up/Pp \times Pcr/Ucr].$$

This obviates the necessity of timed urine collections which may be difficult in children. However, since TRP is partly dependent on the serum phosphorus level, a more precise assessment can be estimated from the nomogram of Walton and Bijvoet[8] for the calculation, from TRP and serum phosphorus, of TmP/GFR which is independent of the latter and which is as applicable to children as to adults[9], although normal values are higher in children[10].

It is now well established that vitamin D is available from two sources, both as vitamin D_2, ergocalciferol, and vitamin D_3, cholecalciferol, which are equipotent in man and which undergo two hydroxylation steps, firstly, to 25-hydroxyvitamin-D (25OHD) in the liver, and, secondly, to 1,25-dihydroxyvitamin-D ($1,25(OH)_2D$) in the kidney before becoming fully active (Figure 1). Several other metabolites are also synthesized and all the major compounds which are known to circulate in man can now be measured either by radioreceptor[11] or radioimmunoassays[12]. Because of cross-reactivity between the binding proteins and the various substrates, clear separation between them must first be obtained using high performance liquid chromatography. This is particularly important since the most active metabolite, $1,25(OH)_2D$, circulates in the lowest concentration of 20–60 pg/ml[12], whilst the circulating concentration of the most abundant metabolite, 25OHD, may be as much as 1000 times greater (3–30 ng/ml)[13].

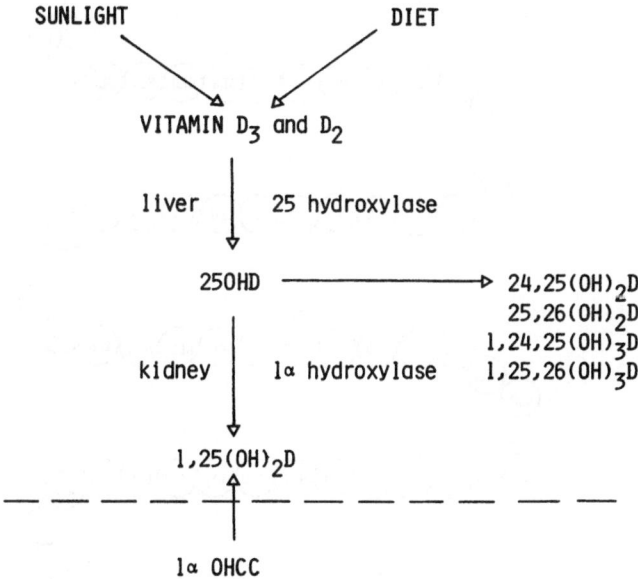

Figure 1 Schematic representation of the major pathways of vitamin D metabolism. The main pathway to the active metabolite, $1,25(OH)_2D$, is shown on the vertical axis, additional pathways horizontally. Below the horizontal interrupted line the synthetic compound 1α-OHCC is shown

The measurement of parathyroid hormone (PTH) in serum is fraught with problems, not least because PTH is a single-chain polypeptide hormone of 84 amino acids (Figure 2), only the first 34 of which are required for full biological activity. Assays of PTH which are routinely available are immunoassays, and the best employ antibodies to human hormone which have been selected for high affinity for one or other part of the PTH molecule[14]. However, the antibodies probably only recognize sequences of six to eight amino acids[15], and it is now becoming increasingly recognized that much of the material which is measured in these assays has no biological activity. Recent studies using bioassays of PTH in plasma, particularly the cytochemical bioassay[16,17], have confirmed the view that, in most situations, at least 90% of the PTH which is measured by immunoassay is inert. Nevertheless, immunoassays remain the clinical yardstick by which PTH secretion is assessed, although the results must be interpreted with caution. As with phosphorus and alkaline phosphatase[18], both $1,25(OH)_2D$ and PTH concentrations are generally higher in children than in adults, particularly during periods of rapid growth[19].

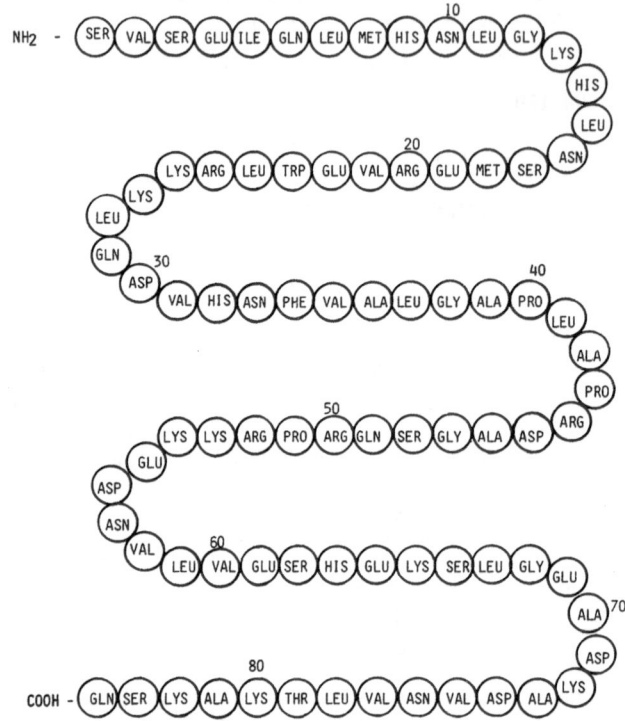

Figure 2   Amino acid sequence of human PTH. The sequence of the intact hormone is shown. Only the first 34 residues are required for full biological activity. The function of the rest of the molecule is not known

In some situations it is necessary to measure the response of target organs, particularly the kidney, to PTH which has been administered exogenously. In the Ellsworth–Howard test[20] changes in urinary excretion or tubular reabsorption of phosphorus are measured before and for 3 hours after giving a standard dose of PTH, usually $200\,U/1.73\,m^2$. During this time phosphate excretion should increase at least three-fold. Alternatively, since PTH is thought to act in the kidneys via adenosine 3'5'-cyclic monophosphate (cAMP) as a second messenger[21], changes in the urinary excretion or plasma concentration of cAMP can be measured in response to a similar dose of PTH[22]. I prefer the latter method as this obviates the necessity of timed urine collections which may be unreliable in children. A normal response is seen if a rise of at least 60 nmol/l in the plasma concentration of cAMP occurs (Figure 3). The peak of this rise is usually 7–10 minutes after the injection of PTH. Urinary cAMP excretion should increase 50–80-fold[22]. Impaired responses are seen as a primary phenomenon in pseudohypoparathyroidism[23,24] or as a result of hyperparathyroidism[25], or in renal failure[22].

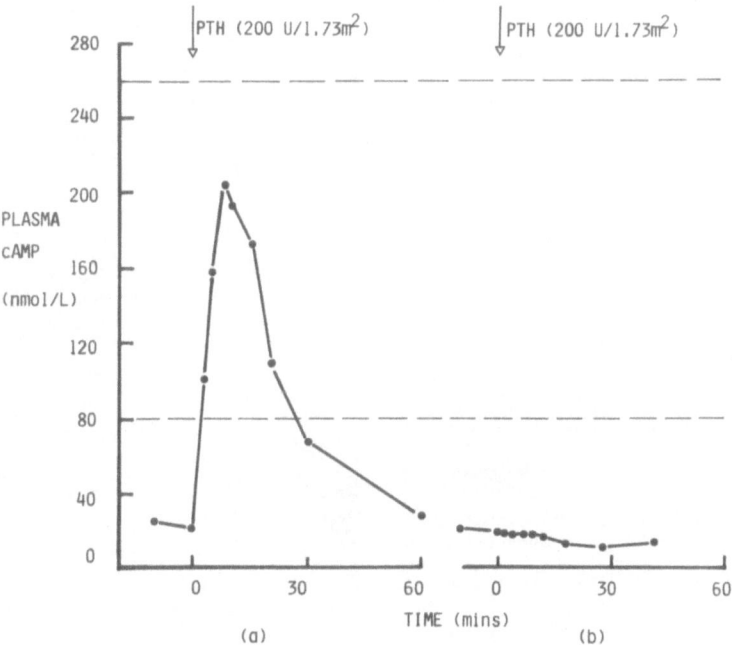

Figure 3 Plasma cAMP responses following intravenous injection of PTH (200 U/1.73 m²). (a) Normal response, (b) patient with pseudohypoparathyroidism. The horizontal interrupted lines represent the limits of the normal response

Radiological studies are frequently of help in the investigation of disorders of mineral metabolism. Some caution must be exercised in interpreting these X-rays in children, particularly since the appearances of hyperparathyroidism and rickets may closely resemble one another[26].

CLINICAL APPLICATIONS

(1) Rickets of very low birth weight (VLBW) infants

In recent years, since the introduction of more effective methods of treating VLBW infants, rickets of prematurity has become increasingly recognized as a problem which may result in respiratory distress, fractures and osteopenia (Figure 4). The aetiology of this condition is not

245

known for certain. It has been suggested that inadequate supply[27] or impaired metabolism or utilization[28] of vitamin D may be responsible, but treatment of these infants with even very large doses of vitamin D, up to 2000 U/day, or its more active metabolites, has not always resulted in resolution of the problem[29], and attention has therefore been focussed on the possibility that deficiency of the substrates for mineralization, particularly calcium and phosphorus, may also be partly responsible[30, 31].

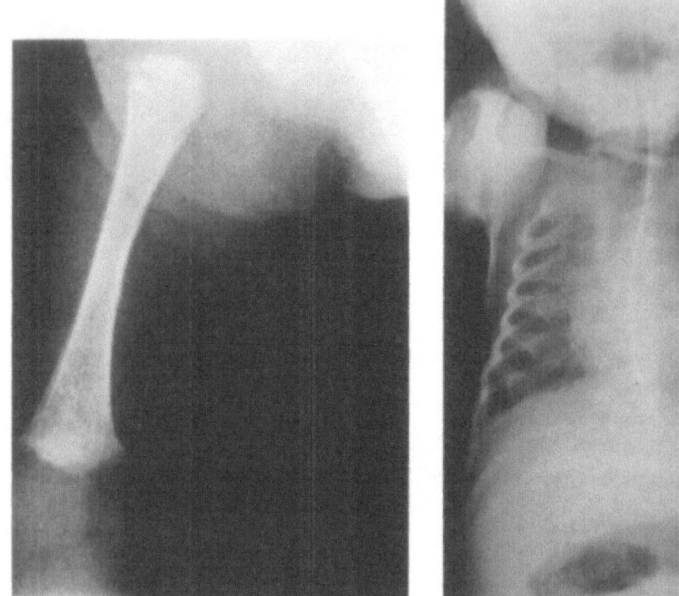
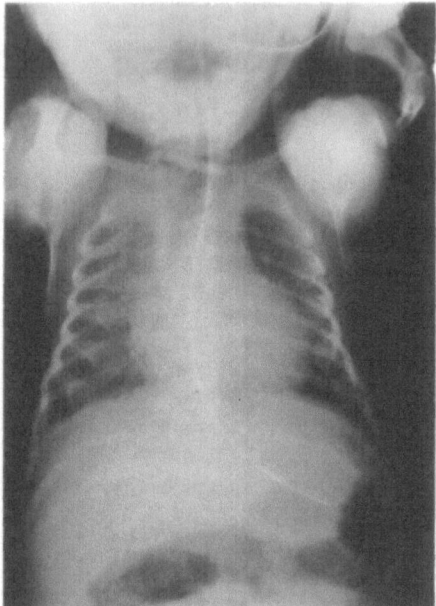

Figure 4   X-ray appearances in rickets of prematurity. (a) Femur, (b) chest. (Films by courtesy of the X-ray Department, Birmingham Maternity Hospital)

Requirements for calcium and phosphorus for normal bone mineralization are considerable and a very good correlation exists between $\log_{10}$ body-weight and $\log_{10}$ total body content of these minerals (Figures 5 and 6.)[32]. Differentiation of the equations for the regression lines yields the following formulae:

$$Ca(mg) = 0.982 \times \text{body-weight}^{0.3093}(g)$$
$$\text{and} \quad P(mg) = 0.906 \times \text{body-weight}^{0.2409}(g).$$

From these formulae the rate of accumulation of calcium and phosphorus per unit gain in weight can be calculated for any given body-weight. If this figure is multiplied by the observed rate of weight gain, an estimate of the daily calcium and phosphorus requirements for normal growth can be made. A logical approach to the treatment of these babies can therefore be taken by ensuring that they have adequate supplies of vitamin D, usually 1000–2000 U/day, to allow optimum gastrointestinal absorption of minerals[33], and by attempting to ensure that sufficient quantities of calcium and phosphorus are supplied in the diet in the right proportions[34]. This itself may be difficult since breast milk does not contain sufficient minerals to satisfy the needs of premature infants, and fortification of milk with calcium and phosphorus may result in insoluble precipitates which are impossible to administer. The current development of suitably fortified artificial milks, formulated especially for premature infants, may help to overcome the problem and reduce the incidence of rickets of prematurity which remains a difficult condition to treat.

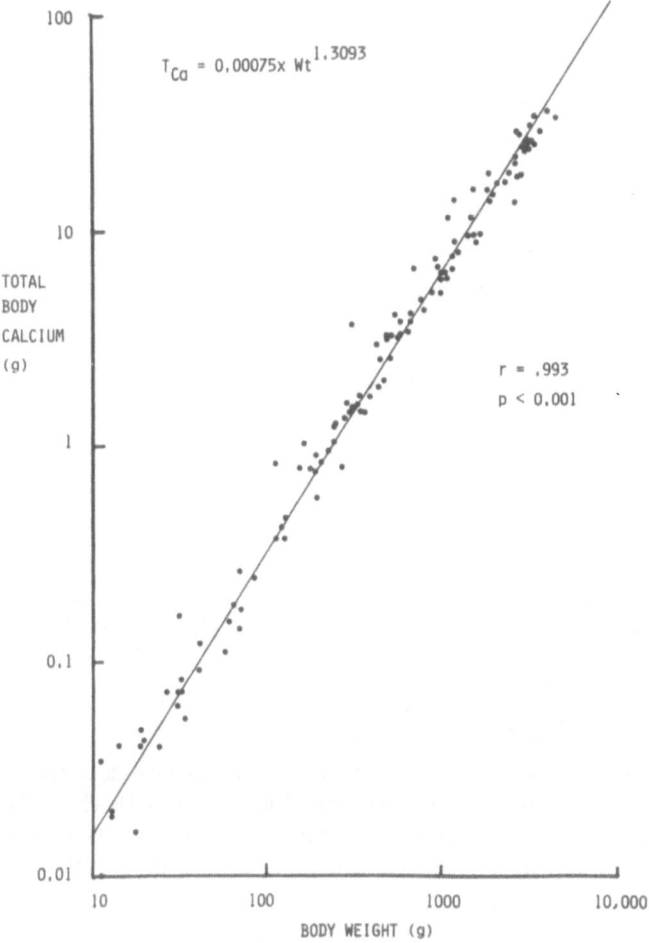

Figure 5 Relationship between total body calcium and body-weight in the 'normal' human embryo and fetus. Data on 117 subjects taken from all 15 available published sources

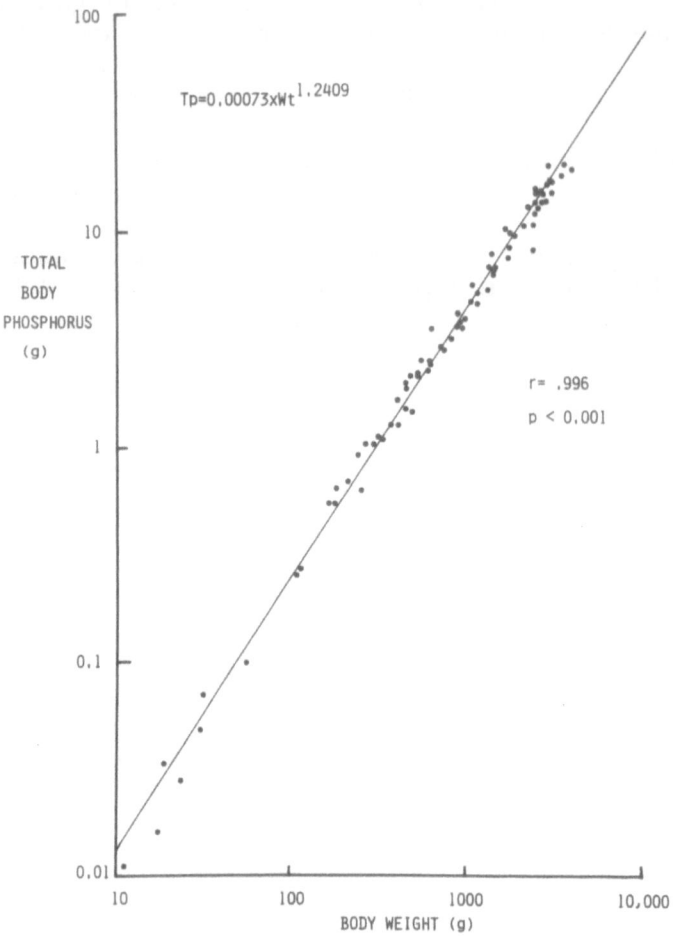

$$Tp=0.00073xWt^{1.2409}$$

$r = .996$

$p < 0.001$

TOTAL BODY PHOSPHORUS (g)

BODY WEIGHT (g)

Figure 6 Relationship between total body phosphorus and body-weight in the 'normal' human embryo and fetus. Data on 78 subjects taken from 13 available published sources

(2) Neonatal hypocalcaemia

Serum calcium in cord blood is high and a positive gradient from mother to fetus occurs during intrauterine life[35]. After birth, this maternal supply of calcium is abruptly and completely withdrawn, resulting in a physiological fall in serum calcium which has a nadir 48–72 hours after birth before rising to a fairly constant level 7–10 days after birth (Figure 7)[36]. Several homeostatic mechanisms operate to limit the fall[37] which, in most instances, is not sufficiently large to cause clinical symptoms. It can be calculated that, in the absence of any such homeostasis, even allowing for alternative supplies of calcium from feeds, if mineralization were to continue to proceed at the same rate after birth as beforehand, serum calcium would fall from 2.7 to 2.0 mmol/l within 12 hours in term infants and within $2\frac{1}{2}$ hours in infants of 35 weeks' gestation—considerably faster than the observed rates of fall. Thus mineral homeostasis in the immediate postnatal period is normally very efficient. Not surprisingly, this physiological fall is greater in premature than in term infants[36], since mineralization rates are larger; but it is also true of those

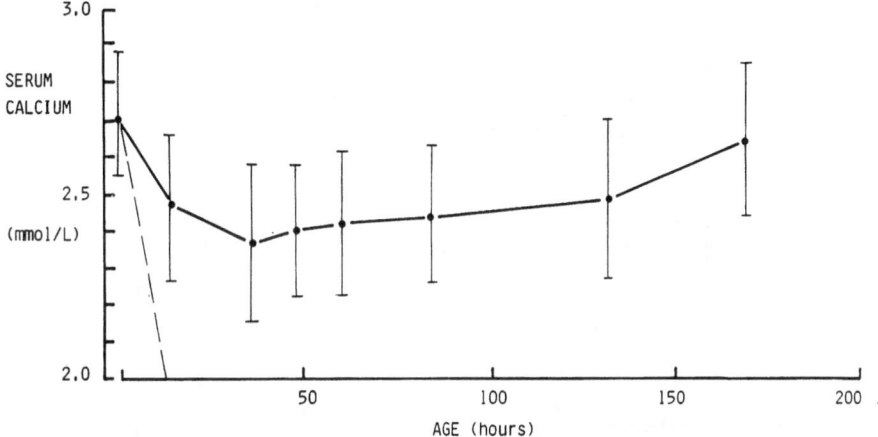

Figure 7   Serum calcium concentrations in full-term infants during the first week of life. Mean values $\pm$ 1 SD. (Data adapted from David and Anast[38] and Hillman *et al.*[36]). The interrupted line shows the theoretical rate of fall of calcium which would occur if bone mineralization were to continue at the same rate after birth as beforehand

infants who have a concurrent problem, such as hypoxia[38], infection[38] or maternal diabetes[39] and leads to 'early' hypocalcaemia (within 3 days of birth). The precise mechanisms by which the system fails in these infants are not fully understood, but are probably related to a combination of poor responsiveness of the parathyroid glands to hypocalcaemia[38], failure or immaturity of end-organ responsiveness to PTH[40], raised serum calcitonin[36], vitamin D deficiency and hypomagnesaemia[41]. In addition, the presence of maternal disease, such as hypercalcaemia, diabetes mellitus or osteomalacia, may be important. These influences are summarized in Figure 8. Some of them can be reversed.

It is therefore self-evident that prevention of hypoxia, infection and hypoglycaemia may reduce the incidence of hypocalcaemia and diagnosis of maternal disease may point to a diagnosis in the infant. Serum magnesium, as well as calcium, should be measured, since hypomagnesaemia may be a factor in the aetiology of neonatal hypocalcaemia. If so, magnesium sulphate (50% solution of $MgSO_4 \cdot 7H_2O \equiv 2$ mmol/ml) in a dose of 0.1 ml/kg body-weight should be given as necessary, by intramuscular injection, to maintain serum magnesium above 0.7 mmol/l.

Vitamin D supplements of 1000 U/day should be given and calcium gluconate (10% solution ≡ 0.225 mmol/ml) 1–2 mg/kg body-weight added to feeds. Intravenous calcium gluconate usually only has a transient effect on serum calcium when given by bolus injection and must be administered with caution as extravasation can cause considerable skin sloughing. If given intravenously it is best administered by slow infusion. If these measures fail, treatment with 1α-hydroxycholecalciferol (1αOHCC) (Alfacalcidol, Rocaltrol) 15–30 ng/kg/day may be necessary, and a more permanent cause of the hypocalcaemia should be sought.

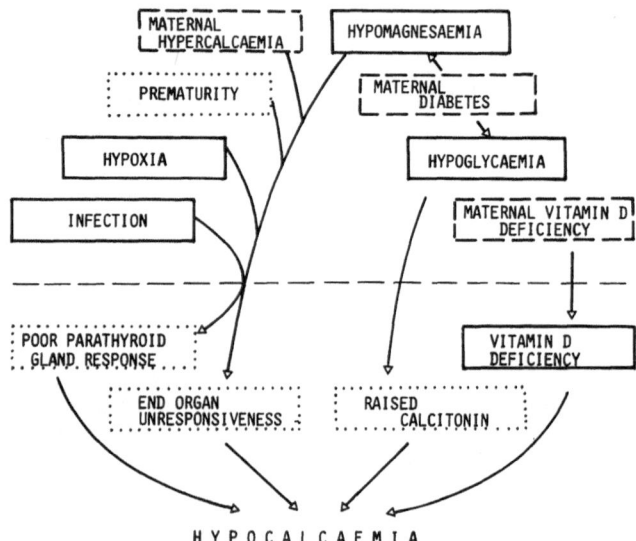

Figure 8 Schematic representation of the pathological causes of neonatal hypocalcaemia. Solid lines enclose the factors which potentially can be reversed; dotted lines enclose those which cannot be altered, and interrupted lines enclose maternal influences

(3) Hypercalcaemia in childhood

Compared with hypocalcaemia, and in contrast to the situation in adults, hypercalcaemia is relatively uncommon in childhood, since primary hyperparathyroidism and malignant disease are unusual. When it does occur it is generally either 'idiopathic' in origin or the result of excessive PTH secretion, increased tubular reabsorption of calcium or vitamin D toxicity.

Idiopathic hypercalcaemia of infancy of the severe type has probably not diminished in incidence recently[42] and measurement of serum calcium should be included in the investigation of any child with failure to thrive, particularly if he is under 1 year of age. Diagnosis can be made from the persistently elevated serum calcium, typical 'elfin' facies and, if present, the cardiovascular abnormalities of supravalvar aortic stenosis or, more rarely, peripheral pulmonary stenosis. Hyperabsorption of calcium can be demonstrated after administration of a standard oral calcium load[43], hypercalciuria is usually present and the bones may be radiologically dense. Treatment consists of correcting any dehydration which may be present and reducing the dietary vitamin D and calcium intake to allow serum calcium to return to normal. An initial course of oral steroids may be of value. The progress of one such patient is shown in Figure 9.

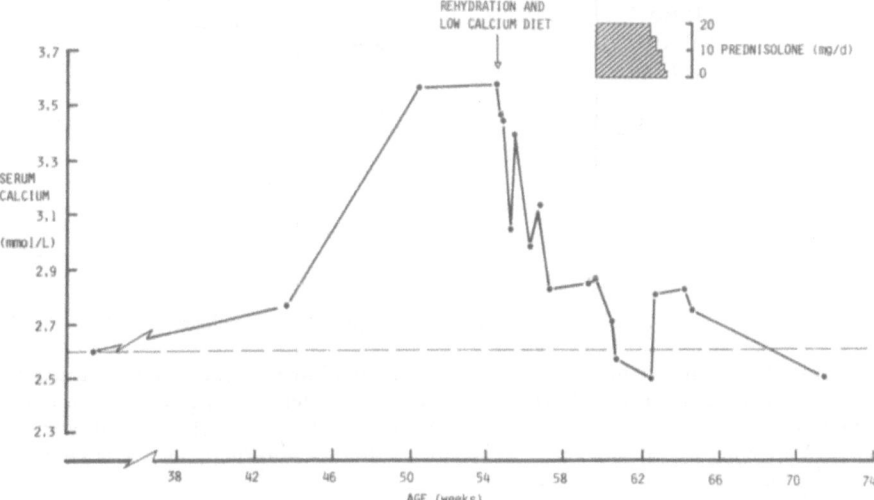

Figure 9 Changes in serum calcium in a patient with idiopathic hypercalcaemia of infancy. An initial fall is seen when rehydration and a low calcium diet were started. Serum calcium returned to normal when steroids were added to the treatment, and remained normal after these were stopped

Primary hyperparathyroidism occasionally occurs in childhood and may be familial in origin, but it must be distinguished from familial hypocalciuric hypercalcaemia (FHH) as a cause of hypercalcaemia[44,45]. Although the degree of hypercalcaemia is similar in these two conditions (Figure 10), they can be distinguished by the very low rate of urinary calcium excretion in the latter (Figure 11)[46]. In addition, the incidence of symptoms in FHH is low, immunoreactive PTH concentrations are normal, or only slightly elevated, and radiological evidence of bone disease is usually absent except during the neonatal period when there may be some overlap between the two conditions. Treatment of FHH is usually not necessary but requires *total* parathyroidectomy to be effective should it become so. In contrast, primary hyperparathyroidism should be treated with subtotal parathyroidectomy, with or without autotransplantation, in order to avoid the problems of worsening bone disease and renal failure.

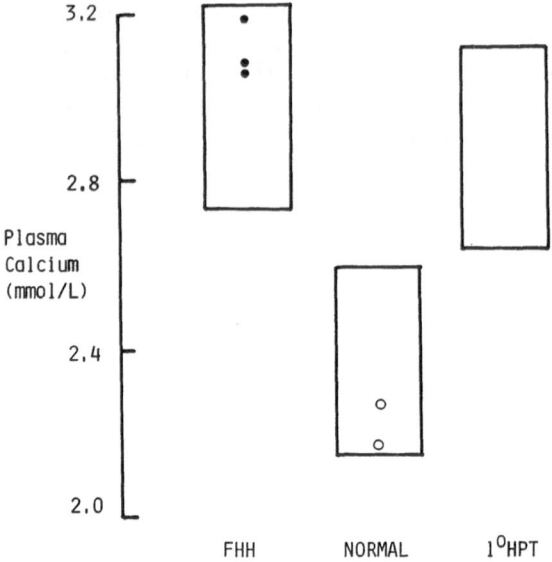

Figure 10 Serum calcium concentrations in familial hypocalciuric hypercalcaemia. Normal values and previously reported ranges for patients with FHH and primary hyperparathyroidism are represented by the rectangular boxes. (Data from Marx *et al.*[45].) Values in three affected members of one kindred are shown in solid circles, normal members in open circles

Hypercalcaemia due to vitamin D toxicity is most frequently caused by overtreatment of other disorders of mineral homeostasis with excessive amounts of vitamin D or its more potent analogues. In most cases the hypercalcaemia settles within a few days of stopping treatment with these analogues[47], since they have relatively short half-lives in serum. Hypercalcaemia due to vitamin D toxicity may take longer to settle and steroids are of value in hastening a return to normal if this is prolonged.

(4) Hypocalcaemia in childhood

Hypocalcaemia in childhood in the presence of normal renal function generally occurs as a result either of interference with the supply or utilization of vitamin D, or of impaired secretion or responsiveness to PTH.

If vitamin D deficiency is the culprit, osteomalacia is present, although rickets may not be clinically apparent. It is not generally appreciated that many cases of nutritional vitamin D deficiency are accompanied by profound hypocalcaemia and a raised serum phosphorus

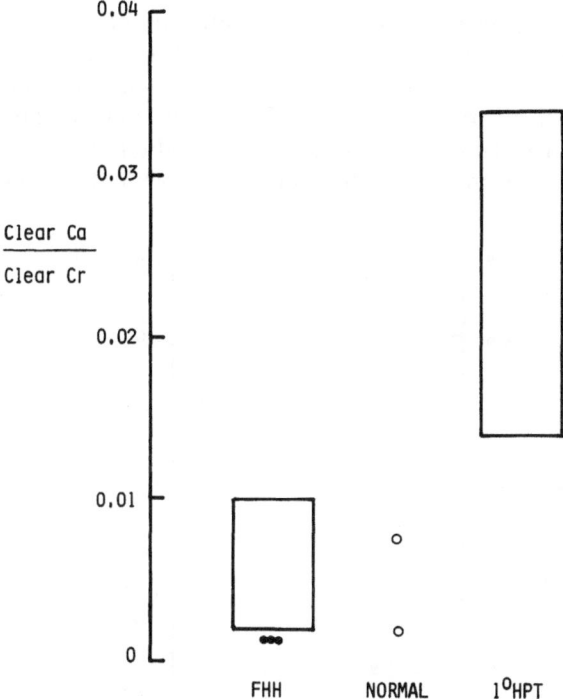

Figure 11 Calcium excretion in patients with familial hypocalciuric hypercalcaemia. Urinary calcium excretion is expressed as calcium/creatinine ratio to eliminate the variable effects of renal function and body size. Symbols as for Figure 10

(Figure 12) with little radiological evidence of osteomalacia. Such patients can be distinguished from those with hypoparathyroidism by their raised concentrations of PTH, low or undetectable levels of 25OHD and $1,25(OH)_2D$ and a satisfactory response to physiological doses of vitamin D. If hypocalcaemia is less profound, the more widely recognized association with hypophosphataemia is usually present when symptoms are more likely to be related to the rickets than to the hypocalcaemia.

Hypoparathyroidism, of whatever aetiology, is usually accompanied by hypocalcaemia and hyperphosphataemia. Failure of the parathyroid glands in children is usually 'primary' in origin, presumably as a result of autoantibody production, and is sometimes associated with cutaneous moniliasis and autoimmune failure of other endocrine glands. It can occasionally be seen as a complication of thalassaemia major[48]. In either case, target organ responsiveness, as shown by the responses of phosphaturia and plasma cAMP, are normal[24].

An important secondary cause of parathyroid gland failure is magnesium deficiency. In children this most frequently results from generalized intestinal malabsorption or from inadequate supplementation during total parenteral nutrition, but may occasionally occur in infants who have a primary defect of magnesium absorption, primary hypomagnesaemia[49]. In these infants oral supplementation with large doses of magnesium may help to overcome the defect. An interesting condition, nephrogenic hypomagnesaemia, which has recently been described, results from an isolated renal tubular leak of magnesium[50].

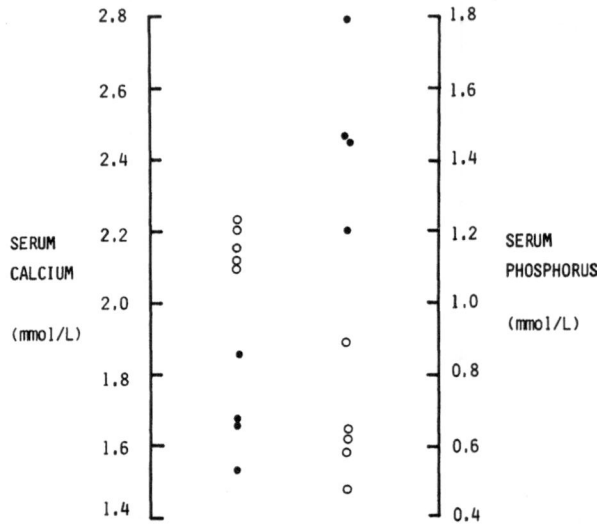

Figure 12 Serum calcium and phosphorus in patients with nutritional vitamin D deficiency. All the patients who had a serum calcium concentration < 2.0 mmol/l had a serum phosphorus concentration > 1.0 mmol/l (open circles). When serum phosphorus was < 1.0 mmol/l, serum calcium was > 2.0 mmol/l (closed circles)

This is associated, in some cases, with nephrocalcinosis and impaired renal function. These are features which it shares with Bartter's syndrome[51,52], but whether or not it is related to that disease is uncertain. It can be distinguished from other causes of hypomagnesaemia by measuring renal tubular excretion of magnesium which is greatly elevated (Figure 13).

Hypomagnesaemia leads to hypocalcaemia by interfering with PTH secretion[3,53]. However, in mild cases PTH levels may be raised, though presumably not high enough to prevent hypocalcaemia, and these cases are complicated by the fact that target organ resistance to PTH may also be present. The latter is probably a reflection of the raised PTH levels rather than of the hypomagnesaemia itself[53]. Treatment of the hypomagnesaemia is usually sufficient by itself to correct all the biochemical abnormalities.

Pseudohypoparathyroidism[54] is probably a heterogeneous group of conditions which are characterized by the biochemical features of hypoparathyroidism, hypocalcaemia and hypophosphataemia, in the presence of raised concentrations of PTH and target-organ resistance to the hormone. In the classical form of the disease, Albright's hereditary osteodystrophy and mental retardation are also present, but diagnosis does not depend on the presence of these features[24]. End-organ resistance to PTH must be demonstrated in order to make a diagnosis, but there is some dispute over whether this is the primary aetiology of the disease[55]. Occasionally there may be dissociation between the phosphaturic and cAMP responses, the latter being normal in Type II pseudohypoparathyroidism[56], and the responses may vary with treatment[57]. In some instances there is radiological evidence of secondary hyperparathyroidism, indicating that a degree of skeletal sensitivity to the

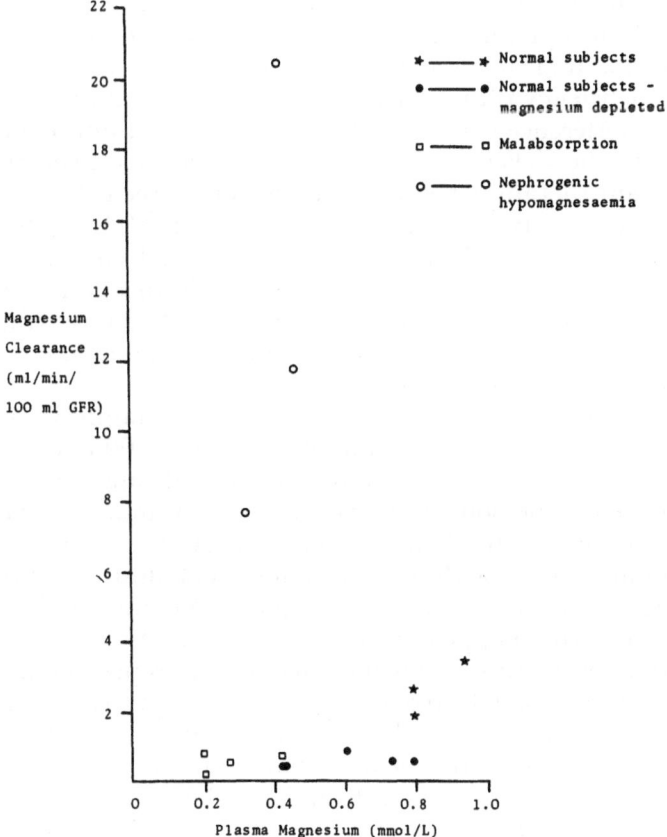

Figure 13 Magnesium excretion in nephrogenic hypomagnesaemia. Clearance values are expressed as ml/min/100 ml GFR to eliminate the effects of body size and renal function. (Data in normal subjects from Dunn and Walser[64])

hormone is preserved[26]. In pseudopseudohypoparathyroidism[58], Albright's hereditary osteodystrophy alone is present, all other parameters of mineral metabolism being normal, but it may occur in the same families as patients with pseudohypoparathyroidism.

The treatment of both hypoparathyroidism and pseudohypoparathyroidism is similar. 1αOHCC is given in sufficient dosage, usually about 30 ng/kg/day, to maintain serum calcium concentrations within the normal range and without causing hypercalciuria.

(5) Rickets

Rickets (Figure 14) almost invariably results either from an interruption to the supply, metabolism or utilization of vitamin D, or from a renal tubular disorder of phosphate transport. In the former there is a tendency to hypocalcaemia, which may be profound, usually, though not always, accompanied by hypophosphataemia; and secondary hyperparathyroidism is present. The various causes can be distinguished by measuring vitamin D metabolites. In the majority, in whom nutritional vitamin D deficiency is the cause, concentrations of all the metabolites are low[59]. Interference with 25-hydroxylase activity is unusual but may contribute to the rickets occasionally seen in chronic liver disease or anticonvulsant therapy when a similar picture is seen. In vitamin D-dependent (Prader type) rickets[60] concentrations of $1,25(OH)_2D$ are usually below 10 pg/ml in the presence of normal concentrations of 25OHD, whereas in the very rare end-organ resistance to $1,25(OH)_2D$, which is sometimes associated with alopecia[61], concentrations of $1,25(OH)_2D$ may be very high (several hundred pg/ml), especially if treatment has already been attempted.

Following the start of treatment of nutritional vitamin D deficiency with 'physiological' doses of vitamin D (1000–3000 U/day), serum $1,25(OH)_2D$ levels rise to well above the normal range before falling back to normal as the bones heal over the next few months[59]. Similarly, it is safe, and may hasten bone healing, to begin treatment of vitamin D-dependent rickets with supraphysiological doses of 1αOHCC, 100–200 ng/kg/day, together with adequate calcium supplements, in order to mimic what happens in vitamin D deficiency. Hypercalcaemia does not develop on this dose while osteomalacia is present and, as the bones heal, the dose can be reduced according to the serum and urinary calcium. Ultimately 20–30 ng/kg/day only are likely to be needed.

A renal tubular disorder of phosphate transport is frequently an isolated phenomenon, which results in hypophosphataemic vitamin D resistant rickets (VDRR), but it may be associated with a more generalized defect in proximal tubular function in the Fanconi syndrome. Whatever the cause, untreated hypophosphataemia is accompanied by a normal serum calcium, and evidence of secondary hyperparathyroidism is lacking unless the Fanconi syndrome is associated with renal dysfunction such as occurs in cystinosis. Diagnosis rests on the demonstration of a low TRP (usually $< 50\%$) and TmP/GFR.

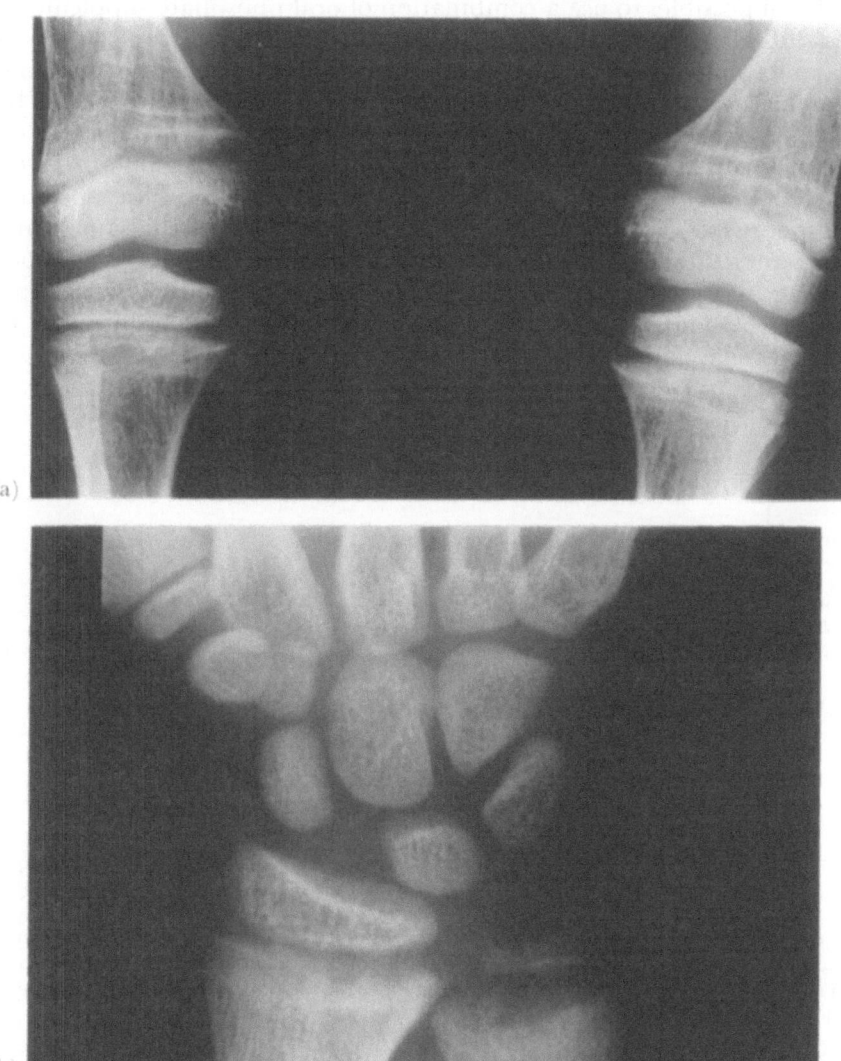

Figure 14 X-ray appearances in rickets. Patient suffering from hypophosphataemic vitamin D-resistant rickets. (a) Lower end of femur, (b) wrist. (Films by courtesy of the X-ray Department, Birmingham Children's Hospital)

The most satisfactory method of treating VDRR has not been properly established. Since excessive renal losses of phosphate are largely responsible for the disease, it is logical to use phosphate replacement in the treatment. However, vitamin D supplementation is also necessary to prevent hypocalcaemia and secondary hyperparathyroidism, and does promote bone healing. Some clinicians rely on vitamin D alone, but I prefer, if possible, to use a combination of oral phosphate supplements and 1αOHCC, particularly in severe cases. The main problem is that oral phosphate supplements are rapidly excreted in the urine, resulting in a 'see-saw' pattern of serum phosphorus (Figure 15), and need to be given, preferably, five times a day, which can lead to problems of drug compliance. The aim should be to maintain serum phosphorus levels above 1 mmol/l throughout the day and 24-hour profiles of serum phosphorus are helpful in this respect (Figure 15). At the same time, sufficient 1αOHCC must be given to prevent hypocalcaemia without causing hypercalciuria. It is therefore essential to monitor serum calcium levels and urinary phosphate excretion at regular intervals to prevent renal damage ensuing.

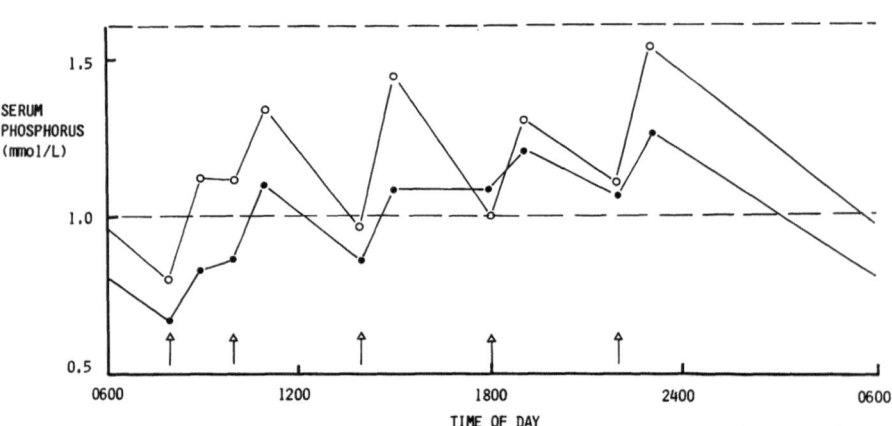

Figure 15   24-hour profile of serum phosphorus in a patient with hypophosphataemic vitamin D-resistant rickets. When dietary phosphorus supplements were increased from 2.5 to 3.5 g/day, serum phosphorus showed a more marked 'see-saw' pattern but rose to > 1.0 mmol/l for most of the 24-hour period

An alternative renal tubular cause of rickets is distal renal tubular acidosis. Biochemically this resembles nutritional vitamin D deficiency, but is associated with hypercalciuria, nephrocalcinosis and impaired renal function. It is important to distinguish this from other causes of rickets as alkali therapy is all that is usually required to prevent progress of the disease, and vitamin D treatment is potentially dangerous, since it increases gastrointestinal absorption and urinary excretion of calcium, thereby making the renal failure worse.

(6) Renal failure

The bone disease of renal failure is complex in its aetiology. It is principally related to phosphate retention, depressed 1α-hydroxylase activity and impaired end-organ responsiveness to PTH, all of which occur as a result of loss of renal tissue mass, together with PTH hypersecretion as a consequence of the hypocalcaemia caused by the other three factors. These together give rise to a combination of hyperparathyroid and osteomalacic bone disease. In addition, other factors, such as osteoporosis, osteosclerosis, aluminium toxicity and disturbances of magnesium homeostasis, may be seen.

Treatment must therefore be directed towards preventing as many of these factors as early as possible. Oral aluminium hydroxide has traditionally been used with some success to limit phosphate retention. More recently, calcium carbonate has been shown to be as effective[62] and has the advantages of reducing the aluminium load and providing additional calcium. The serum phosphorus should be maintained below 1.6 mmol/l. Depressed 1α-hydroxylase activity can be overcome by the administration of 1αOHCC 15–30 ng/kg/day, but caution must be exercised as gastrointestinal absorption of phosphorus tends to increase with this therapy. The effects of loss of renal function on end-organ responsiveness to PTH are difficult to reverse except insofar as they may be exacerbated by the secondary hyperparathyroidism.

SUMMARY

As our understanding of the aetiology of disorders of mineral metabolism in childhood increases, it becomes easier to follow a logical series of steps in their management. Correct diagnosis depends upon the use of the diagnostic tools which have become available in the light of that knowledge, and treatment can follow. However, as it has recently been pointed out[63], it must be remembered that the agents which are now available for that treatment, particularly the metabolites of vitamin D, are powerful and potentially toxic. Adequate monitoring of the response to treatment must therefore be undertaken, particularly in the early stages, so that therapy can be altered as necessary and to ensure that deleterious effects do not arise.

ACKNOWLEDGEMENTS

I am grateful to Dr G. Durbin, Dr P. H. W. Rayner, Dr P. H. Weller and Professor J. L. H. O'Riordan for permission to include data on their patients, and to Mrs P. Jackson for preparing the drawings and manuscript.

References

1. Arnaud, S. B., Goldsmith, R. S., Stickler, G. B., McCall, J. T. and Arnaud, C. D. (1973). Serum parathyroid hormone and blood minerals: interrelationships in normal children. *Pediatr. Res.*, **7**, 485–93
2. Round, J. M., Butcher, S. and Steel, R. (1979). Changes in plasma inorganic phosphorus and alkaline phosphatase during the adolescent growth spurt. *Ann. Hum. Biol.*, **6**, 129–36
3. Rude, R. K., Oldham, S. B., Sharp, C. F. and Singer, F. R. (1978). Parathyroid hormone secretion in magnesium deficiency. *J. Clin. Endocrinol. Metab.*, **47**, 800–6
4. Stanbury, S. W. (1968). The intestinal absorption of calcium in normal adults, primary hyperparathyroidism and renal failure. In Berlyne, G. M. (ed.) *Nutrition in Renal Disease*. pp. 118–32. (Edinburgh: E. and S. Livingstone)
5. Heaton, F. W. and Pyrah, L. N. (1963). Magnesium metabolism in patients with parathyroid disorders. *Clin. Sci.*, **25**, 475–85
6. Ghazali, S. and Barratt, T. M. (1974). Urinary excretion of calcium and magnesium in children. *Arch. Dis. Child.*, **49**, 97–101
7. Marshall, D. H. (1976). Calcium and phosphate kinetics. In Nordin, B. E. C. (ed.) *Calcium, Phosphate and Magnesium Kinetics. Clinical Physiology and Diagnostic Procedures.* pp. 257–97. (Edinburgh: Churchill Livingstone)
8. Walton, R. J. and Bijvoet, O. L. M. (1975). Nomogram for derivation of renal threshold phosphate concentration. *Lancet*, **2**, 309–10
9. Kruse, K., Kracht, U. and Gopfert, G. (1982). Renal threshold phosphate concentration (TmPO$_4$/GFR). *Arch. Dis. Child.*, **57**, 217–23
10. Corvilain, J. and Abramow, M. (1972). Growth and renal control of plasma phosphate. *J. Clin. Endocrinol. Metab.*, **34**, 452–9
11. Eisman, J. A., Hamstra, A. J., Kream, B. E. and DeLuca, H. F. (1976). A sensitive, precise and convenient method for determination of 1,25 dihydroxyvitamin D in human plasma. *Arch. Biochem. Biophys.*, **176**, 235–43
12. Clemens, T. L., Hendy, G. N., Papapoulos, S. E., Fraher, L. J., Care, A. D. and O'Riordan, J. L. H. (1979). Measurement of 1,25-dihydroxycholecalciferol in man by radioimmunoassay. *Clin. Endocrinol.*, **11**, 225–34
13. Preece, M. A., O'Riordan, J. L. H., Lawson, D. E. M. and Kodicek, E. (1974). A competitive protein-binding assay for 25-hydroxycholecalciferol and 25-hydroxyergocalciferol in serum. *Clin. Chim. Acta*, **54**, 235–42
14. Manning, R. M., Hendy, G. N., Papapoulos, S. E. and O'Riordan, J. L. H. (1980). The development of homologous immunological assays for human parathyroid hormone. *J. Endocrinol.*, **85**, 161–70
15. Walsh, J. H. (1978). Radioimmunoassay methodology for articles published in gastroenterology. *Gastroenterology*, **75**, 523–4
16. Chambers, D. J., Dunham, J., Zanelli, J. M., Parsons, J. A., Bitensky, L. and Chayen, J. (1978). A sensitive bioassay of parathyroid hormone in plasma. *Clin. Endocrinol.*, **9**, 375–9
17. Allgrove, J., Chayen, J. and O'Riordan, J. L. H. (1983). The cytochemical bioassay of parathyroid hormone: further experiences. *J. Immunoassay*, **4**, 1–19
18. Chesney, R. W., Hamstra, A. J. and DeLuca, H. F. (1978). Serum 1,25(OH)$_2$ vitamin D levels in children and alteration with disorders of vitamin D metabolism. *Pediatr. Res.*, **1**, 503
19. Lund, Bj., Clausen, N., Lund, Bi., Anderson, E. and Sorensen, O. H. (1980). Age-dependent variations in serum 1,25-dihydroxyvitamin D in childhood. *Acta Endocrinol.*, **94**, 426–9
20. Ellsworth, R. and Howard, J. E. (1934). Studies on the physiology of the parathyroid glands. VII. Some responses of normal human kidneys and blood to intravenous parathyroid extract. *Bull. Johns Hopkins Hosp.*, **55**, 296–308

21. Chase, L. R. and Aurbach, G. D. (1967). Parathyroid function and the renal secretion of 3'5'-adenylic acid. *Proc. Natl. Acad. Sci. USA*, **58**, 518–25

22. Tomlinson, S., Barling, P. M., Albano, J. D. M., Brown, B. L. and O'Riordan, J. L. H. (1974). The effects of exogenous parathyroid hormone on plasma and urinary adenosine 3'5' cyclic monophosphate in man. *Clin. Sci. Mol. Med.*, **47**, 481–92

23. Chase, L. R., Melson, G. L. and Aurbach, G. D. (1969). Pseudohypoparathyroidism: defective excretion of 3'5' AMP in response to parathyroid hormone. *J. Clin. Invest.*, **48**, 1832–44

24. Lewin, I. G., Papapoulos, S. E., Tomlinson, S., Hendy, G. N. and O'Riordan, J. L. H. (1978). Studies of hypoparathyroidism and pseudohypoparathyroidism. *Q. J. Med.*, **47**, 533–48

25. Tomlinson, S., Hendy, G. N., Pemberton, D. M. and O'Riordan, J. L. H. (1976). Reversible resistance to the renal action of parathyroid hormone in man. *Clin. Sci. Mol. Med.*, **51**, 59–69

26. Costello, J. M. and Dent, C. E. (1963). Hypo-hyperparathyroidism. *Arch. Dis. Child.*, **38**, 397–407

27. Bosley, A. R. J., Verrier-Jones, E. R. and Campbell, M. J. (1980). Aetiological factors in rickets of prematurity. *Arch. Dis. Child.*, **55**, 683–6

28. Hillman, L. S. and Haddad, J. G. (1975). Perinatal vitamin D metabolism. II. Serial 25 hydroxyvitamin D concentrations in serum of term and premature infants. *J. Pediatr.*, **86**, 928–35

29. McIntosh, N., Livesey, A. and Brooke, O. G. (1982). Plasma 25-hydroxyvitamin D and rickets in infants of extremely low birthweight. *Arch. Dis. Child.*, **57**, 848–50

30. Von Sydow, G. (1946). A study of the development of rickets in premature infants. *Acta Paediatr. Scand.*, **33** (Suppl. 2), 1–22

31. Roe, J. C., Wood, D. H., Rowe, D. W. and Raisz, L. G. (1979). Nutritional hypophosphataemic rickets in a premature infant fed on breast milk. *N. Engl. J. Med.*, **300**, 293–6

32. Allgrove, J. (1984). Total body calcium and phosphorus in the human foetus: significance for the prevention and treatment of rickets of very low birth weight infants. (In preparation)

33. Santerre, J. and Salle, B. (1982). Calcium and phosphorus economy of the preterm infant and its interaction with vitamin D and its metabolites. *Acta Paediatr. Scand. Suppl.*, **296**, 85–92

34. Brooke, O. G. (1983). Supplementary vitamin D in infancy and childhood. *Arch. Dis. Child.*, **58**, 573–4

35. Pitkin, R. M. (1975). Calcium metabolism in pregnancy: a review. *Am. J. Obstet. Gynecol.*, **121**, 724–37

36. Hillman, L. S., Rojanasathit, S., Slatopolsky, E. and Haddad, J. G. (1977). Serial measurements of serum calcium, magnesium, parathyroid hormone, calcitonin and 25-hydroxy vitamin D in premature and term infants during the first week of life. *Pediatr. Res.*, **11**, 739–44

37. Tsang, R. C., Steichen, J. J., Chan, G. M., Chen, I-W., Whittsett, J. A., Erenberg, A. E., Donovan, E. F. and Brown, D. R. (1980). Recent advances in understanding the neonatal parathyroid and vitamin D jigsaw. In DeLuca, H. F. and Anast, C. S. (eds.) *Pediatric Diseases Related to Calcium*. pp. 323–44. (Oxford: Blackwell Scientific Publications)

38. David, L. and Anast, C. S. (1974). Calcium metabolism in newborn infants. The interrelationship of parathyroid function and calcium, magnesium and phosphorus metabolism in normal, 'sick' and hypocalcemic newborns. *J. Clin. Invest.*, **54**, 287–96

39. Tsang, R. C., Chen, I-W., Friedman, M. A., Gigger, M., Steichen, J., Koffler, H., Fenton, L., Brown, D., Pramanik, A., Keenan, W., Strub, R. and Joyce, T. (1975). Parathyroid function in infants of diabetic mothers. *J. Pediatr.*, **86**, 399–404

261

40. Tsang, R. C., Light, I. J., Sutherland, J. M. and Kleinman, L. I. (1973). Possible pathogenetic factors in neonatal hypocalcemia of prematurity. *J. Pediatr.*, **82**, 423–9

41. Tsang, R. C. and Oh, W. (1970). Serum magnesium levels in low birthweight infants. *Am. J. Dis. Child.*, **120**, 44–8

42. Kershaw, C. R. and Jordan, S. (1980). William's syndrome: what happened to idiopathic hypercalcaemia? Presented at the *52nd Meeting of the British Paediatric Association*, April 15–18, York

43. Barr, D. G. D. and Forfar, J. O. (1969). Oral calcium-loading test in infancy, with particular reference to idiopathic hypercalcaemia. *Br. Med. J.*, **1**, 477–80

44. Foley, T. P., Harrison, H. C., Arnaud, C. A. and Harrison, H. E. (1972). Familial benign hypercalcemia. *J. Pediatr.*, **81**, 1060–7

45. Marx, S. J., Spiegel, A. M., Brown, E. M. and Aurbach, G. D. (1977). Family studies in patients with primary parathyroid hyperplasia. *Am. J. Med.*, **62**, 698–706

46. Marx, S. J., Spiegel, A. M., Brown, E. M., Koehler, J. O., Gardner, D. G., Brennan, M. F. and Aurbach, G. D. (1978). Divalent cation metabolism: familial hypocalciuric hypercalcemia versus typical primary hyperparathyroidism. *Am. J. Med.*, **65**, 735–42

47. Kanis, J. A. and Russell, R. G. G. (1977). Rate of reversal of hypercalcaemia and hypercalciuria induced by vitamin D and its 1 alpha hydroxylated derivatives. *Br. Med. J.*, **1**, 78–81

48. Flynn, D. M., Fairney, A., Jackson, D. and Clayton, B. (1976). Hormonal changes in thalassaemia major. *Arch. Dis. Child.*, **51**, 828–36

49. Paunier, L., Radde, I. C., Kooh, S. W. and Fraser, D. (1965). Primary hypomagnesemia with secondary hypercalcemia. *J. Pediatr.*, **67**, 945

50. Evans, R. A., Carter, J. N., George, C. R., Walls, R. S., Newland, R. C., McDonnel, G. D. H. and Lawrence, J. R. (1981). The congenital 'magnesium-losing kidney'. Report of two patients. *Q. J. Med.*, **50**, 39–52

51. McCredie, D. A., Rotenberg, E. and Williams, A. Z. (1974). Hypercalciuria in potassium-losing nephropathy: a variant of Bartter's syndrome. *Aust. Paediatr. J.*, **10**, 286–95

52. Mace, J. W., Hambidge, K. M. and Gottlin, R. W. (1973). Magnesium supplementation in Bartter's syndrome. *Arch. Dis. Child.*, **48**, 485–7

53. Allgrove, J., Adami, S., Fraher, L., Reuben, A. and O'Riordan, J. L. H. (1984). Hypomagnesaemia: studies of parathyroid hormone secretion and function. *Clin. Endocrinol.* (In press)

54. Albright, F., Burnett, C. H., Smith, P. H. and Parson, W. (1942). Pseudohypoparathyroidism—an example of the 'Seabright–Bantam' syndrome. *Endocrinology*, **30**, 922–32

55. Editorial (1983). Pseudohypoparathyroidism: continuing paradox. *Lancet*, **2**, 439–40

56. Drezner, M., Neelon, F. A. and Lebovitz, H. E. (1973). Pseudohypoparathyroidism Type II: a possible defect in the reception of the cAMP signal. *N. Engl. J. Med.*, **289**, 1056–60

57. Breslau, N. A., Notman, D. D., Canterbury, J. M. and Moses, A. M. (1980). Studies on the attainment of normocalcemia in patients with pseudohypoparathyroidism. *Am. J. Med.*, **68**, 856–60

58. Albright, F., Forbes, A. P. and Henneman, P. H. (1952). Pseudopseudohypoparathyroidism. *Trans. Assoc. Am. Physicians*, **65**, 337–50

59. Papapoulos, S. E., Clemens, T. L., Fraher, L. J., Gleed, J. and O'Riordan, J. L. H. (1980). Metabolites of vitamin D in human vitamin D deficiency: effect of vitamin D or 1,25-dihydroxycholecalciferol. *Lancet*, **2**, 612–15

60. Prader, A., Illig, R. and Heierli, E. (1961). Eine besonde form der primaren vitamin D resisten Rachitis mit hypocalcamie und autosomal dominanten Erbgang: die hereditare pseudo-mangelrachitis. *Helv. Paediatr. Acta*, **16**, 452–68

61. Liberman, V. A., Samuel, R., Halabe, A., Kauli, R., Edelstein, S., Weisman, Y., Papapoulos, S. E., Clemens, T. L., Fraher, L. J. and O'Riordan, J. L. H. (1980). End-organ resistance to 1,25-dihydroxycholecalciferol. *Lancet*, **1**, 504–7
62. Mak, R., Turner, C., Thompson, T., Powell, H., Haycock, G. and Chantler, C. (1983). Treatment of secondary hyperparathyroidism by phosphate restriction in children with uraemia—effect on growth, bone disease, renal function and anaemia. *Eur. J. Paediatr.*, **140**, 200
63. Chan, J. C. M., Young, R. B., Alon, U. and Mamunes, P. (1983). Hypercalcemia in children with disorders of calcium and phosphate metabolism during long-term treatment with 1,25-dihydroxyvitamin D. *Pediatrics*, **72**, 225–33
64. Dunn, M. J. and Walser, M. (1966). Magnesium depletion in normal man. *Metabolism*, **15**, 884–95

INDEX